Success of Homoeopathy
Authentic Cures with Medical Reports before & After Treatment

Success of Homoeopathy

Authentic Cures with Medical Reports before & After Treatment

BY
Dr. Subrata K. Banerjea
Gold Medalist
B.H.M.S. (Honours In Nine Subjects of Calcutta University).
Fellow: Akademie Homoopathischer Deutscher Zentralverein (Germany);
Homoeopathic Medical Association of The United Kingdom
Director: Bengal Allen Medical Institute.
Principal: Allen College of Homoeopathy, Essex, England.

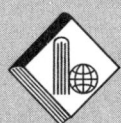

B. Jain Publishers (P) Ltd.
USA — Europe — India

Success of Homoeopathy
Authentic Cures with Medical Reports Before & After Treatment

First Edition: 2012
3rd Impression: 2018

All rights reserved. No part of this book may be reproduced, stored in a retrieval system or transmitted, in any form or by any means, mechanical, photocopying, recording or otherwise, without any prior written permission of the publisher.

© with the Author

Published by Kuldeep Jain for
B. JAIN PUBLISHERS (P) LTD.
D-157, Sector-63, NOIDA-201307, U.P. (INDIA)
Tel.: +91-120-4933333 • *Email:* info@bjain.com
Website: **www.bjain.com**
Registered office: 1921/10, Chuna Mandi, Paharganj,
New Delhi-110 055 (India)

Printed in India by
J.J. Offset Printers

ISBN: 978-81-319-1913-2

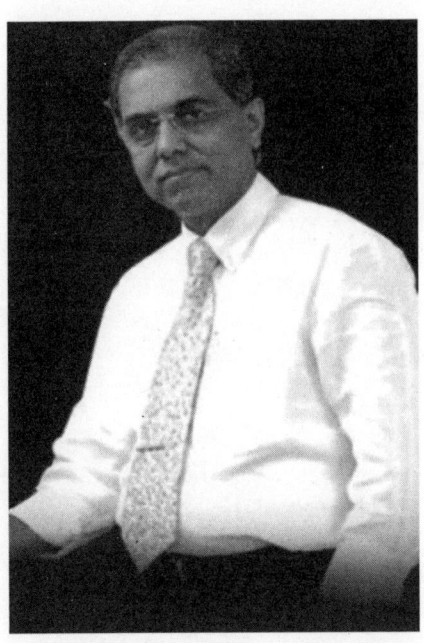

Authentic Cures
with
Medical Reports before & After Treatment

Dr. Subrata Kumar Banerjea was born in Calcutta, India in 1957, the fourth generation of a distinguished and widely respected homoeopathic family. He graduated in Homoeopathy from the University of Calcutta with a record number of honours passes in nine medical subjects and with five gold medals to his name, setting himself on a path to become an internationally acclaimed homoeopathic clinician, lecturer and author. He is now acknowledged to be the world's leading authority on miasmatic prescribing.

Dr. Banerjea is an Honoured Fellow of several academies; Director and Principal Lecturer of the Bengal Allen Medical Institute, Calcutta; Principal and Chief Lecturer of Materia Medica and Clinical Therapeutics at the Allen College of Homoeopathy, Essex, England. When he is not lecturing, he divides his time between his clinical practices in England and in India where he also acts as Clinical Consultant in various rural and slum clinics.

Despite this hectic international scheduling, Dr. Banerjea together with his brother Joy and wife Janet, plays an active role in the Kamala Banerjee Fund, a charity which distributes milk to the poor children of Calcutta.

Students of Dr. Banerjea will testify to the remarkable knowledge and enthusiasm which he generously imparts to all who share his passion for this most rational of healing arts. His dedication to the truth of homoeopathy is regarded as inspiring and unsurpassed.

Author's Dedication

To commemorate the sacred memory of my ancestors, who have dedicated their lives for the cause and development of Homoeopathy and to them Homoeopathy was wealth and honour. The inspiration of this four generations and their "magical cures" are the foundation of all my successes.

Late Dr. Kali Pada Banerjee, my grand-grand father, Proprietor, C. Ringer & Company, Calcutta.

Late Dr. Kishori Mohan Banerjee, my grand father, Founder, Bengal Allen Homoeopathic Medical College & Hospitals, Calcutta.

Late Dr. Naba Kumar Banerjee, my uncle, Principal, Bengal Allen Homoeopathic Medical College, Calcutta; President, Homoeopathic State Faculty, West Bengal and Indian Homoeopathic Association; Author of: A Treatise On Homoeopathic Pharmacy; Practice of Medicine, etc. etc.

&

Late Dr. Ranjit Banerjee, my father, Pathologist & Micro-biologist and then converted to Homoeopathy; Professor, Midnapur Homoeopathic Medical College.

Preface

I am satisfied that this book can be published in the year 2012 as it will mark the celebration of my son, Saptarshi graduating in homoeopathy and continuing the work of this long serving homoeopathic family.

This is also a special year, as my wife and I are planning to enjoy some more time away from clinics and enjoy the peaceful countryside of England.

This book is a tribute to the fraternity of homoeopathy. We can celebrate all the good work homoeopaths throughout the world maintain, despite some adversity and opposition. No science could have survived 200+ years without solid foundation and truth. By publishing success from my consulting room, it is intended to acknowledge the glory of Hahnemann and his beautiful art & science of Homoeopathy.

This book is also a homage to Mahatma Gandhi, who had a message of ahimsa (non-violence). Mahatma Gandhi, was a great supporter of homoeopathy, as it endorses the same philosophy of respecting human life and offering non-violent treatment to the system.

This book is also dedicated to Ramakrishna Paramhansa, who taught that all religions are the same. He said water may be pani in Hindi, Jol in Bengali, water in English but it is all the same. Ramakrishna only used homoeopathy and was treated with Lycopodium by Dr. Mahendra Lal Sircar for his throat cancer.

The credit of the cured cases mentioned in this book does not go to me but to my homoeopathic blood and to Hahnemann who has given us this marvelous rational art of healing for the suffering humanity.

Having published this book of success, I do not like to claim that most of my cases are cured but like everybody else, I do have failures too. I am a humble student of homoeopathy, still collecting pebbles in the shore and always trying to achieve the perfection of prescribing a single dose. I aspire to say to my students "I never repeat".

I love homoeopathy, the homoeopathy which is purely classical, based on solid principles and philosophy. I always prescribe one single medicine, try to give a single dose and wait. In my lectures I do always say, wait and watch with wisdom-www.

Kent mentions perfection of not having to repeat the medicine and curing the patient with a single dose as an aspiration for us all.

As a child, I was brought up with stories of "Magical Cures" in homoeopathy from my ancestors and I always appreciate the wonderful intuition that a Master Prescriber has. I love giving a single dose and watching the flower blossom without interfering.

Most of the long cases are from my Consulting Rooms in India. Due to confidentiality, some of my cases from my consulting rooms in the United Kingdom have to be omitted; however I mentioned many cases in the chapter of short case stories.

Most of the long cases have medical investigations, which you can view in detail in the CD supplied with the book, as well as in my website. The medical evidence of cure is difficult to refute and I have included reports so the authenticity of homoeopathy is beyond doubt.

In some cases, due to culture and lack of education, the patient cannot confirm the exact age, therefore I had to guess. In India, many patients have a habit of doing repeated pathological or radiological investigations therefore they self refer, so my name as the referring doctor might not appear in all the reports.

I am privileged to have a constant source of inspiration, praise and love of my wife, Janet, whom I adore; she gives my mind the deserved peace and tranquility.

I like to say thank you to my graduate Donna Fox, who has painstakingly gone through the manuscripts in order to avoid repetition and confusion of my thoughts, to Debasish Mukherjee for his patience in typing the manuscripts and case notes and to Kuldeep Jain of Jain Publishers who is always there to publish my work.

I also like to acknowledge the support given by my two nice children, Sreyoshee, my daughter and Saptarshi, my son.

I welcome any constructive suggestions towards the improvement of future editions. All the case histories mentioned in this book are directly from the case notes and I did not edit the patient's words, to not only follow Hahnemann's guide 'to listen particularly to the patient's description of his sufferings and sensations' but also to give you the flavour of an un-adulterated version of patient's story.

Preface

I passionately hope that this book will be of immense benefit to the students, as well as practitioners, to carry forward the torch of Homoeopathy in a successful and glorious way.

This book is a celebration of what Homoeopathy can do!

Subrata Kumar Banerjea
Essex, England, 10th April, 2012,
Desk of the Principal,
Allen College of Homoeopathy,
"Sapiens"
382 Baddow Road, Great Baddow,
Chelmsford, Essex CM2 9RA,
United Kingdom.
hahnemann@btinternet.com
www.homoeopathy-course.com

Introduction

I was inspired to write this book by students who have successful practices and encouraged by students who have told me that the fundamentals of good practice lie in the ability to follow a structured approach to homoeopathy. A structured approach that has been verified by many years of understanding and practice by professionals, who follow the intent of Hahnemann, Kent and other such classical masters who practiced in the centuries before us.

I have outlined the structure I follow, below and have referenced the information where relevant. I have the privilege of practicing both in Calcutta, India for many years and also in Essex, Great Britain and use the same method wherever I am. In my experience, patients, whatever their background, culture, ethnicity, gender or age will respond to careful enquiry. It is this that will ensure the most correct prescription. For authenticity I have used the patient's own unadulterated language, in the cases cited throughout the book.

My Case Taking

The phrase *"A case well taken is half cured"* is an example of the wisdom passed from the classical authors. A gem statement.

I always give emphasis on thorough case taking and a classical prescriber should never compromise in that.

All my patients complete a case taking questionnaire prior to their consultation with me. Patients then have the opportunity to think and reflect about their symptoms including the onset and development of symptoms, the chronology, the modalities, character, the emotional features, their temperament and even their hobbies and what is important to them.

By having the case taking form in advance, the patient has ample time to ascertain facts and obtain information from parents or others about their past history and clarify temperament or reactions. I feel in that way the case becomes thoroughly complete in presentation for homoeopathic analysis and evaluation.

Introduction

In India, where the use of homoeopathy is commonplace, I see an enormous number of patients a day and in order to run an efficient clinic, my assistant discusses the case with the patient before I see them. The clinicians ask more questions and clarify the answers on the form, so when the patient enters my consulting room, the case is well taken before I begin the consultation and assessment.

I give lot of emphasis on cause and aetiology of symptoms. This is an important starting place from which evaluation and understanding of the developmental history of the patient can begin, this includes any physical or emotional aetiology. Examples of considerations are below:

- Physical injury, exposure to damp, cold, any incidences from which you have never been well since
- Emotional grief, disappointment, stress which can be attributed to the onset of the current symptoms
- Disease any major illness and you have never been well since
- Medicinal use or abuse of conventional and recreational drugs

For ease and accuracy these questions are divided into 10 years life span, from birth to age 10 years, then 10 years to 20 years and so on.

My Approach

MTEK is an useful memory aid to arriving at a correct prescription and in all cases I ensure the following is included:

M = Miasmatic Totality
T = Totality of Symptoms
E = Essence which includes temperament, posture and behaviour.
K = Keynotes which should encompass peculiar, rare symptoms (PQRS)- refer §153 and §209 of Hahnemann's Organon of Medicine.

Approach-1 - Cases with clarity of symptoms

These cases are usually those which are free from medicinal dependency. These cases present with clear sensations, modalities and aetiology.

When the above criteria are considered and the steps below followed, a correct prescription can be made.

Step-I Make the miasmatic diagnosis of the case i.e. ascertain the surface miasm.

Step-II Assess the Totality of Symptoms, Essence, Keynotes and if any, Peculiar symptoms of the case and decide the indicated remedy.

Step-III Ensure that the indicated remedy covers the surface miasm, as diagnosed in Step I.

Introduction

Step-IV Administer the remedy, which encompasses the miasm as well as the Totality of Symptoms.

Step-I

Make the miasmatic diagnosis of the case, ascertain the surface miasm by

Head to foot miasmatic assessment of symptoms -

Through emotional essence, clinical manifestations, nature and character of the individual case we can diagnose the miasm from different aspects of the patient. e.g.

- **Hair loss** with dry lustreless hair and bran-like dandruff is psora, circular or spotty baldness is sycotic, diffused hair falling is syphilitic, and thick yellow crusts in the hair are tubercular.
- **Taste:** burnt is psoric, fishy is sycotic, metallic is syphilitic and taste of pus is tubercular, **Pulse:** bradycardia is psoric, tachycardia is sycotic and irregular pulse is syphilitic.
- **Bowels:** constipation is psoric, diarrhoea is sycotic, dysentery is syphilitic and malaena is tubercular.
- **Pain:** neuralgic pains are psoric, joint pains are sycotic, bone pains are syphilitic and pains with exhaustion are tubercular.
- *Please refer Miasmatic Prescribing by Subrata K. Banerjea*

Diathesis (tendencies/pre-disposition)

- **Eruptive** diathesis is psoric
- **Rheumatic-gouty**, lithic-uric acid or proliferative diathesis is sycotic,
- **Suppurative-ulcerative** is syphilitic
- **Haemorrhagic, scrofulous** (glandular) diathesis is tubercular.

Secretions

- Psoric secretions are watery, with mucus;
- Sycotic secretions are purulent, thick and yellowish;
- Syphilitic secretions are offensive sticky, acrid, putrid;
- Tubercular discharges are haemorrhagic.

Hobbies

Hobbies can help in the miasmatic diagnosis

Hunting, boxing, wrestling reflects syphilitic taint

Travelling and creative hobbies, cooking, drawing, knitting and acting are tubercular. Gambling is sycotic.

Ask your patient what they would do if they had a week off work and money would be no object. Psora is lazy and will do nothing. Sycosis will go to a casino or the races and Tubercular will go on a round the world trip! All these enquiries assist in enabling you to understand the innate dyscrasia and miasmatic nature of your patient.

Nails

Miasmatic diagnosis can also be made from nail appearance.
- Dry harsh nails are psoric
- Thick, wavy, ribbed, corrugated, convex nails are sycotic.
- Thin, concave nails are syphilitic.
- Glossy and spotted nails are tubercular.

Miasmatic observation of children

- Nervous, anxious, constipated children are psoric
- Restless, hyperactive, colicky, diarrhoeic children are sycotic.
- Withdrawn, dull, extremely forgetful, convulsive, dysenteric children are syphilitic.
- Allergic, haemorrhagic, stubborn, impatient children are tubercular.

By including the miasmatic dyscrasia of the person, the axiom of 'rapid, gentle and permanent recovery' (Hahnemann's Organon §3) is encompassed and the chances of recurrence are eradicated. In cases of one-sided disease with a scarcity of symptoms, the action of the anti-miasmatic remedy is centrifugal, and by bringing the suppressed symptoms to the surface it enables a proper totality to be framed.

The miasmatic consideration is therefore of great importance as demonstrated in the following example:-

A person is suffering from features of gastric ulcer, which has been confirmed by radiography. As ulceration is syphilitic, the surface miasm is therefore syphilitic also. Let us say that the totality of symptoms (physical, emotional and essence) of the person reflects towards Kali Bichromicum, an anti-syphilitic remedy. The choice of remedy is therefore simple, as Kali Bich covers both the totality of symptoms and the surface miasm of this gastric ulcer case. Kali Bich will peel away the outer layer and reveal a second layer underneath. This second layer may perhaps manifest through the appearance of warts or moles on the face, an indication of suppressed sycosis and the next assessment of the case should include this new surface totality. Following Kentian ideology we now know that there needs to be a change in the plan of treatment, that is, the previous syphilitic plan needs to change to a current sycotic plan, and a new anti-sycotic medicine needs to be selected based on the presenting totality.

Step II

Assess the Totality of Symptoms + Essence + Keynotes and PQRS, if any, of the case and formulate the indicated remedy.

Totality of symptoms

- Each of the symptoms must be complete with regard to its location, sensation, modality and concomitant
- The symptoms should have a chronological order of development and progression.
- Environmental, occupational and other exogenous influences on the case must be evaluated.
- Then the background of the case from the past history including any suppression and family history which gives any inherited miasmatic influences.
- The qualitative totality of all the symptoms, 'outwardly reflected picture of the internal essence of the disease' is the sole indication for the choice of the remedy.

Essence

Acquaintance with the psychological essences and personification of drug pictures will assist in the correct choice. As broad examples:

Lycopodium become teachers, doctors and politicians and their personality traits include being careful, cautious, conscientious, conservative, courteous, contained, avoids risk and commitments in other words, safe.

Nux Vomica can become stock brokers, salesmen, and their personality shows they are ambitious, impatient, arrogant, charismatic, aggressive, independent, confident, perfectionists.

Pulsatilla may choose to become nursery nurses, teachers or carers and their personality is emotional, tearful, moody, changeable, pleasing, perceptive, affectionate, caring, forsaken, worriers.

Phosphorus can be an artist, an actor, receptionist or politician and their characteristics demonstrate they are expressive, emotional, social, artistic, impressionable, gregarious, sympathetic and sensitive.

To ascertain a clearer picture for the constitutional medicine ask about the **innate nature** of the person, for example ask the patient to give ten words to describe themselves. Then if patient says I am

Compassionate: medicine such as Argenticum Nitricum, Belladonna, Calcarea Carbonicum, Calcarea Phoshorus, Carcinosin, Causticum, Cocculus, Graphites, Ignatia, Lachesis, Natrum carbonicum, Natrum Muriaticum., Nitric Acid, Nux Vomica., Phosphorus, Pulsatilla,and Sulphur come to mind. Likewise:

Dutiful: Calc. Carb., Calc. Iod., Carcinosin, Cocculus, Ignatia, Kali Ars., Kali Carb., Kali Iod., Lycopodium, Natrum mur., Pulsatilla

Easy Going: Arsenicum, Calc., Carcinosin, Lil.Tig., Lycopodium, Mag. Mur., Natrum mur, Nux vomica, Phos. acid., Phosphorus, Pulsatilla, Rhus tox., Sepia, Silicea, Sulphur, Thuja

Family Oriented: Acetic acid, Anacardium, Arsenicum, Baryta carb., Calc., Calc. Iod., Calc. Sil., Carcinosin, Graphites, Hepar Sulph., Ignatia, Iodium, Kali Brom., Kali Nit., Kali Phos., Lycopodium, Mag Carb., Natrum Carb., Natrum Mur., Petroleum, Phosphorus, Phos. Acid, Pulsatilla, Psorinum, Rhus tox., Sulphur

These of course are all modern interpretations of old proving symptoms, details can be found in "Classical Homoeopathy for an Impatient World" by Dr. Subrata K. Banerjea.

Approach-2 - Cases without clarity of symptoms those which may be on medicinal drugs

It is necessary to perceive the uncontaminated picture of the natural disease according to aphorism §91 of Hahnemann's Organon. However in this drug dependent world the expression of the natural disease may not be visible. By gradual weaning of conventional chemical based drugs it will be possible to unveil the original picture. This can be achieved with homoeopathic organopathic medicines.

In these drug dependent cases, it is very difficult to get a clear picture of the case. The artificial, medicinally induced chronic disease is superimposed on the original natural disease, (ref. §91, Organon) therefore symptoms are contaminated or suppressed and the patient cannot give clear modalities, sensations or concomitants. In such cases, a medicine which has predominant action on the main vital organ that is affected can be prescribed on the basis of few available symptoms (according to §173--§178, Ref. Organon of Medicine) and in this way the conventional pharmaceutical drug is gradually withdrawn. A small organopathic medicine may be suitable for this purpose.

Introduction

In my experience after the patient has weaned off approximately 50% of the conventional medicine, suppressed or previously vague symptoms surface and the patient can be more specific about modalities and sensations. This will lead to making a change in the plan of treatment and using MTEK as discussed in the Approach 1, a constitutional prescription can be made. Through this approach, the patient gains immediate confidence that homoeopathy is acting but has no or little requirement for the conventional pharmaceutical medication.

My experience has shown

In **drug dependent Arthritic cases** medicines such as Actaea Spicata, Angustera Vera, Benzoic Acid, Caulophyllum, Cobaltum Nitricum, Cyclamen Europaeum, Eupatorium Perfoliatum, Formica Ruffa, Franciscea Uniflora, Gettysburg Water, Ginseng (Panax), Gnaphalium, Guaiacum, Hedeoma Pulegioides, Helonias, Kali Iodatum, Lacticum Acidum, Lithium Carbonica, Macrotin, Manganum Aceticum, Natrum Salicylicum, Oleum Jecoris Aselli, Pimpenella Saxifraga, Radium Bromatum, Rhamnus Californica, Rhododendron, Stellaria Media, Viola Odorata and X-Ray can successfully wean the patient off the conventional medication. By using medicine such as that listed above we can start the treatment of steroid dependent arthritic cases which have an absence of clear modalities. Such lesser known organopathic medicines have the capability to alleviate symptoms to a certain extent, thereby the patient is managing the symptoms with homoeopathy as a step to removing the conventional medication. Experience shows that after 40-50% withdrawal of the pharmaceutical drug the uncontaminated, clear symptoms of the natural disease surface and give scope for constitutional prescribing.

In the same way, for **conventional pain killer dependent Migraine cases**, the artificial chronic disease is superimposed on the original natural disease, therefore symptoms are contaminated or suppressed and the patient cannot give a clear picture for a constitutional medicine. In such cases, the following medicines can be selected on the basis of few available symptoms, e.g., Acetanilidum, Anagyris, Bromium, Chionanthus Virginica, Epiphegus, Ferrum Pyro-Phosphoricum, Indium, Iris Versicolor, Kalmia Latifolia, Lac Defloratum, Melilotus, Menispernum, Menynanthes, Oleum Animale, Onosmodium, Saponin, Usnea Barbata, Yucca Filamentosa. Accordingly the conventional allopathic pain killer is gradually withdrawn and after approximately 50% weaning off of the conventional medicine, suppressed symptoms surface and now the patient can give much clearer modalities.

Similarly for **drug dependent Hypertensive cases** where the following medicines Allium Sativa, Crataegus Oxyacantha, Eel Serum, Ergotinum, Lycopus Virginicus, Rauwolfia Serpentina, Spartium Scoparium, Strophanthus Hispidus.

For **drug dependant Hyper-cholesterolaemia cases use of** Adrenalin, Crataegus Oxycantha, Ergotin, Polygonum Aviculare, Spartium Scoparium, Sumbul are capable of gradually weaning off the conventional medication.

For **drug dependent Hayfever cases** where the following medicines Ambrosia, Arundo, Linum usitatissimum, Phleum pratense, Rosa damascena, Skookum Chuck, Wyethia are useful in gradually weaning off the conventional medication.

In **drug dependent Asthma cases**, when the patient is on an inhaler and/or steroids. In such cases it is very difficult to get a clear picture of the case. Medicine such as Aralia Racemosa, Blatta Orientalis, Aspidosperma, Cassia Sophera, Eriodictyon, Pothos Foetidus can be prescribed on the basis of few available symptoms.

Dispensing of the dose of Homoeopathic broncho-dialators

The method that I have found to be most effective is as follows: When the patient requires the conventional bronchodilator when out of breath, to sip the homoeopathic bronchodilator medicine as mentioned above, to be prescribed on the basis of the few available symptoms in drug dependant cases, instead of conventional broncho dialator and in this way tries to defer the conventional medicine as much as possible. In this way, a steroid dependent patient who used to take steroid inhaler 8 hourly, can, with the help of homoeopathic medicine defer the steroids to 12 hourly, then 16, 18, 24 hourly and so on. In this way the conventional medication is gradually weaned off

In my experience after the patient has weaned off approximately 50% of the conventional medicine, suppressed symptoms surface and the patient can give much clearer modalities. *This may lead to making a change in the plan of treatment and on the basis of MTEK a constitutional prescription can be made. Through this approach, not only does the patient gain confidence that homoeopathy is acting, but has also weaned off the conventional medication to a certain extent.*

The patient is often aware of the side effects of the chemicals of the conventional medicine and wants to stop or reduce the dose. I give full control to the patient who often consults with the conventional medicine doctor. By reducing the pharmaceutical drugs in this way empowers the patient and gives confidence to the process, as throughout general well being will improve and the patient's energy level will increase. I do not advise exactly how much to wean off because that should be guided both by the patient together with the prescribing doctor. As the patient tends to make the decisions, so I recommend a disclaimer signed by the patient, especially in my U.K practice.

My Remedy Selection & Dispensing the Dose

Obviously if the case has a clear picture with clear modalities and sensations, I will take Approach 1, as detailed above.

The constitutional prescribing which has the *qualitative* totality, not only a mere quantitative addition of symptoms, the essence, temperament and behaviour of the patient with the miasmatic totality should be present in the final remedy selection.

I prescribe a single medicine, mostly in centesimal potency which I always dispense in water. Ref. Organon §288 5th Edition. By dispensing in water I have observed that aggravation can be avoided and it permits a strong dynamic penetrating action. Ref. Organon §272 6th edition, §288.

I give one single poppy seed Ref. Foot Note §285 5th edition, No.X sized globule. Ref. Organon Foot Note §246 5th edition and §275 6th edition in some sugar of milk Ref. §272 6th edition, to make a medicated sachet. You may note that this dispensing method is heavily referenced from the Organon of Medicine which is the source of the classical method. I instruct the patient to dissolve that powder in half a litre of water which should be shaken and sipped throughout the day, a little should be saved and topped up with fresh water the next morning and shaken and sipped throughout the next day. This process should be continued for 5 to 7 days. So *one single globule of medicine*, without adding any further dose is to be plussed and sipped for 5 – 7 days, then no medication for 1 or 2 weeks.

A second dose may not be required if improvement has commenced however if by chance the recovery has not begun a second dose of the same medicine may be given in the same way, in water, over a series of days, diluting as the days proceed.

Each dose of medicine to sip for 7 days

- When there is a very good similimum with the totality and characteristic symptoms in a clear case.
- When there are more mental symptoms and a good match with personality type.

- When the patient is quick to act and react
- Intellectually keen patients
- Lack of reaction to well indicated medicine
- Lack of vital reaction, lost all susceptibility
- Hypersensitive people on allopathic drugs for a long time
- In sensitive patients who react unfavourably the medicine can be diluted in further, in 3 separate glasses of water and using 50ml from the final glass of dilution in the bottle which will be sipped as described above. To be more clear, the first dose to be dissolved in a litre of water, then take one tea-spoon from that medicated water, put it into a second bottle (half or one litre), top it up with fresh drinking water (tap or mineral), shake and mix, then take one tea spoon from that medicated water, put it into the third bottle (as above), top it up with fresh water, shake and mix and then sip from this third bottle for very sensitive patients.

Each dose medicine to sip for 3–5 days

- Sluggish people who are slow to react
- Drug dependent cases, on regular allopathic drugs
- Terminally ill with gross pathological changes
- Rapid fatal diseases
- Heavy pathology
- Homoeo Prophylaxis
- Acute diseases with clear picture
- Prescription based on NBWS, to clear up the suppression

Each dose medicine to sip for 1–3 days

- Low vitality with high susceptibility those who react powerfully
- Acute
- Gross structural change, when prescribing 6C for example

By dispensing and instructing the patient as above you are following the "Doctrine of Minimum Dose", "Doctrine of Divisibility" and "Doctrine of Plussing" and in my long experience, I have found the centesimal scale has excellent penetrating dynamic power and is capable of uprooting deep seated suppressions of the contemporary world.

LM prescriptions

I rarely use the LM scale even though in fact encouraged to do so by a very famous LM potency prescriber in Calcutta who prescribed only LM scale for over 40+ years, whom I observed in practice for several months after my graduation. Unfortunately, even in this experienced hand I observed aggravation which is meant to be avoided by using the LM scale. I almost exclusively use the centesimal scale and I am confident in this scale of potency. Being a strict classical prescriber, I like to remind you that although Hahnemann mentioned that LM scale is his 'most perfected' method I am of the opinion that if Hahnemann had lived 10 more years, he might have changed his Organon for five more times, Hahnemann was constantly developing and trying make Homoeopathy perfect.

I earnestly encourage my readers to try the above method of water dispensing, diluting, plussing and succussing the single dose of centesimal scale and watch your success with patients grow and flourish.

Advantages of Diluting, Plussing & Dividing the Dose

- The medicine gently stimulates the Vital Force and smoothly overpowers the symptoms
- Ref. Hahnemann's Chronic Disease, P.156 – 157
- Avoids aggravation in hypersensitive patients
- Diminution of the strong power of medicine Ref.§285 thereby avoiding aggravation

For best results- Plus and Succuss

- By modification of every plussed dose, which is given in several different forms, it can best extract the morbid disorder Ref. Foot Note §247

Aggravation from Unchanged, Unmodified Dose

By giving an unchanged dose, the vital force revolts §246

Divisibility of Dose is not addition of the Dose but gradual proportionate liberation of energy

Divided dose is the same quantity which is proportionately divided §287 this leads to a gradual release of energy.

In dosing, think of a pizza, you can finish the whole pizza in one go or you might cut the same pizza into 20 small pieces and eat 2 in the morning, 2 in the afternoon each day, thereby dividing your dose of pizza and at the end of the say 5th day you have finally finished that pizza. Accordingly the patient is having ONE single medicated globule or pizza, fragmented into smaller doses or slices which gives gentle stimulation, without appreciable aggravation of the vital force.

If the case is contaminated through drug dependency I will follow Approach 2 as detailed above and gradually wean off the conventional medicine. Here again I follow §91 of Organon. Generally I have seen after weaning off 40% - 50% of conventional medication, the natural disease surfaces. You will see clear modalities, sensations, character of symptoms and at that stage you follow Approach-1. Do not fire your polychrest until and unless you prepare the case and match with the totality and MTEK. Respect your polychrest and do not prescribe a polychrest when there is scarcity of symptoms such as commonly found in drug dependent cases. By weaning off, when more symptoms come in the surface, then and only then, fire your polychrest and that will overpower the disease. So prepare the patient to receive the polychrest.

My Repetition of the Medicine

I do not repeat the medicine very often. As mentioned above, generally I give a single medicated globule in water, which the patient sips for few days. I might repeat another dose, if there is no change from the very first dose. The reasoning for giving the second dose is
- Many medicines have primary and secondary action, which Hahnemann mentioned in Materia Medica Pura in the Bryonia chapter.
- In this polluted, hectic environment, smoke, fumes, chemicals, the second dose will penetrate the vital force, if, per chance the first dose has been antidoted, lost or spoilt.

Generally after the first prescription, I do a follow-up in 6 – 8 weeks to assess the reaction to the medicine. I may wait at least 3 – 4 months in chronic cases before repeating the dose however if there has been even a 2% positive change on any of the following areas, I will wait and watch with wisdom. WWW. You will never, I repeat never, gain anything by premature repetition; on the contrary you will always lose. This is the most difficult part for any homoeopath to learn. I have found over the years practitioners are enthusiastic and excited, if the patient is 10% better it is too tempting to repeat the medicine to get a 'faster' result this usually means the reverse,

Introduction

the patient's improvement will be slower and might even spoil the case.

In order to be exact, during both the initial consultation and follow-up evaluation, I always ask my patients to evaluate and then grade the main complaints, they might be one or many. e.g. if the patient is complaining of headache, I will ask to put a grade about the intensity and severity of the pain out of 10 or a percentage. Similarly I always ask to put a value out of 10 or a percentage relevant to the following areas

- General sense of well being
- Physical Energy, vigour, strength, co ordination
- Mental Energy, power of focus, motivation, concentration and memory
- Appetite,
- Sleep, quantity and quality, feels refreshed
- Temperament, emotional tranquility and sense of harmony in the patient

In some cases it is useful for the patient to keep a diary of the changes to their symptoms and at their appointment can summarise these details.

By adopting this method, during the follow-up consultation when a patient says 'I am not feeling any change' it is possible to compare with the previous report and can include scrutinising head to foot symptoms, with the scores of suffering, intensity and frequency, this will be clear to both the practitioner and patient the exact condition and you may find in many aspects, patient is 5 to 10% better.

After a successful first prescription, in many cases, I have waited, not prescribed, for over two years. Of course I do the follow-ups in every 6 to 8 weeks or so and I carefully consider how the patient is responding. In some cases it is beneficial for the patient to have a prescription of non-medicated globules which is confirmed by many master Homoeopaths and the medical fraternity alike, including Hahnemann, Organon §91, §281 6th Edition.

As I said above, even if there is 2% positive change

YOU WAIT & WATCH WITH WISDOM -WWW

Please do not repeat the medicine when there is a positive report, when you will become proficient at this you will find yourself amongst the class of very successful prescribers.

The last and final deciding factor is the patient's sense of well being and emotional harmony, from the onset of your homoeopathic treatment up until now. This can be represented in a graph, an ascending curve represents improvement, a straight line represents stand still status and declining curve represents going down hill.

You should WAIT if the curve is either straight line or ascending. You repeat when the curve is declining.

Sometimes my students in different parts of Europe and the United States doubt this long waiting in the haste and hurry of life. I respectfully invite them to any of my teaching clinics both the Allen Teaching Clinic and the Bengal Allen Teaching Clinic where you can see how the methodologies detailed above are successfully implemented in the drug dependent population.

When I Might Change the Medicine

I will change in the following situations:
- No improvement even after reasonable time of waiting (it is difficult to say what is this reasonable time; as many times it's a feeling that the last medicine is not working but generally I will take time to make my first prescription and will wait at least for 3 to 5 months in chronic cases, before I change. In acute situations, of course it will be different.
- The health graph as stated above is in straight line for at least for two consecutive follow-ups meaning there has been no change for a while which represents stand still status or declining curve which represents going down hill only then I will change the medicine. And also if the symptoms show a different picture.
- There is severe aggravation of some symptoms and needs urgent intervention, may be an acute or acute exacerbation of chronic symptom.
- Miasmatic or Aetiological block or cessation of improvement, needs an intercurrent to remove the block.
- The symptoms picture has changed. So to evaluate the new miasmatic totality and totality of symptoms and prescribe accordingly.
- Your last medicine has exhausted all that it could have done, may be you even ascended to CM potency however, sometimes if I still feel it's the same medicine, according to Kent, I will repeat the series again, so you need to change the plan of treatment either according to the presenting totality or a complementary or related or chain of medicine that follows well.

Introduction

Some Interesting Notes from the Organon of Medicine

- **Single Globule to be used :** Foot Note §246 5th Ed.; §275 6th Ed.
- **Size of the globule is of Poppy-Seed :** Foot Note §285 5th Ed.
- **Medicine must be dispensed in Liquid Vehicle water :** §288 5th Ed.; §272 6th Ed.; §246 6th Ed.
  - ▲ Even Centesimal Scale Potencies to be dispensed in water : Appendix. P. 263.
  - ▲ Feeble action if given dry : Chronic Disease P. 159.
  - ▲ Even 30th potency to be dissolved in water : §128.
- **Every Dose should be deviated from the former :** §246 6th Ed., §247 6th Ed., §280 6th Ed.
- **Doctrine of Divisibility :** Appendix. P. 266.
- Even in dilution, the power of the medicine remains the same : §287, §286, §285.
- **Application of Placebo :** §91, §281 6th Ed..
- **Do not Repeat when the Patient is Improving:** §245.
- **Against Polypharmacy :** § F.N. 272.
- **Homoeopathician treats the Miasm, upon which the Malady depends :** §205.
- **No Food restriction in Acute Diseases :** §262, 263.
- **Smallness of Dose :** §277, 278, 284, 285.
- **Divided Dose**
  - ▲ Diminution of strong power of medicine for sensitive patients §285 & F.N.
  - ▲ Effect is increased but actual amount remains same §286.
  - ▲ Every portion of plussing. Smallest portion of diluting fluid receives same quantity of medicine in *proportion* as all the rest §287 and the last selected homoeopathic remedy could best extract the morbid disorder only if applied in several different forms § F.N. 247.
- **Do not prescribe on undefined, non-characteristic, vague symptoms:** §165
- **If two medicines are indicated**: Prescribe the most indicated one, after that's action is over, do not automatically prescribe the second one but re-examine the case: §169.
- **Olfaction of medicines:** § F.N. 288, FN § 247.
- **How long the medicine can last**: Medicinal power stay, upto 20 years → § F.N. 288.

- **Deviation of Dose**: Every potency should be deviated from former or later → §246, 247, 280.
- **No requirement of Antidote**: Next selected medicine antidotes: § F.N. 249
- **Scope of Intercurrent medicine** : Sulph – Hepar Sulph → § F.N. 246.
- **Succussion**: Every dose to be raised by sucussion → §280.
- **Even after discovery of LM potency, Hahnemann did not discarded the centesimal scale**: Mentioning of 30th potency even in 6th edition → §128.
- **Do not repeat when patient is improving:** §245.
- **Minutest employment of dose :** §246.
- **Single globule to be administered not 6-7 globules**: § F.N. 246, 275.

Contents

Authentic Cures with Medical Reports before & After Treatment — v
Author's Dedication — vii
Preface — ix
Introduction — xiii

1. **Cardio-Vascular Diseases - Cured Cases** — 1
   A Case of PALPITATION — 1

2. **Dermatological Diseases - Cured Cases** — 7
   An Obstinate Long Standing Case of Psoriasis, Completely Cured — 7
   A Case of Baldness Miasmatic Approach of Prescribing — 15
   A Diagnosed Case of Atopic Dermatitis — 26
   A Case of Wart on Palm – Mrs R. S. — 34
   A Case of Fistula in Cheek – Mr P.B. — 42
   A Case of Eczematous Ulcer in Cheek — 46
   A Case of Psoriasis: Mr P.D. — 52
   A Case of Wart on Hand & Feet: Mast. U.S. — 56
   A Case of Lip Lipoma: Mr S.M. — 60
   A Case of Atopic Vesicular Dermatitis – Master B.M. — 64
   A Case of Facial Acne – Miss R.D. — 70

3. **E.N.T. Diseases - Cured Cases** — 77
   A Case of Chronic Suppurative Otitis Media (C.S.O.M): Mr N.D. — 77
   A Case of Recurrent Epistaxis (Nose Bleeding): Mr A.B.S. — 84

4. **Endocrinological Disorders - Cured Cases** — 89
   A Case of Diabetes Mellitus - Mr M.M. — 89
   A Case of Hypo-Thyroidism: Mr S. C. — 96
   A Case of Diabetes – Mr M.K.C. — 100
   A Case of Diabetes Mellitus– Mr S.B. — 104
   A Case of Diabetes - Mr M.M. — 110
   A Case of Hypothyroidism – Mrs M.G. — 115
   A Case of Hypo-Thyroidism: Miss R.M. — 122

A Case of Diabetes – Mrs A.D.	127
A Case of Hyperthyroidism: Mrs I.B.	132
A Case of Hyperthyroidism: (49 Year Old Male)	137
A Case of Diabetes: Mr J.K.S.	141

5. Gastro–Intestinal (G.I.) Diseases – Cured Cases — 145

A Case of Salivary Duct Calculus: Mr L.D.	145
A Case of Duodenal Ulcer – Mr M.M.	151
A Case of Cholelithiasis (Gall Bladder Stone) : Mr S.S.	155
A Case of Peptic Ulcer: Mrs R.C.	159
A Case of Hepatomegaly: Mr.R.M.	162
A Case of Fatty Liver: Mr C.M.	167
A Case of Cholelithiasis: Mrs R.K.	171
A Case of Cholecystitis With Thickened Wall of Gall Bladder : Miss B.C.	177
A Case of Duodenal Ulcer: Mrs R.C.	183
A Case of Duodenal Ulcer: Mr T.D.	188
A Case of Giardiasis : Master A.D.	195
A Case of Splenomegaly: Master M.S.	202
A Case of Cholecystitis (Thickened Non Functioning Gall Bladder) :Mr J.S.	206
A Case of Chronic Duodenal Ulcer: Mr J.A.	210
A Case of Salivary Duct Calculi: Mr A.N.	215
A Case of Cholesteoma Of Gall Bladder: Mrs M.D.	219

6. Gynaecological Diseases – Cured Cases — 225

A Case of Bilateral Polycystic Ovaries: Mrs K.B.	225
A Case of Infertility Associated With Pelvic Inflammatory Disease & Bilateral Large Ovarian Cysts Completely Cured By Homoeopathy	229
A Case of Fibroid & Renal Stone Mrs K.S.	237
A Case of Ovarian Tumour: Mrs M.G.	243

7. Uro-Genital (Male) Diseases - Cured Cases — 249

A Case of Abdominal Tumour: Mr A.R.	249
A Case of Oligospermia : Mr S.B.	253
A Case of Urethral Stricture: Mr.A.M	260
A Case of Recurrent Herpes Genitalis: Mr K. C. M.	266
A Case of Hypertrophy Of Prostate With Recurrent– U.T.I.	273

8. Neoplastic Diseases - Cured Cases — 279

A Case of Brain Tumour: Mrs P.R.J	279
A Case of Cystic Hygroma of The Neck: Master S.M.	288

Contents

A Case of Fibrolipoma –Inguinal Region: Mr A. K. C.	293
A Case of Chronic Sub-Mental Lymph Node Enlargement: Ms. B.S.	299
A Case of Sebaceous Cyst In The Neck: Mr T.S.	303
A Case Bronchogenic Carcinoma: Mr S.L.	308

9. Neurological Diseases - Cured Cases — 313
A Case of Long Standing Cerebral Atrophy: Mr R.N.B. — 313

10. Psychiatric Disorders - Cured Cases — 321
A Case of Anxiety Neurosis: Ms. F.K. — 321

11. Respiratory Diseases - Cured Cases — 327
A Case of Pleural Effusion: Dr. S.K.C. — 327
A Case of Emphysema with Bronchospasm: Mr N.C.D. — 332
A Case of Emphysema of Both Lungs — 340
A Case of Eosinophilia: Mr S.H.M. — 345
A Case of Tuberculosis with Bronchospasm: Miss B.K. — 351
A Case of Pulmonary Koch's (Tuberculosis) with Bronchospasm In 30 Year Old Female — 361

12. Rheumatological Diseases - Cured Cases — 367
A Case of Shoulder Joint Dislocation: Miss O. S. — 367
A Case of Rheumatoid Arthritis in A 18 Years Old Female, Arnica Montana Given — 372

13. Urological Diseases - Cured Cases — 379
A Case of Renal Calculi: Mr R.C. — 379
A Case of Renal Calculi: Mr P.G. — 384
A Case of Renal Calculi : Mr S.P.M. — 388
A Case of Renal Calculi in 48 Years Old Female — 393
A Case of Renal Calculi and Hydronephrotic Kidney : Mr G.D. — 397
A Case of Renal Calculi in 41 Year Old Male: Mr D.P.M. — 402
A Case of Renal Calculi: Mr J.H. — 407

Short Case Stories — 412

CHAPTER 1

Cardio-Vascular Diseases-Cured Cases

1. A Case of PALPITATION

Case No. C001

Age : 31 year-old as on 28.11.1988.
Sex : Female.
Weight: 50 kgs.

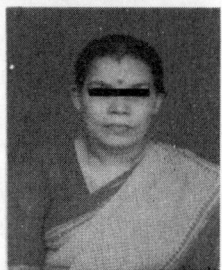

Photo of the patient Mr. S.D.

Presenting Complaints

- Palpitation of heart, it can get so much that she becomes senseless. Problem started after the death of her sister 6 months ago. She is still grieving.
- Relapses: 4-5 times, every week.
- Pain in both legs to ankle, loin, elbow to wrist joint; aggravated from lying down, aggravated by rest; aggravated at bed time; aggravated by 1st motion, ameliorated by massage and gentle movement.
- Patient feels uneasy from any gas.
- Disturbed sleep, for last 6 months.
- Itching in skin, but no visible eruption – buttocks, abdomen and chest, gradually moving upwards. Excessive itching, aggravated by perspiration, in summer; no discharge, began in 1988.
- Toothache → in decayed teeth; better gurgling with cold water, aggravated by taking hot water or tea.
- Hesadache – from bus (coach) journey, congestive sensation, aggravated in a smoky room; ameliorated by massaging, sleeping.

- Menses – early (10 days advanced) for last 5 months. Excessive pain in lower abdomen during menses. Weakness (++) during menses.
- Quantity – normal but excessively large clots; the more the flow the less the pain. Amelioration after passing clots, associated with diarrhoea.
- Discharge: thick, sticky white, after menses.
- Profuse gas formation, rumbling sound in abdomen, profuse flatus.
- Morning diarrhoea – once or twice, offensive smelling, undigested food particles.
- Quantity – Scanty; yellowish; pain before stool, aggravated from irregular diet, rich and spicy food; better from having less spicy food.
- Nervous temperament. Easily hurt. Jealous
- Moody (+++), changeable mood.
- Anger ++, Indifferent ++.
- Demanding, high expectations.
- Very sensitive.
- Thirst: average.
- Perspiration: Medium to profuse (++)
- Thermal: Chilly patient.

Investigations Carried Out Before/After Dr. Banerjea's Treatment

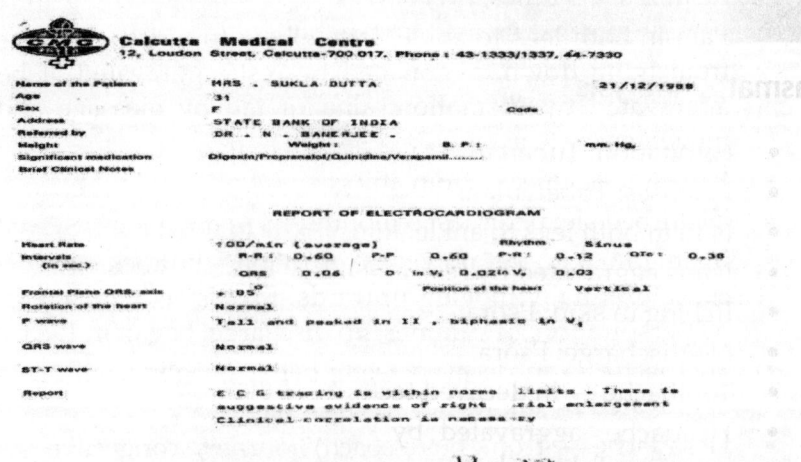

ECG Report of Mrs. S.D. before Homoeopathic treatment

Cardio-Vascular Diseases-Cured Cases

ECG Report of Mrs. S.D. 12 months after treatment

11th Aug'88: Blood Eosinophil-6, Erythrocyte Sedimentation Rate 30, Red Blood Cell 4 x10^6

Culture urine: No growth. BSPP (Blood Sugar Post Prandial): 104.

21st Dec'88: Electro Cardio Gram (ECG): Evidence of right atrial enlargement.

19th Jul'89: Chest X-ray: Nothing Abnormal Detected. Electro Cardio Gram (ECG): Nothing Abnormal Detected.

4Th Mar'90: Electro Cardio Gram (Ecg): Electro Cardiogram Tracing Is Normal

CASE ANALYSIS, MIASMATIC DIAGNOSIS AND FINAL PRESCRIPTION

Miasmatic Analysis

- Palpitation: Tubercular.
- Relapses: Tubercular.
- Pain in both legs to ankle, loin, elbow to wrist joint: Sycosis.
- Pains aggravated by rest, ameliorated by gentle rubbing: Sycosis.
- Itching in skin: Psora.
- No discharge: Psora.
- Toothache → in decayed teeth: Syphilis.
- Headache, aggravated by riding in a carriage (bus or coach journey): Tubercular.

- Headache ameliorated by rest: Psora-tubercular.
- Menses – early: Tubercular.
- Weakness (++) during menses: Psora-tubercular.
- Excessively large clots: Tubercular.
- White discharge thick, sticky: Syphilis.
- Profuse gas formation, rumbling sound in abdomen: Psora.
- Morning diarrhoea: Sycosis.
- Lienteria (undigested food particles): Syphilitic.
- Stool: yellowish: Sycotic.
- Nervous temperament: Psora.
- Jealous: Sycosis.
- Moody (+++), changeable mood: Tubercular.
- Indifferent ++: Tubercular.
- Very sensitive: Psora-sycosis.

Mixed Miasmatic with Tubercular preponderance.

Prescription Made on the Basis of

- Palpitation of heart: problem started after death of sister 6 months back: grief.
- Patient feels uneasy from any gas. Rumbling in abdomen, much flatulence.
- Disturbed sleep, for last 6 months.
- Toothache → aggravates after taking hot water or tea.
- Headache – congestive sensation following grief, aggravated in a smoky room.
- Menses – early (10 days advanced) for last 5 months.
- Excessive pain –during menses. Weakness (++) during menses.
- Itching of skin.
- Nervous temperament.
- Easily hurt. Jealous.
- Moody (+++), changeable mood.
- Indifferent ++.
- Demanding, high expectations.
- Very sensitive.

The miasmatic breakdown of Ignatia is Psora +++, Sycosis ++, Syphilis +, Tubercular +++, which covers the case as well.

Final Prescription and Remedy Reaction

I started the case with Ignatia 200 C followed by 1M (2 potencies were given, as prescribed on the basis of Aetiology (NBWS). Patient improved dramatically and finished the case with 50M, in just over 12 months. Unfortunately a detailed prescription chart is not available for this case.

This is a wonderful case where Ignatia has been prescribed though six months after the grief incident but as the grief was still raw, reason therefore Ignatia has been selected. I have even prescribed Ignatia two years after the bereavement, if the grief is still fresh and patient thinks about this at least 3-4 times in a week.

Authenticity of Cure

CD Reference: C001-PALPITATION-SD

CHAPTER 2

Dermatological Diseases-Cured Cases

1. AN OBSTINATE LONG STANDING CASE OF PSORIASIS, COMPLETELY CURED

Case No. D001

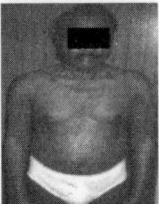
Mr. A.L. Psoriasis

Mr. A.L. 52 yrs. old, came to me first on 11th April, 1987, complaining as follows:
- Eruptions all over the body, skin dries and peels off, no discharge of blood, fluid or pus. No itching, no pain.
- Scaly in character with profuse bran like scaling.
- The skin disease started in 1970, at the seaside in Goa, and since then the patient has consulted various dermatologists without any appreciable change.
- It started on the trunk, chest and back, and slowly spread over almost all parts of the body covered by clothes.
- The face and scalp were clear from the beginning.
- Previously there was nothing on the palms but around 1978, one circular spot appeared near the wrist. The patient tried to conceal that during his office hours, so he put on gloves and subsequently it broke virulently in the palm and dorsum of both the hands.
- The patient also tried various Ayurvedic and Homoeopathic medicines and ointments without any permanent improvement.
- Occasional cough during winter.
- Appetite - Normal.
- Sweat - Profuse.
- Stool and urine - Normal.
- Sexual organs - Nothing abnormal is noted.
- Skin heals in normal time; does not suppurate.
- Temperament - Mild, quiet and non communicative, sympathetic, depressed, occasionally weepy.

- Memory - Normal.
- Fears - Nothing particular.
- Past History (i) Typhoid in 1964. (ii) Asthma in 1985. (iii) Psoriasis since 1970.
- Patient had allopathic treatment for typhoid and asthma, including steroids for asthma.
- Vaccinations - No adverse reaction.
- Chilly patient who also catches cold easily.
- Likes spicy food, salt ++, salty +, cold food ++. Likes meat, but after eating red meat there is unusual irritation and discomfort in the skin.
- Though chilly, likes winter, which is better for skin. Dislikes rainy weather and damp. Easily affected by changes in weather.
- Thirst - Normal.
- Perspiration- Heavy and oily.
- Sleep and dreams - Nothing abnormal noted.
- Married with four children.
- Family History
  - Father died at the age of 45 with asthma.
  - Mother died of hepatitis at the age of 48.

(a) Provisional Diagnosis: Psoriasis.

(b) Miasmatic Diagnosis: Mixed miasmatic (preponderance of psora-sycosis).

Miasmatic Interpretation of the Psoriasis Case

Psora	Sycosis	Syphilis	Tubercular,
• Skin dry and harsh • Mild, silent temperament	• Skin peels off • Skin scaly in character • Circular spots appeared near the wrist • Oily skin with thickly oozing perspiration • Psoriasis • Tendency to conceal the symptoms • H/O Asthma is Psora-sycotic • Desire for salt & salty foods • Meat causes uneasiness • Hates rainy weather & damp • F/H of asthma with father • Fish scale eruptions are tri-miasmatic	• Depressed	• Chilly • Catches cold easily • Desires salt

Psora 2   Sycosis 12   Syphilis 1   Tubercular 3

Dermatological Diseases-Cured Cases

In this case there is a clear Sycotic preponderance in the history and the presenting symptoms reflect Sycosis as a surface miasm. On the basis of the totality of symptoms Thuja was chosen, which covered the surface miasm and the family history. Thuja also covers the surface symptoms as well as the surface miasm and therefore it is capable of peeling off this presenting layer. In this case there was no need to compare remedies miasmatically as the case was clearly Thuja (presenting symptoms and the surface miasm supports the prescription), however in few other cases below you will see how the miasmatic analysis helped to differentiate the remedy choice as the case was confused by excessive suppression.

This is a wonderful example of how miasmatic interpretation of a case helps the certainty of chronic prescribing as Thuja covers the miasmatic totality as well as the totality of symptoms therefore one can be confident to watch and wait for the movement of symptoms. In this case, you can see from the illustrations that after 50% improvement of the case, the appearances of the skin lesions were circular which confirmed that the patient still required a Sycotic medicine; therefore no change in the miasmatic plan of treatment was required. This reflects that miasmatic understanding helps in management and prognosis of the case and confirms any need for a change in the plan of treatment.

Note: Generally in psoriasis, one may find the dryness of Psora, squamous character of Syphilis and thickened skin with fish scale eruptions of Sycosis.

Thuja has the miasmatic breakdown: Psora ++, Sycosis +++, Syphilis ++, Tubercular ++.

Prescription Chart

Dates	Points in favour of the Prescription	Prescribed Medicine
11th Apr'87	(i) Eruptions are only in the covered areas; (ii) Oily & shiny appearance of the face; (iii) Change of weather affects the patient; (iv) Chilly patient but desires cold food; (v) Averse to rainy season (hydrogenoid); (vi) Sycotic coverage.	Thuja 30 1 dose followed (48 hours later) by Thuja LM 3 1 globule in a bottle of water to be sipped --- top up – sip --- top up continue like this for 1 week.
12th May'87	Severe <aggravation.	Thuja LM 5 1 globule in a bottle of water to be sipped --- top up – sip --- top up continue like this for 1 week.

Dates	Points in favour of the Prescription	Prescribed Medicine
11th Jun'87	Entire layer of skin from the sole came off, patient feeling better on the whole.	Thuja LM 7 1 globule in a bottle of water to be sipped --- top up – sip --- top up continue like this for 1 week.
10th Jul'87	Patient complaining of nocturnal fever, night sweats, hot flushes. No change in skin. Change in the plan of treatment. Anti-tubercular coverage.	Ars. Iod. 30 2 doses (1 globule in water to be divided into two doses) (alternate mornings)
25th Jul'87	Feeling better of the nocturnal fever. Wait and watch before any change.	Sac lac 15 doses (alternate mornings).
31st Jul'87	Patient came back with severe dyspnoea (a return of an old symptom suppressed by allopathic medicine). Patient is having attacks at midnight and better in orthopnoea (bending forward with piled up pillows to lie on).	Ars. Alb. 30 2 doses (daily morning).
10th Aug'87	Dyspnoea is much better. Change of plan of treatment. Complementary of Arsenicum album, i.e. Thuja being prescribed again.	Thuja LM 9 1 globule in a bottle of water to be sipped --- top up – sip --- top up continue like this for 1 week.
8th Sep'87	As a whole psoriasis is better again and the patient feels well.	Thuja LM 11 1 globule in a bottle of water to be sipped --- top up – sip --- top up continue like this for 1 week.
26th Sep'87	Feeling better. Psoriasis disappearing from above downwards. Upper part of the trunk, palms, soles and the back are 50% better.	Thuja LM 13 1 globule in a bottle of water to be sipped --- top up – sip --- top up continue like this for 1 week.
29th Oct'87	Entire layer from the shin-bone came off. As a whole feeling better. Appetite increased. Depression is much less.	Thuja LM 15 1 globule in a bottle of water to be sipped --- top up – sip --- top up continue like this for 1 week.
3rd Dec'87	The eruptions are slowly disappearing. No new scales or patches have appeared.	Thuja LM 17 1 globule in a bottle of water to be sipped --- top up – sip --- top up continue like this for 1 week.

Dermatological Diseases-Cured Cases

Dates	Points in favour of the Prescription	Prescribed Medicine
4th Jan'88	The eruptions are slowly disappearing. No new patches have appeared.	Thuja LM 19 1 globule in a bottle of water to be sipped --- top up – sip --- top up continue like this for week.
4th Feb'88	The eruptions are slowly disappearing. No new patches have appeared	Thuja LM 21 1 globule in a bottle of water to be sipped --- top up – sip --- top up continue like this for 1 week
7th Mar'88	Patient is much better. I have changed the scale and potency, to finish the case.	Thuja 10M 1 globule in a bottle of water to be sipped --- top up – sip --- top up continue like this for 10 days.
5th Apr'88	Much better. Wait and watch.	
19th May'88	Much better. Wait and watch.	
13th Jul'88	Much better. To finish the case and to observe if there is any residue to resolve and see if anything new appears.	Thuja 50M 1 globule in a bottle of water to be sipped --- top up – sip --- top up continue like this for 10 days.
5th Sep'88	Much better. To finish the case and to observe if there is any residue to resolve and see if anything new appears.	Thuja CM 1 globule in a bottle of water to be sipped --- top up – sip --- top up continue like this for 10 days.
21st Nov'88	Nothing noted to complain about. Overall very well. Still I asked him to visit, so that he can be prescribed a deep acting anti-tubercular to close.	
30th Jan'89	Total cure. To finish the case deep acting Syco-tubercular remedy.	Bacillinum 200 1 globule in a bottle of water to be sipped --- top up – sip --- top up continue like this for 10 days
	Instruction to the patient - only visit if any symptoms re occur.	

Miasmatic Approach in Psoriasis Treatment

- Dr. H. Roberts says, Psoriasis is the marriage of all miasms, but its characteristics are predominantly Psoric and Sycotic.
- My approach for the treatment of chronic cases is always from the miasmatic point of view, the heritage that I have descended from, my three generations of homoeopaths. I do take up the whole case and from the totality of symptoms, I make a miasmatic totality and thereby arrive at a miasmatic diagnosis of the case. Then, I like to ensure that the remedy which is indicated by the totality of the symptoms, should cover the miasmatic totality too. Or in other words, the remedy should also cover the miasmatic background of the patient. In this way I am confident my prescribed remedy always covers both the totality of symptoms and the miasmatic dyscrasia of the patient and the cure becomes permanent as discussed in §3 of Hahnemann's Organon of Medicine.
- In this case of Psoriasis, I started with a deep acting anti-sycotic remedy, as there was sycotic preponderance, but one should also remember, that polychrests like Thuja, do cover most of the miasms in greater or lesser degrees. So in this tri-miasmatic case of Psoriasis, Thuja not only covered the sycotic preponderance but also touched the other miasms.
- I've learnt from the collective experience of 106 years of my ancestral homoeopaths, who passed their gems of wisdom from one generation to the next, that in Psoriasis cases at any stage or at the end, you will find tubercular miasmatic state will surface and a deep acting Anti-Tubercular remedy will be needed on the basis of the presenting totality of symptoms. This will ensure the cure is permanent. The 'Medicine of Experience'! **I never prescribe for miasm but prescribe for miasmatic state and their presenting symptoms**. It is the ability of the physician to skilfully elicit the symptoms from the patient, in order to assess the surface and the latent miasms.
- In this case, Bacillinum was prescribed as a completing remedy which is a Syco (++) Tubercular (+++) remedy; and also, Bacillinum has the capacity to throw out to the surface the eruptions, which were suppressed previously by the use of allopathic steroid medicines. This property of Bacillinum has also been recognised by Dr. Burnett in terms of ringworm - repercussion.

CONCLUSION

This was a very interesting case of long-standing Psoriasis and through my miasmatic approach of prescribing; the patient has not only found relief from his problem but still over twenty years later enjoys permanent good health.

*Readers may view the pictures of the case (before and after treatment) in our website under Dermatological Diseases (**Case No. D001**- A case of Psoriasis in a middle aged man, completely cured by Thuja).*

Authenticity of Cure

CD Reference: D001-PSORIASIS-LAZ

Cured Cases

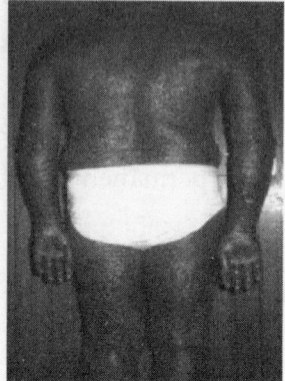

Mr. A.L. Psoriasis, before treatment of Dr. Banerjea.

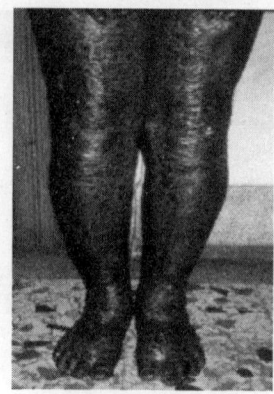

Mr. A.L. Psoriasis, before treatment

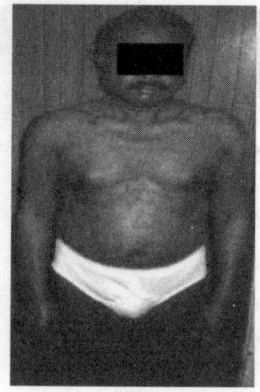

Mr. A.L. Psoriasis, before treatment

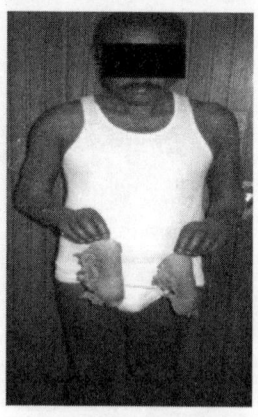

Sloughing of a layer (de-toxification), 2 months, after treatment

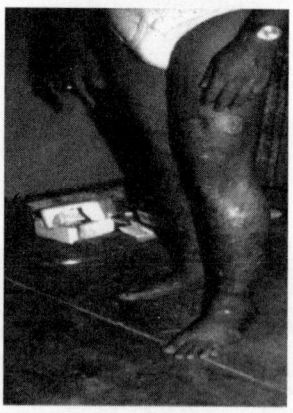

16 months of homoeopathic treatment

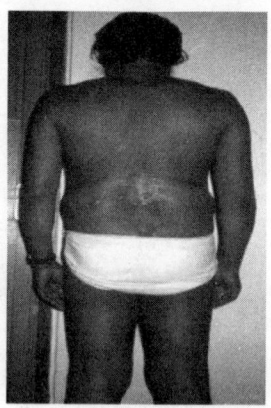

20 months of homoeopathic treatment

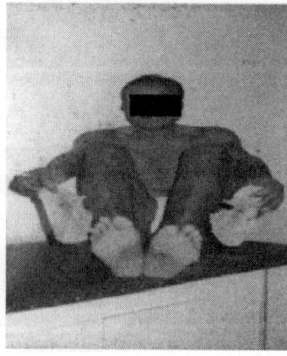

Sloughing of skin from both leg, towards the end (22 months) of treatment

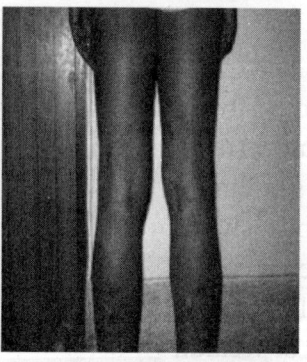

22 months of homoeopathic treatment

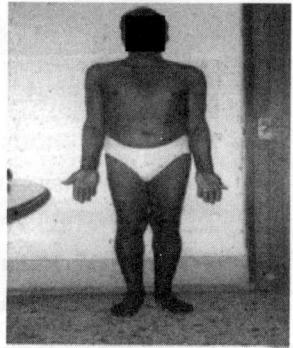

Not a single spot in the whole body. Treatment stopped but the case monitored for 85 months, nothing returned

2. A CASE OF BALDNESS MIASMATIC APPROACH OF PRESCRIBING

Case No. D002

Name of the Patient Mr. G.M., 20 years.

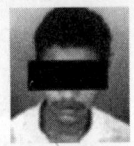

Mr. G.M., a case of total Baldness

Presenting Complaints

- Complete hair loss, almost shiny baldness.
- Hair started falling out about nine years ago, which patient thinks was after delayed convalescence of typhoid fever (enteric fever).
- For about the last fourteen months, there has been complete baldness.
- At the initial stage of hair falling, it used to aggravate (increased hair falling) after showering, and during rainy season.
- Gas and distension of abdomen, since typhoid fever, aggravates from rich and spicy food. Appetite has also become poor.
- Extreme weakness, easy fatigue ability, from least exertion.
- Bouts of nausea come on during the day, more after heavy meals, since typhoid fever.
- Weakness aggravated by exertion and motion, better by complete rest.
- Head- Hot flushes from vertex with occasional burning when gets irritated, ends up with headache which is long lasting.
- Eyes - Nothing particular.
- Ears - H/O (History of) glue ear (discharge from ear) during childhood. Now better.
- Nose - Catches cold easily. It starts with a runny nose → sneezing.
- Mouth - Apthous ulcer (recurrent). Foetor oris.
- Teeth - Occasional swelling of the gums from cold.
- Tongue - Thick, moist, slight imprint of the teeth.
- Throat - When catches cold, pain left side of the throat.
- Lungs - Occasional dry cough.
- Heart - As a result of weakness, occasional palpitation, < while fast walking, < from exertion, < from emotional upsets.
- Abdomen - (i) Distension of abdomen, especially. upper and middle portion. (ii) Eructation ameliorates. (iii) Since typhoid fever, his

digestive capacity has become extremely poor.
- Stomach - Appetite poor.
- Sweat - Average, no specific odour.
- Urine - Regular, no odour.
- Stool - (i) Stool not clear. (ii) Mucus +. (iii) Offensive odour +(iv) Sensation as if not finished so has to wait a long time in the bathroom.
- Upper Extremities - Nothing particular.
- Palms- Occasional perspiration in palms when he feels extremely frustrated.
- Lower Extremities - Nothing particular.
- Male Genital Organs - Sexual desire strong. Prolonged History of masturbation, which he thinks has weakened him. Wet dreams - occasionally.
- Anus - Nothing particular.
- Skin (i) Delayed healing. (ii) Pityriasis - more in the trunk, for the last two years, aggravates during summer.
- Temperament - Extremely irritable, objects to parental guidance in every way. Whimsical, suicidal. Likes to leave home (escape).
- Tendencies - Suicidal tendency.
- Habits (i) Silent habits. (ii) Dirty habits.
- Life and Hatred - Desire for death, disgusted with life.
- Memory - Weak, gradual loss of memory.
- Weeping - Weeping mood, involuntary sighing.
- Sympathy - Sympathetic - average.
- Actions - Slow.
- Perceptions- Dull.
- Fears - Fear of darkness, thunderstorms, incurable diseases, failure.
- Causative Factors/Aetiology - Bad effects of masturbation; he thinks weakness since loss of semen; profuse loss of vital-fluids; weakness. Bad effects of typhoid fever delayed convalescence. Hair falling started thereafter. N.B.W.S - excessive mental labour; mental worries, anxiety, memory weakness since. Has suffered from a skin condition, Pityriasis and has applied some lotions. (vi) Habits- Alcohol, smoking, takes opium. No such bad effects from them.
- Past Medical History - Typhoid, skin disease, measles.

- Vaccination History- Regular vaccinations. Has not suffered from chicken pox or any other infective/childhood disorders.
- What is the first cause of breakdown of health? Typhoid fever - N.B.W.S.
- Homoeopathic Generalities:
- Heat and cold relationship - Chilly ++. Hates rain. Catches cold easily.
- Desire and aversion for foodstuffs - Sweet ++, sour +, pungent and hot ++, salt +, salty ++, bitter +. Bread +, milk – aversion to, potato +, vegetables and spinach +, onion +, fruit +, fish ++, meat and chicken ++, egg (boiled and fried) +. Rich, spicy and fat food ++, warm food- no, cold food +++ Warm drinks - no, cold drinks +. Thirsty ++.
- Sleep - Disturbed sleep, wakes up 4 a.m. and cannot sleep again. Dreams of robbers, dead people.
- Discharges - Stool, urine, sweat, only stool has offensive odour. Sweat and urine are normal.
- Family history (i) Uncle - cancer of the stomach. (ii) Maternal aunt - diabetes.
- History of treatment - Has had lots of allopathic, Ayurvedic and homoeopathic medicines without any lasting improvement. Patient cannot name the medicines, oils, and lotions applied, but there were plenty.

Case Analysis, Miasmatic Diagnosis and Final Prescription

I started the case with Typhoidinum considering the bad effects being caused by the enteric (typhoid) fever and as the patient mentioned that he is N.B.W.S. (never been well since). According to Dr. D.M. Foubister's approach, Typhoidinum was given in order to clear up the bad effects caused by the disease and to restore the vitality. The patient had improved to a certain extent with Typhoidinum and I presume that the block from the disease had been removed. After a considerable period of waiting (W.W.W. = Wait, Watch with Wisdom) with the indicated remedy, there was no further movement of symptoms, so I decided to make a change in the plan of treatment and according to the totality, Thyroidinum was prescribed and the result was extremely satisfying.

Miasmatic Analysis

Psora	Sycosis	Syphilis	Tubercular
• Gas in the abdomen • Appetite poor • Caches cold easily • Dry cough • Silent habits, dirty habits • Fear of thunderstorms • Fear of darkness • Fear of incurable disease • Fear of failure • Desire for pungent and hot foods • Extreme weakness, easy fatigue, from least exertion (Tubercular miasm joins) • Weakness aggravates from exertion, motion, ameliorates from complete rest • Weak, gradual loss of memory • Weeping mood, involuntary sighing (Sycosis can join) • Actions slow • Food desires- sweet++, sour +, pungent and hot++	• Hot flushes from vertex • Thick tongue • Strong sexual desire • Dreams of robbers • Hair falling, used to (at the initial stage) increase during rainy season • Sexual desire strong	• Burning in head • Apthous ulcer, recurrent (Tubercular joins) • Foetor oris • Mucous in stool with offensive odour • Delayed healing of skin • Dull perception • Complete hair loss, almost shiny baldness • History of glue ear (discharge from ear) (Tubercular miasm joins) • Pityriasis more in the trunk, for last two years which aggravates during summer • Suicidal • Desire for death, disgusted with life • Dull	• Swelling of the gums from cold • Palpitation • Extremely irritable, objects to parental guidance (Syco-tubercular) • Whimsical • Likes to leave home • Weakness from loss of semen • Prolonged history of masturbation, which he thinks weakens him so much • Catches cold easily; starts with a runny nose, and sneezing • When catches cold, pain in left side of the throat (recurrent) • Chilly ++, Catches cold easily • Desires cold food +++

Psora 16 Sycosis 6 Syphilis 12 Tubercular 11

This is an interesting case of hair falling though considering the extreme bald appearance of the scalp it feels like the case has Syphilitic preponderance, but interestingly we can see other miasms are present as well. Thyroidinum is a deep acting mixed miasmatic medicine; it has wonderfully taken care of the maladjustment aspect of the case as well as the totality and covers the miasmatic status of the patient. We see wonderful improvement through the action of Thyroidinum in this case.

So, it is a mixed miasmatic case with Syphilo-tubercular preponderance (or surface miasm). Therefore the selected medicine should cover the symptomatic totality as well as the miasmatic totality.

Final Prescription

- Thyrodinum was selected on the basis of maladjustment, hormonal and emotional, resulting in impaired coordination, metabolic, nervous and vascular, resulting altered growth and development, in this case hair falling.
- Hair falling started about nine years ago, which patient thinks commenced after delayed convalescence from typhoid fever (enteric fever). I took this as a shock to the system resulting in impaired growth and development of hair.
- Extreme weakness, easy fatigue from least exertion.
- Nose - Catches cold easily and starts with a runny nose, and sneezing.
- Mouth - Apthous ulcer (recurrent). Foetor oris.
- Teeth - Occasional swelling of the gums from cold.
- Throat - When catches cold, pain left side of the throat.
- Male Genital Organs - Sexual desire strong.
- Skin Disease - Delayed healing.
- Temperament - Extremely irritable, objects to parental guidance in every way. Whimsical, suicidal. Likes to leave home.
- Tendencies - Suicidal tendency.
- Life and Hatred - Desire for death, disgusted with life.
- Memory - Weak, gradual loss of memory.
- Weeping - Weeping mood, involuntary sighing.
- Fears - Fear of darkness, thunderstorms, incurable diseases, failure.
- Excessive mental labour, mental worries, anxiety, memory weakness since.
- Chilly ++. Hates rainy season. Catches cold easily.
- Desires sweet ++.

THYROIDINUM Miasmatics - Psora++, Sycosis+++, Syphilitic++, Tubercular+++ Chilly

- In this case, there are Psora + Syphilitic preponderances → so Psora + Syphilis = Tubercular miasm, according to John Henry Allen, (Ref. Psora-Pseudo Psora).

- Thyroidinum does cover Tubercular miasm.
- Basically I was looking for a deep acting mixed miasmatic medicine. Therefore, Thyroidinum came in my mind for its mixed miasmatic status as well as being deep in action and it covers the aforesaid symptoms of the case and also:
  - Emotional maladjustment → In-coordination → Temper tantrums.
  - Altered development → maladjustment → In-coordination → Hair falling.
  - Mental in-coordination e.g. manic depression.
  - Vital in-coordination e.g. low energy.
  - Maladjustment acts as a trigger (aetiological factor) → results in-coordination → which can be hormonal.

I have started the case with Typhoidinum, 200C, went up to 1M and 10M consecutively with proper wait and watch. Then Thyroidinum was prescribed and the result was simply marvellous. The medicine was given in water to sip for 7 days as usual.

INTERESTING CLARIFICATIONS

- Thyroidinum is listed as multi-miasmatic in my book, the dominance is sycotic and tubercular with sycotic having L (Leading) status. This was obviously a successful case and the miasmatic weightings would have been considered in the light of the totalities, but it would be of interest to readers why the seeming anomalies in weightings did not direct me away from Thyroidinum.

  THYROIDINUM : Miasmatics :- Psora++, Sycosis+++L, Syphilitic++, Tubercular+++; Chilly patient

  In this case, there are Psora + Syphilitic preponderance à so Psora + Syphil = Tubercular Miasm, according to John Henry Allen, (Ref. Psora-Pseudo Psora).

  Thyroidinum does cover Tubercular Miasm (which is +++). Basically I was looking for a deep acting Mixed Miasmatic medicine. Therefore, Thyroidinum came in my mind for its Mixed Miasmatics status as well as deep in action.

- I have mentioned about 'incoordination' above and would like to expand on this:

⅄ Maladjustment → Incoordination.

   e.g. :-
   (a) Physical maladjustment → Incoordination → Obesity.
   (b) Emotional maladjustment → Incoordination → Temper tantrums.
   (c) Sexual maladjustment → Incoordination → Pre-mature labour.
   (d) Hormonal maladjustment → Incoordination → Pre-menstrual syndrome/swelling of breast, etc.
   (e) Growth maladjustment → Incoordination → Nodules and tumours.
   (f) Altered development → maladjustment → Incoordination → (a) Emaciation/Obesity, (b) Mental incoordination e.g. maniac depression, (c) Vital incoordination e.g. low energy.

Maladjustment acts as a trigger (aetiological factor) → results incoordination → which can be

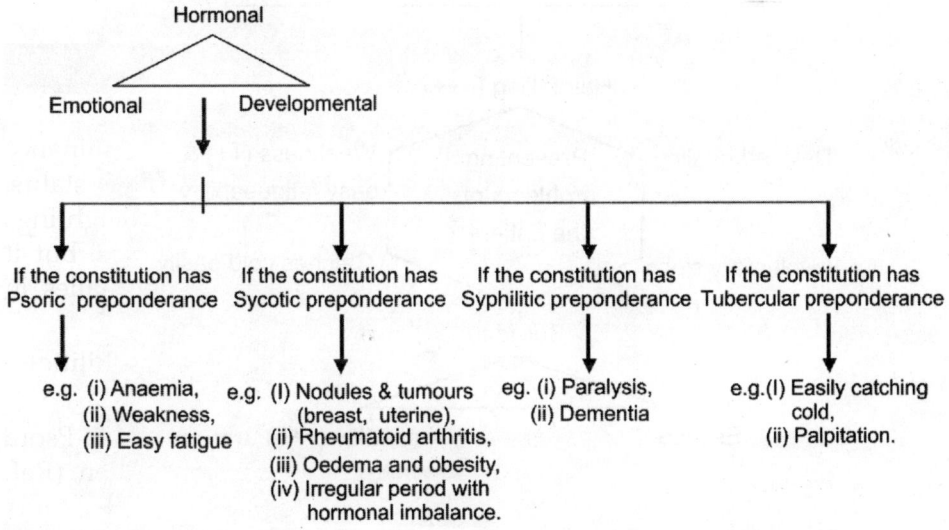

I have successfully treated cases of young women in their late teens and twenties → maladjustment → at home surrounding/new jobs/new adult life → so maladjustment acts as a trigger → Incoordination → resulting the triad of (i) irregular menstruation, can be 45 – 80 days interval, (ii) started putting on weight, (iii) puffiness & oedema.

Cured Cases

Thyroidinum rescues such cases.

- When I refer to shock being a trigger for the move to Thyroidinum in this case, reader might think that the shock referred to is the enteric fever and consequent slow recuperation? Reader might think that the shock has resulted the hair loss, but that was a consequence, surely, rather than a cause.

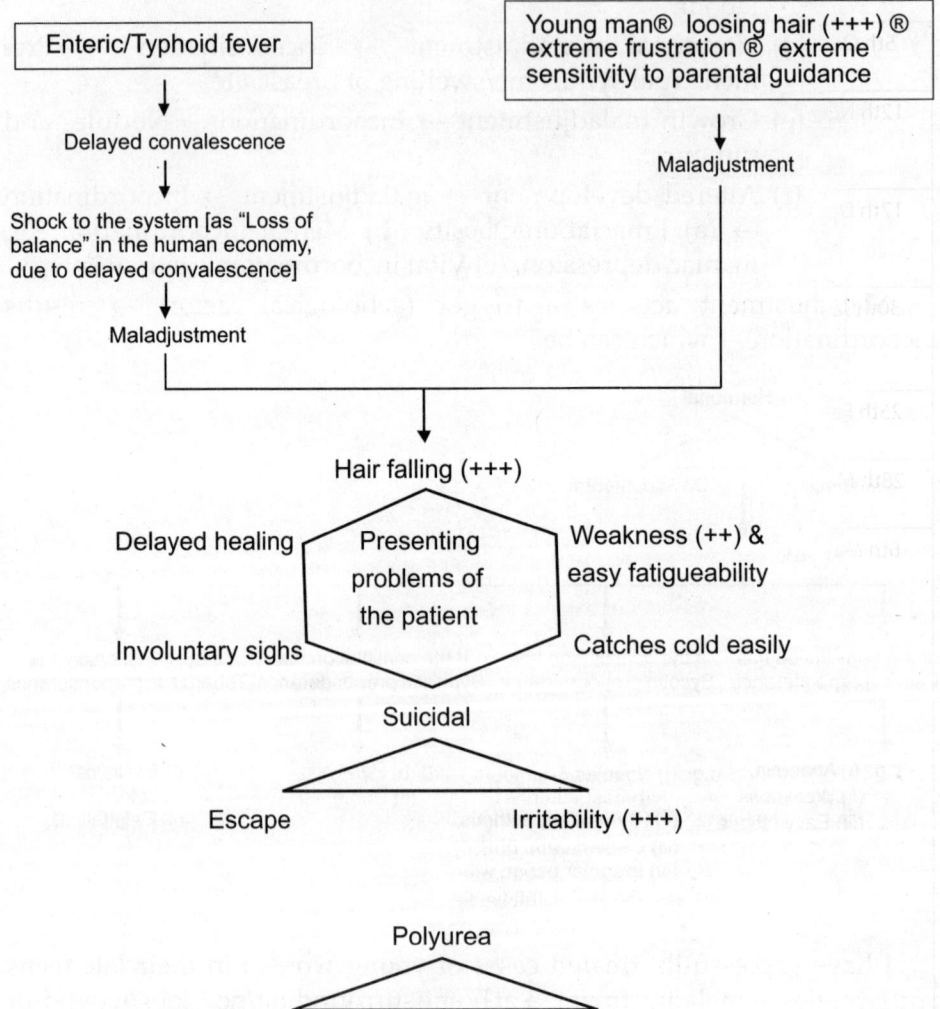

Dermatological Diseases-Cured Cases

Prescription Chart

Date	Prescription Done on the Basis of	Treatment
7th Sep'90	Considering the bad effects of typhoid fever N.B.W.S. (His entire vitality deranged since). Gas and distension and lowered digestive function.	Typhoidinum 200C 2 doses. To sip (with water) the 1st dose for 7 days; 7 days off; then the 2nd dose to sip for 7 days.
5th Oct'90	No appreciable change. Standstill. Wait.	Sac Lac, 15 doses alternate days.
12th Nov'90	No appreciable change. So went higher.	Typhodinum 1000 (1M), 2 doses (Same way as mentioned above)
17th Dec'90	Digestion better, gas and distension as little less, but no change in bald hair, weakness etc. Wait for further movement of symptoms.	Sac Lac, 15 doses alternate days.
30th Jan'90	Digestive power has improved to a certain extent and then standstill. Absolutely no other changes. Wait for any further reaction.	Sac Lac, 15 doses alternate days.
25th Feb'91	Standstill, went higher.	Typhoidinum 10,000, 2 doses
28th Mar'91	No further change. Wait and watch.	Sac Lac, 15 doses alternate days.
6th May'91	Absolute standstill. Change in the plan of treatment. Considering conditions which point towards loss of balance in the human economy due to strain, during some particular period of development, due to climatic variations or due to some other mental or emotional factors, Thyroidinum to be thought of. Want of metabolic adjustment - Thyroidinum exercises a general regulating influence over the mechanism of the organs of nutrition, growth and development. Chilly, sensitive to cold, and catches cold easily. Deep syphilitic miasmatic preponderance (for generalised shining baldness). Mental irritability, whimsical moods. Temperamental disturbances of adolescence. Generalised and profound weakness, easy fatigue. Decided craving for sweets. Palpitation from emotion, exertion. Flatulence, distended abdomen. Long lasting headache from irritability. Suicidal tendencies.	Thyroidinum 1M 2 doses.

Date	Prescription Done on the Basis of	Treatment
10th Jun'91	Started feeling better but no change in bald hair. Wait and watch.	Sac Lac, 15 doses alternate mornings.
8th Jul'91	Weakness much better. Temperament better, calmer. Gas and distension much improved. Digestive process improved. Nausea better.	Sac Lac, 15 doses alternate days.
10th Aug'91	Improved but standstill. Repeat.	Thyroidinum 1000 (1M) 2 doses (procedure as above).
26th Sep'91	Hair growth started. Doing better n every way. Temperament much better. Wait and watch.	Sac Lac, 15 doses alternate days.
2nd Nov'91	Hair is growing. Temperament and suicidal thoughts much improved.	Sac Lac, 15 doses alternate days.
22nd Dec'91	Hair growth steadily improving.	Sac Lac, 15 doses alternate days.
3rd Jan'92	Hair growth improving.	Sac Lac, 15 doses alternate days.
14th Feb'92	Sudden attack of depression and suicidal thoughts. Patient appears to be standstill, so went higher in potency.	Thyroidinum (10M), 2 doses (same way as mentioned above)
26th Mar'92	Again temperament, whimsical thoughts and depression is much improved. Hair growth steadily improving.	Sac Lac, 15 doses alternate days.
20th Apr'92	Much better. Almost normal appearance of the hair.	Sac Lac, 15 doses alternate days.
26th May'92	Cured.	Stopped treatment.

Remedy Reaction: Thyroidinum 1M and then I went gradually up to 10M and cured the case in about twenty months.

*Readers may view the pictures of the case (before and after treatment) in our website under Dermatological Diseases (**Case No. D002** - A case of total Baldness in a 24 years aged person, completely cured by Thyroidinum).*

Authenticity of Cure

CD Reference: D002-TOTAL BALDNESS-GM

Dermatological Diseases-Cured Cases

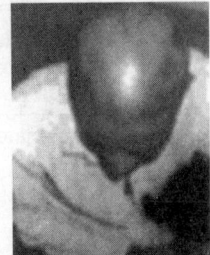

Mr. G.M., a case of total Baldness; before treatment

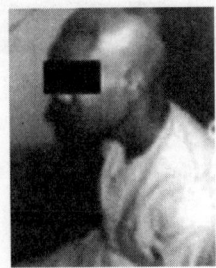

Before treatment

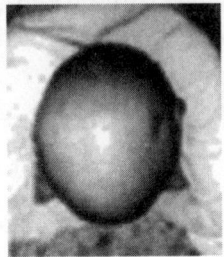

Before treatment

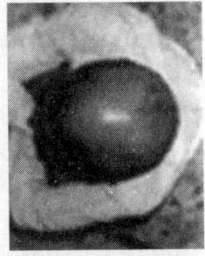

Hair growth starts 6 months after treatment

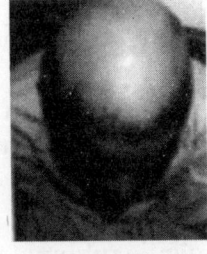

Hair growth 10 months after treatment

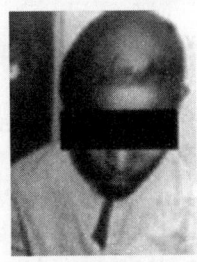

Hair growth 16 months after treatment

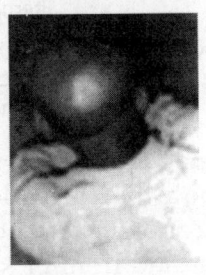

Hair growth 18 months after treatment

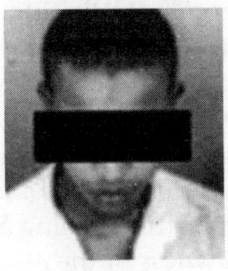

Hair growth 20 months after treatment.

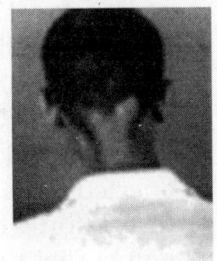

Hair growth 24 months after treatment

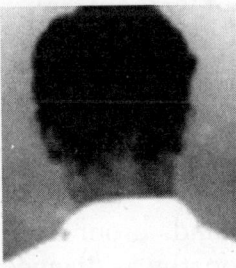

Total growth of hair 26 months after treatment

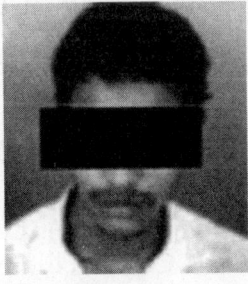

Total growth of hair 26 months after treatment

3. A DIAGNOSED CASE OF ATOPIC DERMATITIS

Case No. D003

Name of the Patient Mast. S.K.S, boy born in 1983

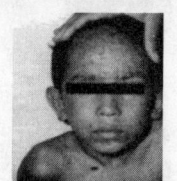

Mast. S.S. Atopic Dermatitis

Presenting Complaints

- Skin eruption especially on the face, since six months of age (now 6 years old).
- Multiple small, red eruptions; pustular and vesicular in type, for last five and half years Oozing fluid and pus. Cycle of pustules → oozes → pus and blood → becomes crusty → child picks and scratches → bleeds → pus → dries → crust again.
- Itching (+++), better by gentle rubbing confirmed by observation and also confirmed by the parents. Hard scratching made the eruption bleed, feels a little better from gentle rubbing. (i) Itching of the skin aggravates at night, from warmth. (ii) Itching aggravates in summer, from heat of the sun. (iii) Itching aggravates by washing; hot or cold. (iv)Skin discomfort aggravation from sour foods and fruit. (v) Skin discomfort aggravation from sweat.
- Stinging and cutting pains (++) with occasional burning in the affected areas of skin. The boy weeps and cries due to the tremendous discomfort which results from itching à bleeding and pus formation with a sensation of rawness of the affected areas and from picking the crusts.
- Had lot of allopathic treatment, including cortisone ointments; and Ayurvedic (naturopathic) treatment without any appreciable or permanent change.
- Chronic loose stool 4-5 times per day with froth and mucus (++) for last two years. This diarrhoea aggravates from motion, eating. Urging initiated after meals or any light food.
- Occasional right sided abdominal pain.
- Extremely painful (+++). Lymph glands around neck swollen for last 3 years (? Cervical lymphadenopathy as diagnosed by medical doctor). Aggravation from cold, touch, pressure; better from warm application.
- Head - Occasional pain in forehead; aggravated in the sun and better by rest.

- Ear - Otorrhoea (discharge from ear) with itching.
- Throat - Occasional throat pain, sore throat from cold, better by warm gargling.
- Lungs - Occasional dry cough; aggravates at night.
- Abdomen – (i) Gas and distension in abdomen. (ii) Gurgling sound in stomach aggravation after full meals. (iii) Occasional right sided abdominal colic, which is aggravated by warm milk.
- Stomach - Appetite decreased.
- Urine - Nothing abnormal.
- Stool - (i) Ineffectual urging, aggravated after eating, with heavy feeling in abdomen. (ii) Profuse, yellowish stool with mucus (++), watery (++), frothy (++), less faecal matter. (iii) Loose, 4-5 times a day; aggravates after meals. (iv) Cramps in right side of abdomen, with urging, before evacuation; better after passing stool. (v) Due to profuse expulsion of stool, child exhausted after each evacuation.
- Mental Symptoms - angry, irritable temper (+), quarrelsome (+), fault-finding (+), obstinate and stubborn. Suspicious (+). Jealous of his friends as they can enjoy normal life whilst he can't. Silent, absent-minded (+), gloomy, timid, broods in silence. Likes to be alone (+). Fear of death (+). Disgusted with life as if the enjoyment of the entire childhood has been lost. Memory weak. Gradual loss of memory (+). This is mainly due to his absent-mindedness. Gloomy and morose (perturbed by the discomfort of the skin). Weeping mood (+). Involuntary sighing. He cries when reprimanded (+). The child is intensely sympathetic (++). He does everything slowly (+). He has a fear of ghosts (+), darkness (+), incurable diseases (+) and accidents (+).
- Has applied a profuse quantity of allopathic creams and lotions, and also tried herbal oils. Feels relieved for some period of time; thereafter it comes back again and generally returns worse than the previous state so he is afraid of trying anything, any more. Totally frustrated. Gonorrhoea of father.
- Past History - Skin disease from the age of 6 months, measles at the age of 3.
- First cause of breakdown of health (N.B.W.S. Never Been Well Since) - Skin disease. Cervical glands.
- Homoeopathic Generalities:
- Heat and cold reaction - Hot patient; likes open air; catches cold easily.
- Desires and aversions for food - Sweet +, pungent and hot +, salty +. Potato, meat and chicken +, rich, spicy and fatty food +, warm food +, cold drinks +, ice cream +. Thirsty.

- Sleep and dreams - Sleeps well during the later part of night. Disturbed sleep and difficulty in falling asleep due to skin discomfort. No recurrent dreams.
- Perspiration - Profuse sweat on face and axillae. Sour smelling. Stains the clothes yellow.
- Family History - Father had asthma, bronchitis; Mother had eczema during pregnancy with this child; cured by ointment.
- Previous Treatment - Allopathic or Pharmaceutical prescriptions. Ayurvedic or Naturopathy, including herbal oils. Homoeopathic medicines prescribed by colleagues. Bacillinum, Graphites and Sulphur in LM and different Centesimal scales all without any appreciable change.
- Provisional diagnosis- Exfoliative dermatitis with cervical lymphadenopathy, Atopic dermatitis.

Miasmatic Analysis

Psora	Sycosis	Syphilis	Tubercular
• Itching+++	• Multiple vesicular eruptions	• All sorts of boils, ulcers, which do not heal fast.	• Oozing of blood
• Itching << washing	• Skin stinging	• Discharge of pus, which is offensive.	• Swollen lymph glands around neck
• Itching << by eating sour fruit or food	• Chronic loose stool	• Itching < at night, from warmth	• Exhaustion after evacuation
• Sun headache	• Yellowish stool	• Itching < summer	• Fault finding, critical
• Headache better by rest	• Cramp in right side of abdomen	• Skin discomfort < by sweat	• Stubborn
• Dry cough	• Quarrelsome	• Skin burning	• Recurrent and obstinate boils and pimples with profuse pus
• Gas and distension in abdomen	• Suspicious	• Sensation of rawness	
• Silent, timid	• Sympathetic	• Stool with mucus	• Skin problem < at night, warmth < after itching and cold washing
• Unhealthy skin represents Psora. Also Psora creates irritation in general → physical itching → over the skin	• Profuse sweat	• Discharge from ear	• Cervical lymph-adenopathy
	• Stains the clothes yellow	• Sore throat from cold	
		• Disgusted with life	• As a result of suffering from severe diseases suppurative otitis media appears
• Desires sweet, pungent and hot foods		• Chronic loose motion dysentery (Recurrent problem Tubercular - Syphilitic)	
• Various fears - darkness, ghosts, accidents, incurable diseases		• Desires spicy ++	
		• Desires to be alone	

Psora 11   Sycosis 10   Syphilis 13   Tubercular 9

This is a mixed miasmatic case with Psora-Syphilo-Tubercular preponderance. As the young boy had such a long history of suppression and therefore the symptoms were quite complicated, Croton Tig was indicated on the basis of the totality with special emphasis on a very peculiar modality, *itching better by gentle rubbing*. It covers the multi-miasmatic background with Psoric preponderance so once again it was a wonderful example of prescribing a medicine which covers the surface symptoms, as well as the surface miasm. By including the miasm in the prescription one can become more confident about the correct selection of the medicine and stay with the medicine with confidence. *The same principle will apply when, by virtue of repertorisation, you have finally ended with four or five top ranking medicines and are now feeling confused about the final selection. In such a case, evaluate the miasmatic background of the case and make sure your final indicated medicine not only covers the symptoms but the miasmatic expression of the case as well.*

Final Prescription and Remedy Reaction

I started the case with Cortisone in homoeopathic potency with an idea to use tautopathy and remove the prolonged bad effect caused by Cortisone (pharmaceutical preparation). I think Cortisone had initially removed the bad effect and thereafter I switched on to Sulphur which I will confess was a mistake and there was no appreciable change. Also it was a case with Syphilo-psoric preponderance. Finally, I realised the presence of Croton Tig symptoms and re-visited the miasmatic analysis. The reasons for the prescription of Croton Tig have been given below in the chart.

This is an interesting case and I must honestly share with you that I was really affected by the condition of this young boy, suffering from his six months of age. I prescribed Sulphur considering the itching and the apparent totality but no improvement. One day, in the consulting room I saw, his mother was gently rubbing over his face and as a Homoeopath, you should be always very observant. Reason therefore I asked, why is she doing that? Mother replied, while itching, scratching aggravates but gentle rubbing gives him some relief. That immediately gave me the clue and I prescribed Croton Tig. You can see the wonderful action of this medicine.

Time and again I have learnt that it not the quantitative totality but the qualitative totality that counts. The qualities of the person should match with the qualities of the medicine.

Croton Tig has the miasmatic breakdown: Psora ++, Sycosis +, Syphilis +, Tubercular +.

Date	Report After Last Medication	Prescription done on the Basis of	Treatment
12th Dec'89		To remove the bad effects of the prolonged use of Cortisone group of ointments.	Cortisone, 200C 1 globule Organon, F.N. §246 (5th ed); §275 (6th ed)]; globule size number X [Size of the poppy-seed i.e. the exactly classical way, F.N. §285 (5th ed)]; to be dispensed in 4 ounce bottle or in a glass with distilled water [vide §272 (6th ed), §288 (5th ed)]; to be taken in sips throughout the day (approximately in every hour), stir thoroughly before every sip [vide §246, §247 & §280 (6th ed) every dose should be deviated from the former].
27th Jan'90	No appreciable change; skin conditions same.	Wait and watch with patience for movement of symptoms.	Sac Lac 15 doses (Placebos) to be taken on alternate mornings.
28th Feb'90	No appreciable change. Absolute stand-still but no deterioration of the status.	I had already waited for two and a half months and there was no appreciable change but no deterioration, even so I planned to repeat the same potency.	Cortisone 200C This time the same medicated water, being divided into two equal halves 2 doses made from that single poppy-seed sized globule; and the patient was asked to sip the 1st dose on the first day, throughout the day, stir and take in sips; whilst the 2nd dose to be taken after 48 hours of the completion of the 1st dose (viz. alternate day, if the 1st to be taken on Monday, the 2nd dose on Wednesday).

Dermatological Diseases-Cured Cases

Date	Report After Last Medication	Prescription done on the Basis of	Treatment
2nd Apr'90	There was absolutely no change.	As it was already four months since the first prescription was made and there had been no changes, I planned to change the remedy.	Sulphur 0/1 (LM1), 8 doses (One globule in water divided into 8 doses). Each to be taken alternate mornings.
4th May'90	No change in these four weeks, rather, the skin is getting more dry and itchy.	Changed the plan of scale.	Sulphur 1000 1 dose in water.
9th Jun'90	Absolutely no change and patient is as a whole no better; discomfort, itchy, more stubborn and gloomy.	I was feeling with my experience that the medicine was not holding him. Anyway, I thought it is better to wait about four weeks more before making another final decision to change the plan of treatment (i.e. the remedy). I always try to be sure before making a change of the remedy.	Sac Lac, 15 doses to be taken on alternate mornings.
6th Jul'90	No change.	So a change in the plan of treatment considering; (i) Pustular eruptions on face. Dr. N.M. Chowdhury in his Materia Medica says Croton eruptions are also vesicular in type. (ii) Itching (+++) → desire to scratch → but skin gets raw, sore, and hypersensitive and bleeds → so better by gentle rubbing. Itching aggravates at night as any symptoms of Croton also aggravate at night. (iii) Burning and smarting pain. (iv) Profuse watery, yellowish stool, urging aggravates after meals. (v) Crampy pain in abdomen, before stool; and gets exhausted from passing of profuse quantity of stool. (vi) Dr. Guernsey mentions about otorrhoea (as quoted by Dr. Clarke). (vii) Warm milk aggravates the abdominal pain (Ref. Dr. Clarke). (viii) Gloomy, morose, weakness of memory; these features of this patient are also covered by Croton. (ix) The strong psoric background (with the features of itchy skin) on which tubercular components are superimposed.	Croton Tig. 30C 2 doses in distilled water.

Date	Report After Last Medication	Prescription done on the Basis of	Treatment
8th Aug'90	Face clearing up. Cervical glands are also better.	Wait and watch.	Sac Lac 15 doses.
6th Sep'90	Improved but now standstill.	Repeat the same potency.	Croton Tig. 30C 2 doses in water.
16th Oct'90	Standstill.	Higher potency given.	Croton Tig. 200C 2 doses in water.
22nd Nov'90	Face almost cleared up. Glands diminished. Much better in all aspects, mentally and physically.	Wait and watch.	Sac Lac 15 doses.
5th Jan'91	All eruptions disappeared. Glands also completely diminished.		Sac Lac 15 doses.

Readers may view the pictures of the case (before and after treatment) in our website under Dermatological Diseases (Case No. D003- A case of Atopic Dermatitis in a young 5 years old boy, completely cured by Croton Tiglium)

Authenticity of Cure

CD Reference: D003-ATOPIC DERMATITIS-SS

Dermatological Diseases-Cured Cases

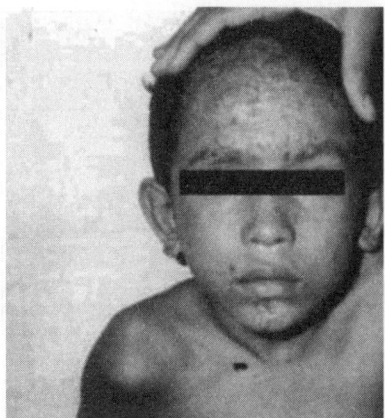

Mast. S.S. Atopic Dermatitis, before treatment of Dr. Banerjea

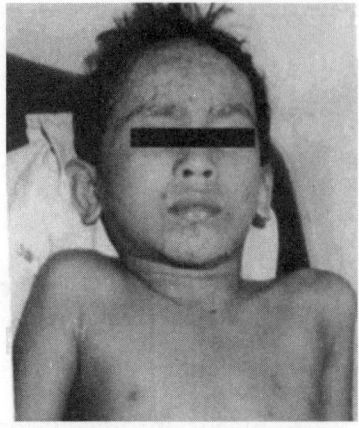

Before homoeopathic treatment

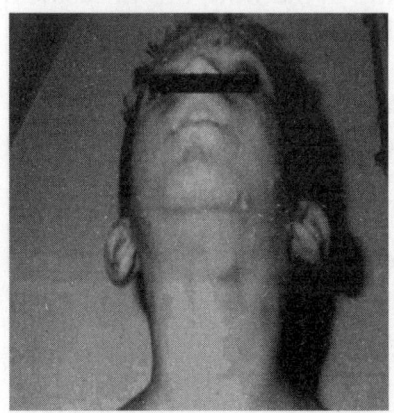

Before homoeopathic treatment

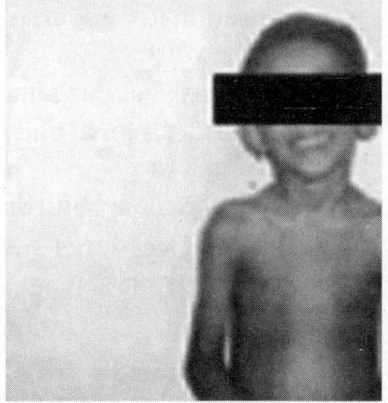

5 months after treatment

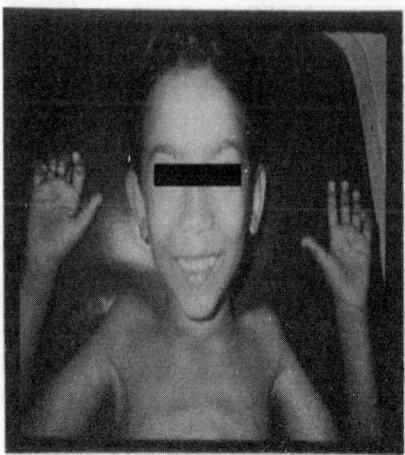

6 months after treatment

4. A CASE OF WART ON PALM - MRS R. S.

Case No. D004

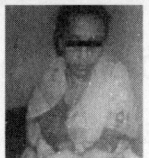

Mrs. R. S., Wart on Palm

Presenting Complaints

- Wart on right palm: for last 3 years: started as a fleshy soft mass, gradually hardened.
- Bleeds profusely on friction, followed by stinging pain with numbness down the right arm.
- Sensation of constriction and squeezing in the wart, this uneasiness sensation in the wart is aggravated while concentrating her attention on the wart.
- Modality: Patient cannot relate anything.
- Head: Occasional burning vertex. Occasional spells of vertigo, better during a meal.
- Eye: Occasional blurring in near vision. Sight better in distant vision,
- Throat: Occasional swelling of left tonsil from exposure to cold.
- Heart: Palpitation aggravates on motion.
- Abdomen: Distention, gas: entire abdomen, ameliorated by eructation.
- Stomach: Loss of appetite.
- Sweat: Profuse, especially on face and axilla. Sweat also on abdomen.
- Urine: Occasional burning.
- Stool: Occasional white mucus, two times daily, clear.
- Upper Extremities: Pain in fingers, especially aching, during new moon & full moon. Periodic contraction of right hand especially of palm.
- Lower Extremities: Occasional severe pain in knee especially during new moon & full moon. While walking cracking in the joints.
- Menses: Hysterectomy done in 1982 due to fibroid uterus.
- Mentals: (a) Irritable, silent habit, desires to be neat & clean, likes company. (b) Memory - extremely weak. Loses the thread of conversation while talking. (c) Weeping mood, having involuntary sighing; sympathetic, cannot tolerate blood letting. (d) Wants to do everything slowly. (e) Discontented and displeased with the affairs of life. (f) Inclination to sit; slowness on motion; indolence.

(g) Illusions see accidents. (h) Lack of religious consciousness, spirituality. (i) Fear of ghosts, failure.

Onset of the Presenting Problem

Exciting Cause of Present Disease:
Nothing particular. She thinks that profuse bleeding from the wart was not so much there at the beginning, but with profuse intake of Homoeopathic medicines from various other homoeopathic practitioners, and the application of Thuja tincture (before coming to me), the wart hardened up. For the last year, it has been bleeding profusely on friction.

Past History
Diseases with which she suffered before:
Severe Typhoid (at the age of 6 years), Malaria, Measles, Chickenpox in childhood, Jaundice twice (7 years & 12 years of age).

First Cause of Break Down of Health
Hysterectomy.

Homoeopathic Generalities

(a) Hot and Cold Relationship: Hot patient, does not like to sleep in closed room. She does not catch cold easily.
(b) Food Desires: Sweet ++, salt, salty, bitter, vegetables, spinach, fish, warm food, cold drinks.
(c) Sleep: Disturbed. Wide awake during the first part of night, sleeps better during mid part of the night.

Marital Relationship

Patient is married; one son, two daughters.

CASE ANALYSIS, MIASMATIC DIAGNOSIS AND FINAL PRESCRIPTION

Miasmatic Analysis

(1) Scanning of Symptoms and their Miasmatic Breakdown thereof:
   (a) Fleshy wart, gradually hardened: Sycotic preponderance.
   (b) Sense of constriction and squeezing within wart: Psora-sycotic.
   (c) Wart: bleeds profusely on friction: Syco-tubercular (as haemorrhage comes under tubercular miasm).

(d) Swelling of tonsils from cold: Psora-tubercular.
(e) Periodic contraction of right hand: Tubercular (as periodicity is one of the feature of tubercular miasm).
(f) Loses the thread of conversation while talking: Syco-psoric.
(g) Discontented, displeased Tubercular.
(h) Inclination to sit, indolence: Psoric.
(i) Cannot tolerate blood letting: Psoric.
(j) Worse for thinking about complaints: Sycotic.
(k) Desire for sweet: Psoric.
(l) Head: Occasional burning – Syphilitic.
(m) Abdomen: Distention, gas: Psoric.
(n) Sweat: Profuse: Sycotic.
(o) Urine: Occasional burning –Syphilitic.
(p) Stool: Occasional mucus: Sycotic.
(q) Lower Extremities: Joint pains: Sycotic. Aggravation motion: Syphilitic.
(r) Fibroid uterus: Sycotic.
(s) Fears of ghosts and failure: Psoric.

(2) Miasmatic Sum-up:
Mixed miasmatic with Tubercular preponderance (haemorrhagic, periodic complaints).

Remedy Selection of Anacardium

- Repertorial Basis:

What made me Look into the Repertory?

Basically I do not open the repertory very often, mainly because of the heavy pressure of patients (approximately an average of 70 patients in a day); and furthermore because of my understanding of Materia Medica!

TWO starting points: which made me open the repertory?

Illusion: sees accidents: since the wart appeared, the bleeding started, this woman started thinking of it as a curse given by God (because she had a vague idea that warts are of gonorrhoeal origin, as she disclosed to me once). She did say, that previously she was a religious and spiritual person, but since the wart (which she thinks a gonorrhoeal sin!) appeared, she started philosophising that even after leading a religious and pious life, God has given this to her. She lost the faith in God, and moreover she felt that the next curse would be an accident; so whenever her chauffeur used to brake hard, whilst she was in the car, she had illusions of an accident; or even when something fell from the top of the cupboard, she would have illusions that it would fall upon her!

I considered this a very important key to open up the case, had a look at Kent, could not find it; got it in Boger Boenninghausen's Repertory (P.205).

Emotional Aspects:

(i) Illusion: sees accidents: Ref. Dr. Boger - Boenninghausen's Repertory; P-205.

(ii) Lack of Spiritually: Ref. Dr. Boger - Boenninghausen's Repertory; P-217.

Contraction of right hand, which is a PQRS (as I give profound emphasis and importance on any PQRS in accordance with Hahnemann's Organon 153 & 209).

Whenever there is prominence of physical generals as well as physical symptoms, I generally look for Drs. Boger - Boenninghausen's or N. M. Chowdhury, Repertory; if at all I'm looking into any repertory!

Physical Aspects:

(i) While walking, cracking in the joints: Ref. Dr. Boger - Boenninghausen's Repertory, P-849.

(ii) Sweat on abdomen: Ref. Dr. Boger - Boenninghausen's Repertory, P-1081.

(iii) Contraction of right hand: Ref. Dr. N. M. Chowdhury's Repertory, P-972.

- Materia Medica Basis:
  - Wart on palmar surface.
  - Sensation of constriction, squeezing in wart.
  - Vertigo ameliorated during a meal.
  - Sweat in abdomen.
  - Periodic contraction of right hand.
  - Discontented, displeased with the affairs of life.
  - Weakness of memory.

Anacardium has the miasmatic breakdown: Psora ++, Sycosis ++, Syphilis ++, Tubercular +.

Miasmatic Discussion of the Remedy

- It is a Psoric and Tubercular remedy. Anacardium inherits the Syphilitic miasm but it represents the features of Tubercular remedies/miasms; so after the use of Anacardium, a dose of Syphilinum is required to complete the cure.
- I won't give the patient a dose of Syphilinum until and unless there is any left over symptoms or traces of syphilitic miasmatic indications. Let me explain this in terms of Kent's approach of `changing the plan of treatment':- which I have followed from my ancestors:
- In Gastrointestinal tract problems, so long as the patient is under the Psoric miasm, there is appetite and the patient feels better after eating; but after sometime there is no amelioration after eating; at this stage the Anacardium patient reflects the Tubercular miasm in the surface.
- There is also a great desire for things which make them sick (craves things which make the person sick); which is also a feature of the Tubercular miasm.
- While scanning the symptoms of Anacardium from Keynotes and Characteristics with Comparisons of Some of The Leading Remedies of the Materia Medica by Dr. H. C. Allen, the following miasmatic dissection (MIASMATIC MATERIA MEDICA) is given for better miasmatic understanding of Anacardium:-
  - Sudden loss of memory; everything seems to be in a dream:- Sudden is dramatic, rapid: so PSORIC, but loss of memory with everything seeming to be in a dream is more of incoordination, so SYCOTIC.
  - Disposed to be malicious, seems bent on wickedness:- SYPHILITIC.
  - Irresistible desire to curse and swear:- A feature characterised by incoordination in behaviour, SYCOSIS. When this is coupled with destructive tendencies, SYPHILITIC miasm comes in.
  - Feels as though he had two wills, one commanding him to do what the other forbids:- Characterised by incoordination in perception, SYCOSIS.
  - When walking, is anxious, as if someone were pursuing him:- Anxiety is more PSORIC, whereas as if someone were pursuing can be highlighted in the aspect of suspiciousness, which is SYCOTIC.

- ▲ Strange temper, laughs at serious matters and is serious over laughable things:- SYCO-PSORIC.
- ▲ Sensation: as of a hoop or band around a part:- As if sensations come under PSORA as well SYCOSIS. This sensation can also be explained in terms of incoordination.
- ▲ Headache: relieved entirely when eating: PSORIC.
- ▲ Gastric and Nervous Headaches:- PSORIC.
- ▲ "All-gone" Sensation:- PSORIC.
- ▲ Warts on palms:- Warts can be explained in terms of proliferation, (as all HYPERS are SYCOTIC; ABSENCE - LACK - SCANTY denotes PSORA; all DYSES like Dystrophy, Dysplasia are SYPHILITIC and One Sided Diseases with absolute scarcity of symptoms associated with Periodicity are TUBERCULAR miasm). So warts are SYCOTIC.

Prescription Chart

Dates	Points in favour of the Prescription	Prescribed Medicine
6th Aug'91	I always prescribe one single globule [Ref. Organon: Foot Note →246 (5th edition); and →275 (6th edition)] of the size of the poppy seed [Ref. Organon: Foot Note →285 (5th edition)] and to be taken with water [Ref. Organon: →288 (5th edition); →272 (6th edition); →246 (6th edition)] for · faster dynamic action.	ANACARDIUM 200 C.: 1 globule (of No.X) in one ounce of distilled water. Divide into 2 doses. To be taken in sips, stirring the medicated water each time; to be consumed on alternate mornings.
9th Oct'91	No appreciable change: [Wait & Watch]	Sac lac given.
20th Dec'91	Dramatically improved. No constrictive pain in the wart and size reduced to half; no bleeding; joint pains also better.	Sac lac given.
6th Feb'92	Wart disappeared. Patient feeling totally better.	No Medication (CURED)

Discussion about the Developments in the Case

(1) As wart was one of the main presenting complaints of the case, and Sycosis is the corresponding miasm thus, Sycosis has 'slowness of recovery' (Ref. Dr. H. Roberts, Art of Cure, P-230). So, even Miasmatic Diagnosis helps to understand the prognosis and remedy reactions and makes you to wait with patience!

(2) Waiting for 2 months is no time at all for a problem for which the patient has been suffering for last three years, and especially with my miasmatic knowledge. I understood Sycosis was the surface

miasm to start with, corresponding to the wart as the presenting feature; so the remedy reaction will be slow. Many times after a prescription, if the patient is improving even slightly. I wait even six months, such is the teaching of Dr. Kent, vide his Lesser Writings and Clinical Cases.

(3) I do exactly follow the Hahnemannian guide-lines regarding dispensing the remedy, and my experience confirms its brilliant results!

(4) After the November 1991 visit of this patient, the warts tended to get smaller and smaller before eventually disappearing totally by mid-February,1992; in addition the

- Irritability → got better, much calmer.
- Most surprisingly, the illusion disappeared and some trust upon God has been restored!
- Memory → much improved.
- Involuntary sighings and discontentment → disappeared.
- Indolence and illusions → were no more present.
- Stool symptoms → had no change, but considering the 'spicy curries' together with intake of excess of sweets, cookies and 'late-dinners', the diet and habit which she had not changed nor she intended to; I did not expect much change in those aspects, until and unless she avoided the 'maintaining causes' completely.

I hope the above information will serve the following purposes:

(a) Elucidation of my approach to miasmatic prescribing;
(b) Clarify the utility of understanding the miasm;
(c) Judgement in favour of change of remedy and change in the plan of treatment (from miasmatic point of view).

Authenticity of Cure

CD Reference: D004-WART ON PALM-RS

Dermatological Diseases-Cured Cases

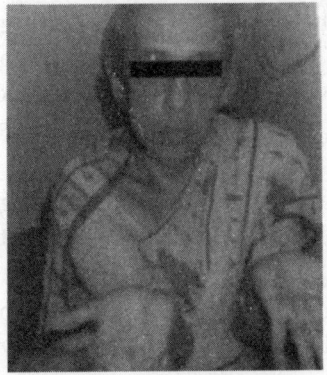

Mrs. R. S., Wart on Palm,
before treatment of Dr. Banerjea

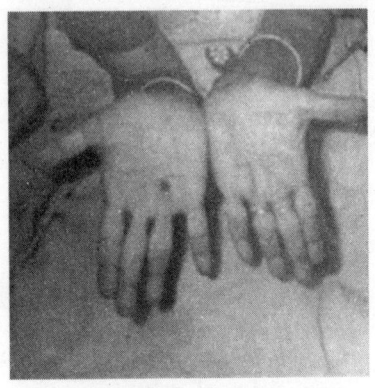

Before homoeopathic treatment

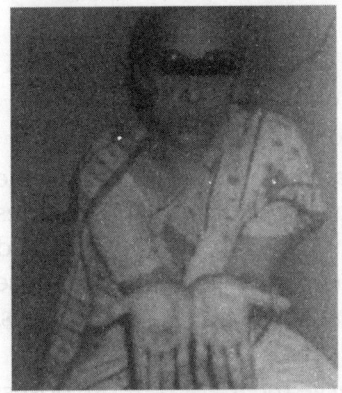

4 months after treatment

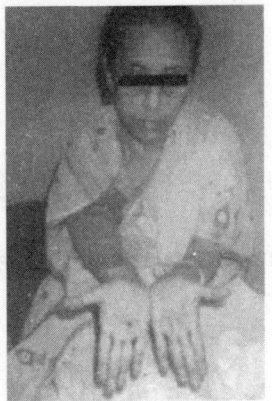

5 months after treatment

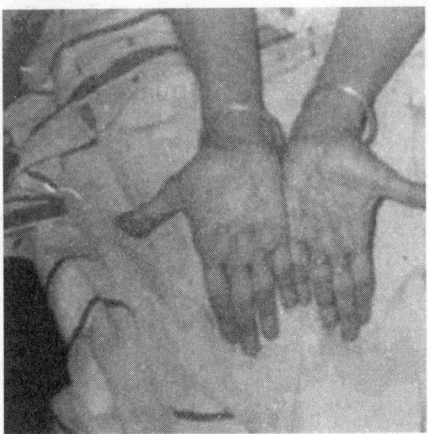

6 months after treatment

5. A CASE OF FISTULA IN CHEEK - MR. P.B.

Case No. D005

Age : 20 years as on 2.9.95.
Height : 5'7"

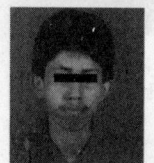

Mr. P. B. before treatment

Presenting Complaints

- Cellulitis in cheek for 2 yrs.
- It burst out after allopathic treatment.
- Thereafter a mole appeared from that wound, adjacent areas are very stiff.
- During shaving it bleeds. Blood: dark
- Bleeds (+++) easily, with stinging pain and soreness of the affected part.
- Pain and bleeding on pressing.
- Catches cold easily, from every time he is in open/draft of air.

Homoeopathic Generalities

- Tendency to catch cold easily – watery discharge followed by white mucoid discharge.
- Appetite: Poor.
- Burning sensation in throat followed by nausea & vomiting.
- Stool: Normal.
- History of allergic manifestation.
- Mentals: Obstinate, talkative, desires to be neat & clean.
- Memory: Consolation ameliorates. Sympathetic. Very active.
- Patient is chilly. Catches cold easily.
- Desires: Sweet+, salt+, salty, fish, chicken++, egg, warm food. Thirst: Less.
- Family History:
- Mother: Rheumatism.
- Father: Expired – Heart attack.

CASE ANALYSIS, MIASMATIC DIAGNOSIS AND FINAL PRESCRIPTION

Miasmatic Analysis

- Cellulitis – Psora: Sycotic.
- Mole growth: Sycotic.
- Bleeds easily (haemorrhagic diathesis) +++: Tubercular.
- Stinging pains: Sycotic.
- Catches cold easily, from every time he is in open/draft of air: Tubercular.
- Burning sensation in throat: Syphilitic.
- History of allergies: Tubercular.
- Mental: Obstinate: Tubercular-syphilitic, Talkative: Sycotic, desires to be neat and clean: Sycotic.
- Desires: Sweet: Psora; Salt – Syco-tubercular; Warm food – Sycotic.
- Family history: Rheumatism – Sycotic.

Final Prescription Made on the Basis of

- Haemorrhage from affected part, with bruised soreness.
- Tubercular nature of the case: catching cold easily, allergic and haemorrhagic diathesis.
- Dark (passive) blood.
- Soreness of the affected part.
- 5) Appetite – Poor.
- 6) Desires – Salt, Salty – Warm food.

Hamamelis has the miasmatic breakdown: Psora ++, Sycosis +, Syphilis +, Tubercular +++.

Remedy Reaction

The case was started with Hamamelis 1M on the basis of vitality and the complaint concerned; 1M is a good potency for haemorrhage. The case was finished with Hamamelis 50M and the patient was cured in just less than one year of treatment.

Prescription Chart

Date	Prescription Done on the Basis of	Treatment
2nd Sep'95	Mole bleeds during shaving (haemorrhagic diathesis). Blood: dark (passive); Bleeds (+++: profuse) with stinging pain and soreness of the affected part. Catches cold easily, from every time he is in open/ draft of air.	Hamamelis ver. 1M, 2 doses.
10th Oct'95	Bleeding has improved. No pain. Doing better.	Hamamelis ver. 1M
12th Dec'95	75% amelioration, improvement in respect of bleeding, but stand still.	Hamamelis ver. 1M
27th Jan'96	80% ameliorated.	Sac lac.
21st Feb'96	Had one day of bleeding otherwise okay.	Hamamelis ver. 10M, 2 doses.
16th Apr'96	99% better.	Sac lac.
4th Jun'96		Sac lac.
16th Jul'96	Standstill – prescription made to finish the case.	Hamamelis ver. 50M, 1 dose
30th Jul'96	Sac lac.	
20th Aug'96	CURED	Sac lac.

Authenticity of Cure

CD Reference: D005-FISTULA-PB

Dermatological Diseases-Cured Cases

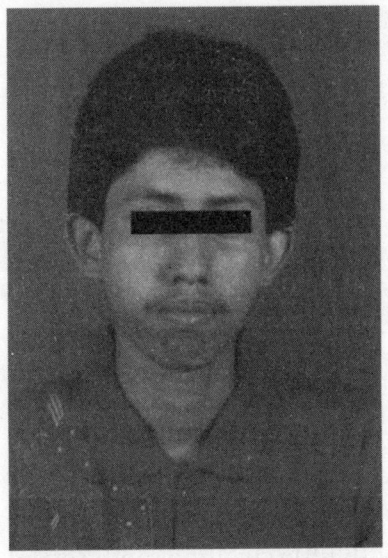

Photo of Mr. P. B. before treatment

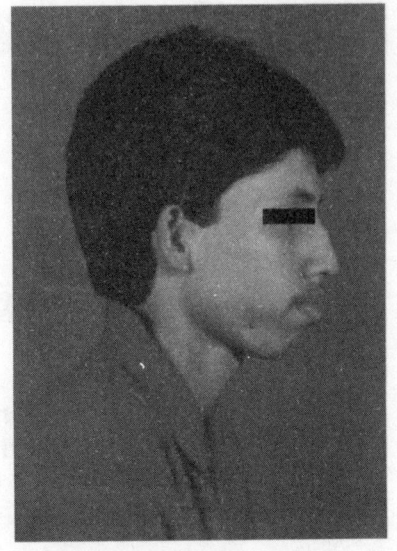

Photo of Mr. P.B. 9 months after treatment

Comments of the patient, before and after treatment

6. A CASE OF ECZEMATOUS ULCER IN CHEEK

Case No. D006

Ms. S. J., 24 years.

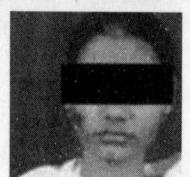

Ms. S. J. before treatment

Presenting Complaints

- Skin lesion: Appeared as pimple on right lower cheek and upper cheek in small circular shape. Duration - 4-5 months. Within a month started spreading and both the upper and lower points joined – gradually become large in size, red in colour. Oozing of thick creamy material.
- Now dark colour patch in the cheek with little swelling, with severe pain.
- On close examination, appears some ulceration.
- After conventional medicine for Herpes, creamish material came out and whole area becomes blackish red.
- Now all affected area become hard to touch. Then it appeared to be bigger in size, looks like cluster of bigger pimples.
- From starting to now, there is acute pain, burning sensation, itching. Now it spreads all over the face. Symptoms > by warm application. Agg-at night.
- Second problem:- is in her right hand, which was partially senseless with a white spot in that area White spot disappeared – but the senseless area is there till now. Duration: since 1996.
- Nature of symptoms:- In starting, pain, burning sensation, itching and oozing. Firstly situation was tolerable, but now cannot.
- Aggravates in sunshine and damp.
- Increases after cold bathing.
- Covering with a thin cloth gives relief for sometimes, > by warmth.
- Problem increases while sweating.
- Warm water on face gives relief.
- Used Betnovate-C for black spots and white heads. Those spots were due to white heads. This may cause the present problem.
- White heads were appearing for two years. But present problem first seen in 2003. And it is till now. (I started treatment in September 2003).

- Other chronic ailments – Left sided headache, constipation (always).
- Heat or burning head; vertigo and giddiness present. One sided headache once or twice in a month.
- Nose: Occasional burning sensation.
- Sometimes Salivation while sleeping.
- Mouth Ulcers:- Once in 2 or 3 months.
- Cough – Dry.
- Appetite – Good. Always feel hungry.
- Distension – Abdomen.
- Gas in middle of abdomen.
- Passing flatus gives relief.
- Stool – with putrid odour; no satisfactory evacuation. Constipated.
- Urine – Acidic, 4-5 hours interval.
- Nail – Thick – Not breakable; dry ridge. Convex.
- Skin Diseases:- Senseless area on right hand.
- Menstrual Cycle – Duration – 5 days. Quantity – Normal. Regular – clotted and with odour. Waist and lower abdominal pain.
- Menses first started 14 years of age.
- Leucorrhoea present.
- Temperament:- Angry+++, Indifferent+++, Introvert++, Sentimental+++, Talkative+++, Sympathetic.
- Fear of thunderstorm, incurable diseases.
- Memory – Can remember the events of past.
- Concentration – Very poor.
- The patient is hot. Desire humid rainy climate.
- Likes to enjoy holidays in cold weather.
- Likes Spring and Winter seasons.
- Food Desire:- Sweet+++, Egg+++, Spice, Fat+++, Ice Cream, Warm food.
- Like hot drinks. Short drinks at long interval.
- She sips at frequent interval.
- She is thirst less.
- Sleep – More than general – always feels sleepy. No dream.
- Peculiar symptoms – Menses – Stain does not go away.
- Bleed easily. Takes time to heal.
- Whenever goes into sunshine gets irritation on her face and hands.
- Past Medical History:- Skin diseases. Addiction to Tea, Coffee.
- Regular mile stones.

- Hepatitis – B – 1 year before.
- Family History:- Mother – Uterine problem. Father – Pneumonia, bronchitis. Grandfather – Cough, cold. Grandmother – Liver trouble.
- Family Tendencies:- Asthma, Allergy, Piles, Blood Pressure, Venereal Diseases.
- Every year eyes become yellow; yellow sweating, yellow urine, and a yellowish appearance.
- Never Been Well Since:- In 1999 taken conventional medicine to get rid of the white spot. Since then some thing happens always, fever, cold, headache, boils, etc.

CASE ANALYSIS, MIASMATIC DIAGNOSIS AND FINAL PRESCRIPTION

Miasmatic Analysis

- Skin: Blackish red, hardening of skin (hyper pigmentation): Syco-Tubercular.
- White spots: Syphilitic.
- Itching, burning sensation: Psora-Syphilitic.
- Pricking pains: Sycotic.
- Symptoms > warm application, < cold bathing: Psora,
- Agg. sweating: Syphilitic.
- Burning pain agg-night: Syphilitic.
- Ulceration of the skin: Syphilitic.
- Mouth ulcers: Syphilo-Tubercular.
- Wounds bleed easily: Tubercular.
- Take time to heal: Syphilitic.
- Constipation: Psora.
- Abdomen – Distension, gas: Psora.
- Menses-clots: Tubercular.
- Temperament – Angry, talkative: Sycotic.
- Introvert: Syphilitic.
- Indifferent: Tubercular.
- Thirst less: Psora.
- Desire sweet: Psora.
- Warm food: Sycotic.
- Addiction to tea, coffee: Syphilitic.

- Dry cough: Psora.
- Urine acidic: Psora.
- As the presenting complaint is a skin lesion with ulcerous manifestation and also delayed healing therefore, I have to think of a mixed miasmatic medicine with syphilitic preponderance.

Final Prescription Made on the Basis of

- Burning in spots > by warmth, warm application (this is a Tarentula symptom).
- Pricking pain. Itching.
- Ulcers: Black taint. Dark colour with itching and burning agg-night.
- Constipation: Putrid odour.
- Indifferent +++, Introverted ++, Angry +++, Talkative+++.
- Poor concentration.
- Wounds take time to heal.
- Aggravation: Cold bathing. Amelioration: Warm water on face.
- Mouth ulcers.
- Head: Burning, heat and vertigo, left sided headache.
- Sleep: Always feels sleepy.
- NBWS - In 1999, taken medicine for dim white spot. Since then – fever, headache, cold, boils etc.
- Every year eyes become yellow, yellow sweating, yellow urine and a yellowish appearance.
- The Miasmatic breakdown of Tarantula Cubensis is Psora ++, Sycosis +, Syphilis +++L, Tubercular ++.
- Tarentula Cubensis covers the case miasmatically as well.

Prescription Chart

Date	Prescription Done on the Basis of	Treatment
20th Sep'03	Burning in spots, > by warmth; pricking pain. Appearance -ulcerous. Black taint.	Tarantula Cubensis, 30C, 2 doses.
14th Oct'03	Slightly better. Burning better, pain slightly better. Pus discharge aggravates better after discharge. Pricking pain aggravate.	Sac lac.
13th Dec'03	As a whole 50% better. Discharge is less. Pus formation much better.	Sac lac.
10th Feb'04	Old rashes are better. Pain better, burning better.	Sac lac.

Date	Prescription Done on the Basis of	Treatment
10th Apr'04	New rashes appear on the affected area. Burning – Nil. Pain – Little. Itching++. Burning only new spots. To take care of Black Spot. Tarantula Cubensis, 200C, 1 dose. I felt 30C was not holding and the colouration of the cheek was not changing; that is the reason without repeating 30C another time, what I generally do (repeat the same potency twice to exhaust it's action, before going to the next potency);	Sac lac.
26th Jun'04	Burning better. Occasional itching. Blackening started getting better. Wait and watch	I prescribed 200C.
11th Sep'04	As a whole 90% - 95% better. Wait and watch.	Sac lac.

Authenticity of Cure

CD Reference: D006-ECZEMATOUS ULCER IN CHEEK-SJ

Dermatological Diseases-Cured Cases

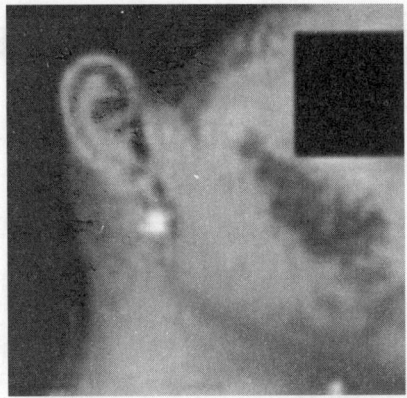

Photo of Ms. S. J. before treatment

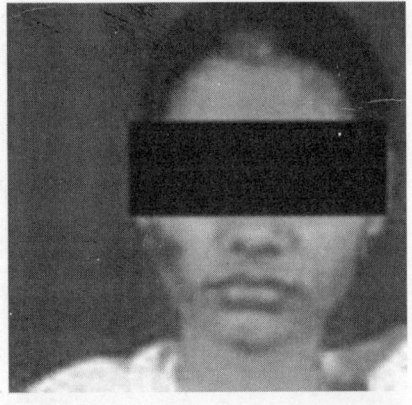

Photo of Ms. S. J. before treatment

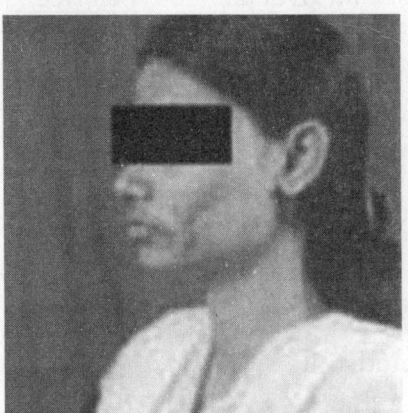

Photo of Ms. S. J. 2 months after treatment

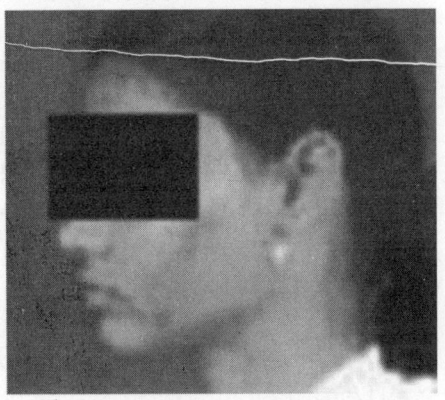

Photo of Ms. S. J. 5 months after treatment

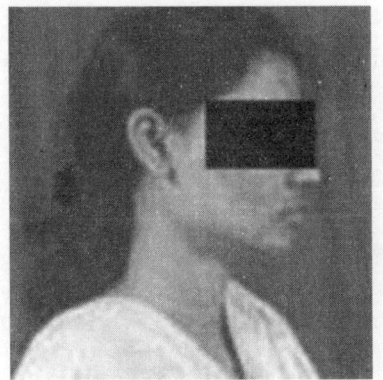

Photo of Ms. S. J. 5 months after treatment

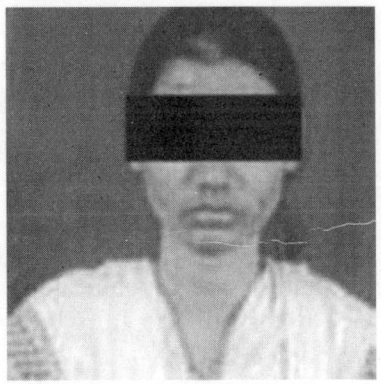

Photo of Ms. S. J. 5 months after treatment

7. A CASE OF PSORIASIS: MR. P.D.

Case No. D007

Age   : 30 year-old as on 28.11.1998.
Sex   : Male.
Weight : 48 kgs.

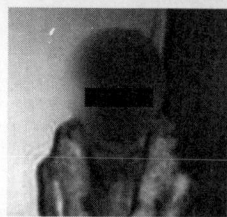

Mr. P. D. with Psoriasis
before treatment

Presenting Complaints

- Skin disease, diagnosed as Psoriasis, all over the body; started 11 years ago. Itching ++, worse from touching and scratching, better by cold application and wash. Occasional burning in spots of the psoriasis, amel. by cold.
- After scratching à bleeds easily.
- Oversensitive to noise, odour.
- Tendency of chronic loose stool and diarrhoea.
- Nervous, weak.
- Feeble constitution.
- Frail constitution, weak ++.
- Anxious, restless, cannot remain standstill.
- Fearful.
- Afraid in the dark.
- Dislike of being alone but gets terrified in a crowded room.
- Artistic and creative.
- Intelligent.
- Likes sympathy and also very sympathetic.
- Talkative.
- Open minded.
- Enthusiastic, responsive.
- Nervous, startle easily.
- Empty sensation in the entire abdomen.
- Craves: Ice-cream; cold food and drinks, juicy, refreshing things. Likes salt and salty food. Craves cucumber, spicy food. Aversion to egg & fish.
- Appetite increased alternating with loss of appetite. Reasonably slender built, flat chest.
- Grew rapidly during puberty.
- Chilly patient; but likes cold air.

Dermatological Diseases-Cured Cases

CASE ANALYSIS, MIASMATIC DIAGNOSIS AND FINAL PRESCRIPTION

Miasmatic Analysis

- Psoriasis: Marriage of all miasms: Tri-miasmatic, it has dryness of Psora, fish scale eruptions and thickened skin of sycosis, ulceration and oozing of fluid à scab formation of syphilis and itching à bleeding and periodical recurrence of tubercular miasm.
- Itching ++: Psora.
- Burning in spots of the psoriasis: Syphilis.
- After scratching à bleeds easily: Tubercular.
- Oversensitive to noise, odour: Sycosis.
- Tendency of chronic loose stool and diarrhoea: Sycosis.
- Nervous: Psora.
- Frail constitution, weak ++: Psora-Tubercular.
- Anxious: Psora.
- Restless, cannot remain standstill: Sycosis.
- Fearful: Psora.
- Afraid in the dark: Psora.
- Dislike of being alone: Psora.
- Artistic and creative: Tubercular.
- Intelligent: Tubercular.
- Talkative: Sycosis.
- Nervous, startle easily: Psora.
- Empty sensation in the entire abdomen: Psora.
- Appetite increased alternating with loss of appetite: Tubercular.
- Chilly patient; but likes cold air: Tubercular.

Prescription Made on the Basis of

- Psoriasis, itching ++, worse from touching and scratching, better by cold application and wash.
- Occasional burning in spots of the psoriasis, amel. by cold.
- After scratching → bleeds easily.
- Oversensitive to noise, odour.
- Tendency of chronic loose stool and diarrhoea.
- Nervous.
- Frail constitution, weak ++.

- Anxious, restless, cannot remain standstill.
- Fearful.
- Afraid in the dark.
- Dislike of being alone but gets terrified in a crowded room.
- Artistic and creative.
- Intelligent.
- Likes sympathy and also very sympathetic.
- Talkative.
- Open minded.
- Enthusiastic, responsive.
- Nervous, startle easily.
- Empty sensation in the entire abdomen.
- Craves: Ice-cream; cold food and drinks, juicy, refreshing things. Likes salt and salty food. Craves cucumber, spicy food. Aversion to egg & fish.
- Appetite increased alternating with loss of appetite. Reasonably slender built, flat chest.
- Grew rapidly during puberty.
- Chilly patient; but likes cold air.
- Phosphorus has the miasmatic breakdown: Psora +++, Sycosis ++, Syphilis +++, Tubercular +++.

Final Prescription and Remedy Reaction

I started and finished the case with Phosphorus, started with 30 C and finish with 10M.

Patient improved gradually and there was a steady progress and finished the case (11 years of suffering from Psoriasis) in 2 years time.

Authenticity of Cure

CD Reference: D007-PSORIASIS-PD

Dermatological Diseases-Cured Cases

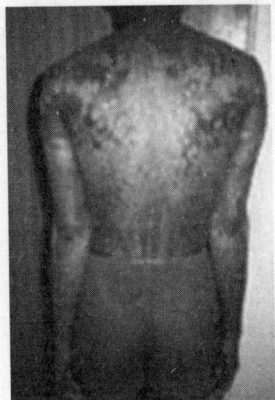

Mr. P. D. with Psoriasis before treatment of Dr. Banerjea

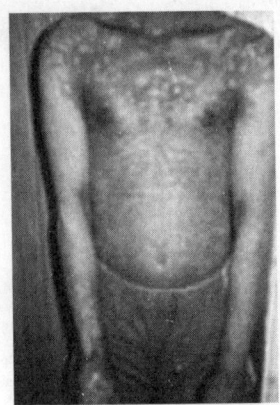

Mr. P. D. with Psoriasis before treatment

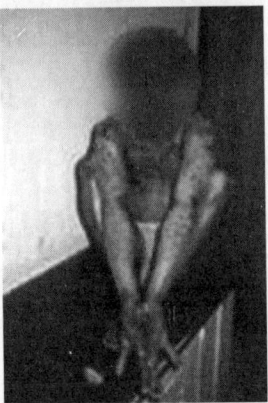

Mr. P. D. with Psoriasis before treatment

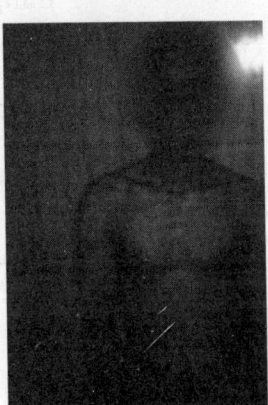

Mr. P. D. 2 months after treatment

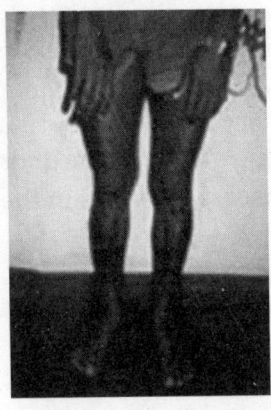

Mr. P. D. 2 months after treatment

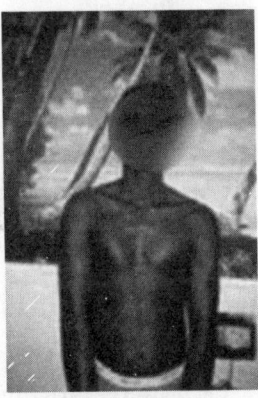

Mr. P. D. 12 months after treatment

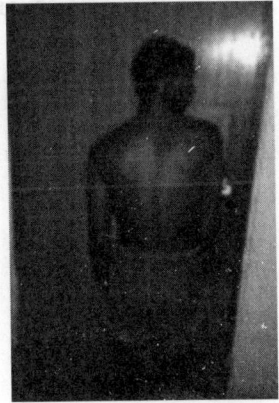

Mr. P. D. 12 months after treatment

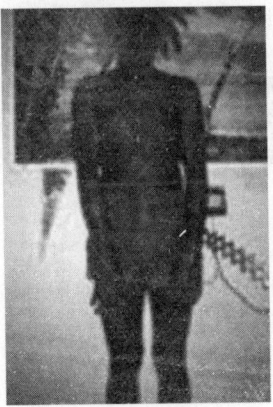

Mr. P. D. 24 months after treatment

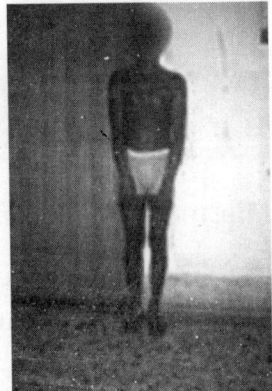

Mr. P. D. 24 months after treatment

8. A CASE OF WART ON HAND & FEET: MAST. U.S.

Case No. D008

Age : 8 year-old as on 31.03.1998.
Sex : Male

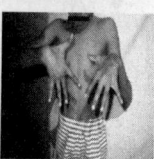
Master U. S.

Presenting Complaints

- Multiple Warts → Cauliflower like growth. First started on back of hands then spread all over the body. Itching+. Operated twice – since last 10 years.
- Stomach:- Acidity++. Sour eructation < morning.
- Sweat:- Sweat more face and back of head. Sour smelling++ especially in neck.
- Skin Disease:- Multiple Warts operated twice. No bleeding.
- Mental Symptoms:- Angry. Obstinate. Very talkative. Desire for company. Memory - active. When reprimanded gets more angry. He wants to do everything slowly. Fears ghost, darkness, thunderstorm.
- Suffer from:- Skin disease; Measles in the past.
- Chilly++ patient. Catches cold easily++.
- Desire: Foods:- Sweet++; Salt+; Egg+++; Sour+; Bread+; Ice Cream++; Cold Drinks+++; Milk; Potato; Cold Food+.
- Generally thirsty for cold drinks.
- Sleep:- Normal.
- Family History:- Blood pressure; Tuberculosis (both side of parents).
- Bowels constipated. 3 times in a week but no discomfort.
- Gets tired (++) easily.

CASE ANALYSIS, MIASMATIC DIAGNOSIS AND FINAL PRESCRIPTION

Miasmatic Analysis

- Multiple warts; Cauliflower like growth: Sycotic.
- Acidity++, sour eructation: Psora.

Dermatological Diseases-Cured Cases

- Sweat; Sour smelling++: Psora-Sycotic.
- Angry: Psora-Sycotic.
- Obstinate: Tubercular.
- Very Talkative: Sycotic.
- Desire for company: Psora.
- Wants to do everything slowly: Psora.
- Fears; Ghosts. Darkness. Thunderstorm: Psora.
- Chilly patient, catches cold easily:Psora.
- Desire Sweet: Psora. Potatoe:Tubercular.
- Desire Cold Drinks+++: Syphilitic.
- Constipation: Psora.
- Gets tired easily: Psora.

Miasmatic Sum-up (Miasmatic Totality)

It is a mixed miasmatic case with Syco-psoric preponderance (or surface miasm). Calcarea calcinata is a remedy for warts, so covers the Sycotic miasm.

Prescription Made on the Basis of

- Multiple warts- Cauliflower like growth – all over the body.
- Stomach:- Acidity++. Sour eructation < morning.
- He wants to do everything slowly. Fears ghost, darkness, thunderstorm.
- Chilly++ patient. Catches cold easily++.
- Desire: Foods:- Sweet++; Salt+; Egg+++; Sour+; Bread+; Ice Cream++; Cold Drinks+++; Milk; Potato; Cold Food+.
- Bowels constipated. 3 times in a week, but no discomfort.
- Gets tired (++) easily.

Calcarea Calcinata has the miasmatic breakdown: Psora+++, Sycosis+++, Syphilis+, Tubercular++.

Final Prescription and Remedy Reaction

The case was started with Calcarea Calcinata 200C, because of the multiple warts in a Calcarea constitution. Then followed by 1M potency, with wonderful results.

Prescription Chart

Dates	Points in Favour of the Prescription	Prescribed Medicine
31st Mar'98	Warts in Calcarea Constitution.	Calcarea Calcinata, 200C: 2 doses
14th May'98	No appreciable change. Wait and watch.	Sac Lac
4th Jul'98	Little better. Few warts have shrunken. Wait.	Sac Lac
14th Aug'98	Little more progress. 50% of the warts have gone. Wait and Watch with wisdom (WWW)	Sac Lac
19th Sep'98	Stand still. Repeat (No further progress).	Calcarea Calcinata, 200C: 1 dose.
31st Oct'98	No further progress. Wait and Watch.	Sac Lac
24th Dec'98	No further progress. Repeat goes higher.	
13th Feb'99	Calcarea Calcinata, 1M: 2 doses in water.	All warts gone. Glory goes to Hahnemann and his beautiful homoeopathy.

Authenticity of Cure

CD Reference: D008-WART ON HAND & FEET-US

Dermatological Diseases-Cured Cases

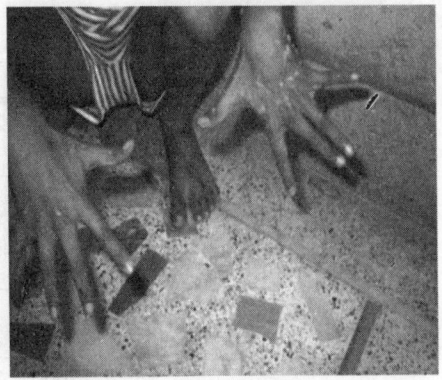

Master U. S. Wart on hand and feet before treatment

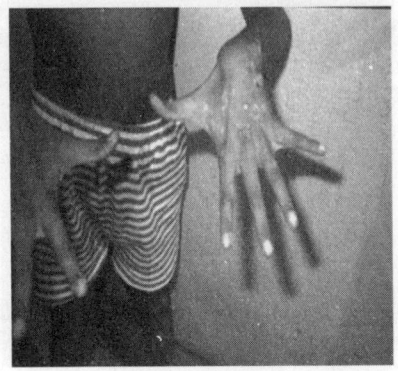

Before treatment

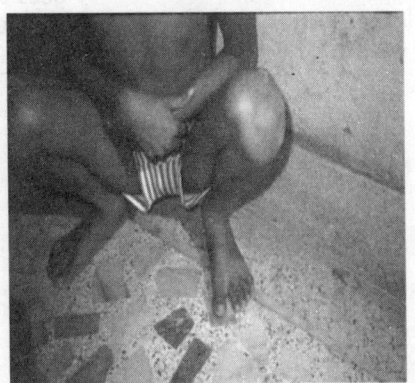

6 months after treatment

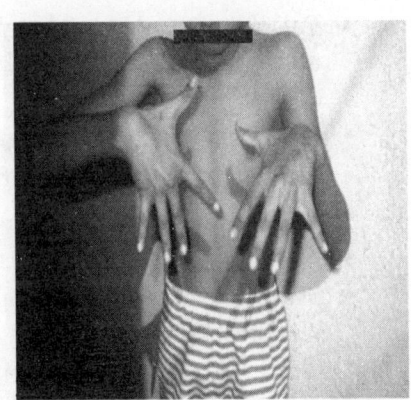

10 months after treatment

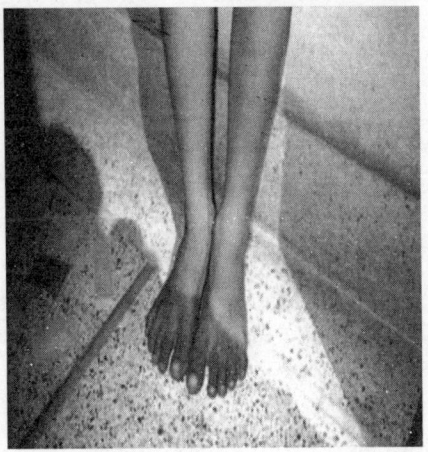

10 months after treatment

9. A CASE OF LIP LIPOMA: MR S.M.

Case No. D009

Age : 15 years as on 21/9/90
Height : 5 ft.
Weight : 39 kgs.

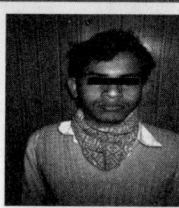

Mr. S. M 16 months after treatment

Presenting Complaints

- A fleshy growth on the right side of upper lip; began in 1989. Very hard, gradually increasing in size, painless, reddish, and moveable. Easily fatigued especially in the outdoors, has profuse sweat with weakness afterwards.
- Past History: Normal delivery, milestones – regular, vaccination – all regular doses, I.U.L (Intra-Uterine Life: Pregnancy history) – no significant history.
- Tongue: Whitish Coating.
- Lung: Occasional cough from cold exposure.
- Abdomen: Okay.
- Stomach: Normal.
- Sweat: Profuse ++ especially in covered areas followed by excessive weakness.
- Stool: Occasionally constipated, 1 – 2 days interval.
- Anus: Itching due to small worms.
- Food Desires: Sweet++, salty ++, hot & pungent food++, sour+, salty, meat, egg, fish, cold food, ice cream++.
- Dislikes: Bitter, vegetable & spinach (does not like green vegetables at all).
- Mental Symptoms: Mild. Desires to be neat and clean: quite fastidious; likes company. Low self-esteem. Dad says he has a tendency to conceal and lie.
- Memory: poor and thinks gradually getting worse.
- Wants to do everything in a hurry.
- Fear of ghosts. Chilly patient but prefers to lie with doors & windows open, likes open air.
- Thirst: Average.
- Sleep: Cannot sleep well (insomnia).
- Urine: Not clear, occasional flow in fork stream.

CASE ANALYSIS, MIASMATIC DIAGNOSIS AND FINAL PRESCRIPTION

Miasmatic Analysis

- A fleshy growth (very hard): Sycosis.
- Gradually increasing in size: Sycosis.
- Easily fatigued: Psora.
- Profuse sweat: Sycosis.
- Occasionally constipated: Psora.
- Small worms: Tubercular.
- Dislikes: Vegetable & spinach (does not like green vegetables at all): Hydrogenoid: Sycosis.
- Mild: Psora.
- Quite fastidious: Sycosis.
- Low self-esteem: Psora.
- Dad says he has a tendency to conceal and lie: Sycosis.
- Memory: poor: Psora.
- Wants to do everything in a hurry: Sycosis.
- Fear of ghosts: Psora.
- Chilly patient, but prefers to lie with doors & windows open, likes open air: Tubercular.
- Mixed miasmatic with sycotic preponderance.

Prescription Made on the Basis of

- A fleshy growth; very hard gradually increasing in size.
- Easily fatigued especially in the outdoors.
- Sweat: Profuse ++ especially in covered areas followed by excessive weakness.
- Stool: Occasionally constipated, 1 – 2 days interval.
- Food Desires: Salty ++, hot & pungent food++, meat, cold food, ice cream++.
- Dislikes: Bitter, vegetable & spinach (does not like green vegetables at all).
- Mental Symptoms: Desires to be neat and clean: quite fastidious.
- Dad says he has a tendency to conceal and lie.
- Chilly patient, but prefers to lie with doors & windows open, likes open air.

- Sleep: Cannot sleep well (insomnia).
- Urine: Not clear, occasional flow in fork stream.
- Sycotic preponderance.
- Thuja is a leading sycotic remedy with miasmatic breakdown of Psora ++, Sycosis +++, Syphilis ++, Tubercular ++.
- Thuja also covers the case miasmatically.

Final Prescription and Remedy Reaction

I started the case with Thuja 30 C and finished with 10M. The 30 C potency was begun with, as this is a growth on the lip; the 30 C potency works well for dermatological cases. Unfortunately a detailed prescription chart is not available for this case, but the lipoma was completely cured after 20 months of treatment.

Authenticity of Cure

CD Reference: D009-LIPOMA OF LIP-SM

Dermatological Diseases-Cured Cases

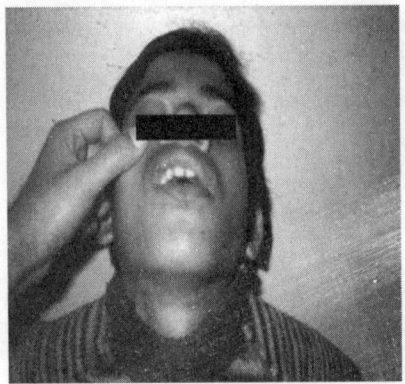

Mr. S. M with Lipoma of lip before treatment

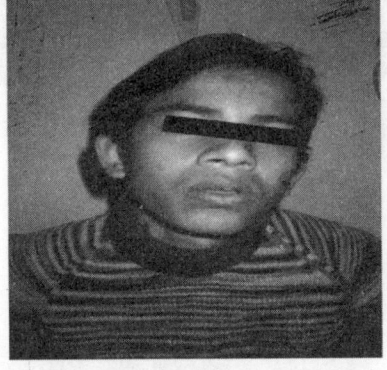

Before treatment

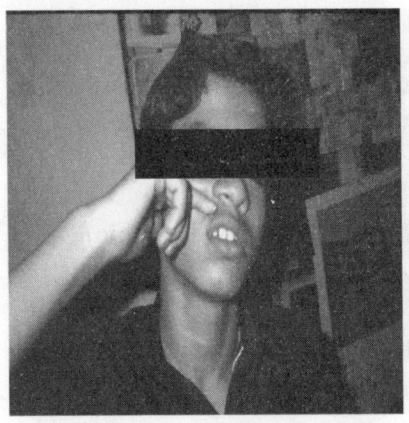

10 months after treatment

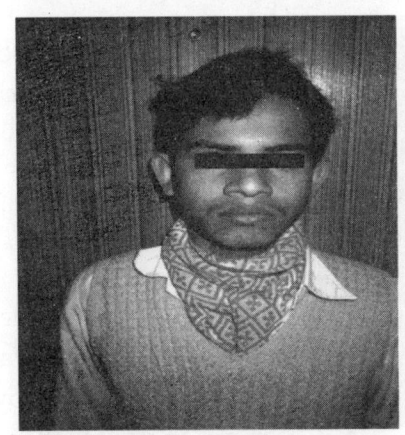

16 months after treatment

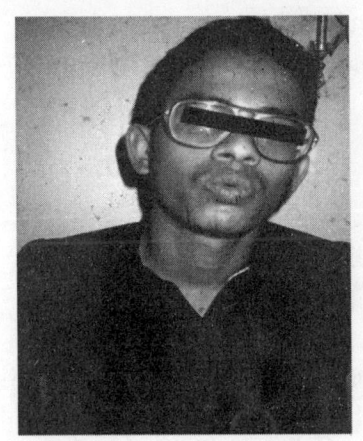

20 months after treatment

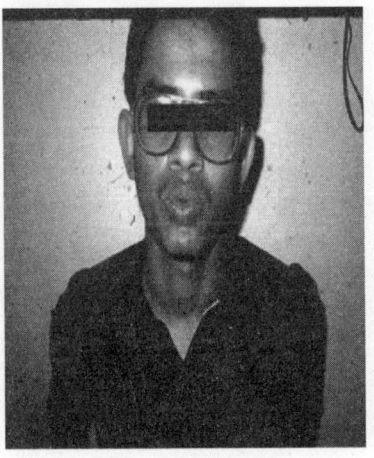

After treatment

10. A CASE OF ATOPIC VESICULAR DERMATITIS - MASTER B.M.

Case No. D010

Age : 21 years old (as on 7th December, 1999)
Height : 5 ft. 6 inches
Weight : 58 kgs.

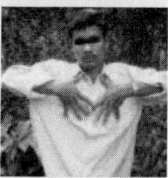

Mr. B. M. with vesicular dermatitis

Presenting Complaints

- Skin disease, vesicular, mainly on fingers of left hand – since 4 years back.
- Aggravates in rainy season.
- Vesicular eruptions à itching à formation of ulcer à suppurates à sticky yellowish pus with fishy odour à occasionally bleeds.
- Occasional burning after scratching, ameliorated by application of coconut oil.
- Previous treatments – both conventional (allopathic) and homoeopathic.
- Hereditary cause – mother has skin disease.
- History of irregular diet and habit of taking rich++ spicy food.
- Indigestion aggravated by taking meat and rich food.
- Gas forms in abdomen, aggravated in the morning, ameliorated by passing of stool.
- Acidity: Sour taste in mouth. Sour eructations.
- Stool: Regular; not clear; diarrhoeic stool; occasional mucus, occasional bad smell.
- Gas and acidity.
- Acidity – Sour eructation.
- Delayed healing.
- Mental Symptoms: Mild, obstinate, talkative, desires company.
- Fear of: Ghosts, darkness.
- Hot patient. Likes open air.
- Desires: Sweet++, pungent and hot++, salt++, milk+, potato+, vegetables and spinach++, onion+, fruits+, meat++, rich, spicy and fat food++, luke warm food++, cold drinks++. Aversion. to sour, bitter.
- Dreams of various kinds.

- Sleep - Normal
- Appetite – Normal
- Thirst – cold drinks++.

Investigation Carried Out before Treatment

Atopic vesicular dermatitis.

CASE ANALYSIS, MIASMATIC DIAGNOSIS AND FINAL PRESCRIPTION

This case is another good example about how Classical Homoeopathy can take care of an advanced Dermatological problem and heal the skin completely.

Miasmatic Analysis

- Skin disease, vesicular: Sycotic.
- Aggravates in rainy season: Sycotic.
- Formation of ulcers: Syphilitic.
- Sticky yellowish pus: Syphilo-Sycotic.
- Fishy odour: Sycotic.
- Acidity: Sour taste in mouth: Psora.
- Delayed healing: Syphilitic.
- Mental Symptoms: Talkative: Sycotic.
- Fear of: Ghosts, darkness: Psora.
- Desires: Spicy: Psora; Pungent and hot: Psora-tubercular; Sweet: Psora; Salt: Syco- tubercular; Meat: Tubercular; Warm food: Sycotic.
- Indigestion aggravated by meat and rich food: Sycotic.
- Distension from gas: Psora.
- Diarrhoeic stool, occasional mucus: Sycotic.

This is a predominantly sycotic case with elements of Psora and Syphilis.

Final Prescription Made on the Basis of

- Skin disease, vesicular. Mancinella has the largest vesicular eruptions in our Materia Medica.
- Aggravates in rainy season.

- Vesicular eruptions → itching → formation of ulcer → suppurates → sticky yellowish pus with fishy odour à occasionally bleeds.
- Occasional burning after scratching.
- Indigestion aggravated after taking meat and rich food.
- Gas forms in abdomen: aggravated in the morning, ameliorated by passing of stool.
- Acidity: Sour taste in mouth. Sour eructations.
- Delayed healing.
- Mental Symptoms: Mild, obstinate, talkative, desire for company.
- Fear of: Ghosts, darkness.
- Hot patient. Likes open air.
- Desire: Sweet++, salt++. Thirst for cold drinks (++).
- Mancinella also has melancholia and depression around the period when the hormonal balance is upset (e.g. puberty, pregnancy and the menopause).
- The miasmatic breakdown of Mancinella is Psora ++, Sycosis +++, Syphilis ++, Tubercular +.
- Mancinella also covers the case miasmatically.

Final Prescription

MANCINELLA, 30 C: 1 globule (No. 10: poppy seed size) in sugar of milk sachet, dissolved in water and sipped for 10 days. Then 10 days of no medicine, followed by another dose to be shaken and sipped for 10 days.

Remedy Reaction

The case was begun with Mancinella 30C to avoid any aggravation. The potency was ascended to 1M over a period of 16 months and the skin completely healed.

Date	Prescription Done on the Basis of	Treatment
7th Dec'99	Strongly sycotic+++. Fishy discharge, yellowish discharge. Vesicular, crust formation. Swelling. Aggravation damp and rainy weather.	Mancinella, 30C, 2 doses
12th Feb'00	Doing better (regarding skin). Stool not clear regularly. Occasional mucus. Occasional indigestion. Gas+ aggravates at night, ameliorated by passing of flatus. Rumbling of abdomen. Nauseatic tendency after eating at night. Appetite - less; Thirst – scanty; sleep – average. History of falling of hair.	Sac lac.

Dermatological Diseases-Cured Cases

Date	Prescription Done on the Basis of	Treatment
27th Mar'00	Occasional itching in (R) little finger. Stool – regular. Health deteriorated. Weakness. Had history of fever. Dimness of vision. History of falling++ of hair. Occasional earache. Dry with roughness of skin in extremities (R).	Sac lac.
15th May'00	Skin disease better than before, occasional itching → vesicular eruptions. Indigestion – gas forms in abdomen, aggravates at night, ameliorated by passing of flatus; Stool: not clear. Occasional water brash; Foetor oris; Hair falling. Ear aching (R) – Standstill. Appetite - average. Sleep – ok.	Mancinella, 30C, 2 doses
3rd Jul'00	History of Skin diseases. Aggravated rainy weather → itching. Stool: not clear regularly. History of: Falling of hair. Occasional gas forms in abdomen. History of: Water brash --. Occasional Itching (R) ear; History of: Night pollution (spermatorrhoea). Appetite – Average; Sleep: disturbed due to itching.	Mancinella, 200C, 2 doses
28th Aug'00	Skin diseases ; Occasional pain in (R) ear --. Stool: not clear; loose stool; History of: Falling of hair. Appetite: average; Sleep: good. Occasional bleeding from gums aggravated by brushing. Occasional water brash in early morning. History of: Night pollution. Burning eyes aggravated when reading a book.	Sac lac.
3rd Oct'00	History of Fever – took Homoeopathic medicine à slight improvement; aggravates in evening; pain on forehead and vertex. Aggravates on movement, aggravates during temperature, with reeling in head and vertigo. Water brash++ à bitter taste in mouth. Foetor oris. Nausea. Stool: irregular with bad odour, mucus; Thirst++; Pain in waist, yellow colour in urine; Sleepless. Skin diseases aggravate; Earache; Appetite – poor.	Mancinella, 200C, 2 doses
20th Nov'00	Had Typhoid. Gastric discomfort rumbling. Had history of Typhoid à since 2½ months back. Took Allopathic medicine. Presenting complaint: Occasional itching all over the body – Occasional buzzing in right ear. Earache. Stool: not clear à evacuation at night, after taking meal à since fever. Occasional mucus. Gas++; rumbling of abdomen; aggravates at night, ameliorates by passing of flatus. History of falling of hair – Occasional pain at root of the hair. Occasional burning eyes --. Occasional night pollution. Aggravation by taking fish, meat and spicy food. Appetite – ok; Thirst normal; Sleep: average.	Sac lac.
26th Dec'00	Itching à. Slightly better. Occasional pain in internal ear, aggravates with pressure. Buzzing in ear ameliorated. History of Falling of hair++ à worse after suffering typhoid fever. Stool: Not clear properly. Gas+ aggravates at night – rumbling of abdomen. Burning eyes. Occasional night pollution. Change in plan of treatment – Mancinella again.	Mancinella 1M, 1 dose

Date	Prescription Done on the Basis of	Treatment
7th Apr'01	Stool not clear; irregular, no mucus. Appetite; Thirstless; Sleepless. Pain in body better; Occasional burning eyes. Memory. Weak. Skin much better.	Sac lac.

Authenticity of cure:

CD Reference: D010-ATOPIC VESICULAR DERMATITIS IN HAND-BM

Dermatological Diseases-Cured Cases

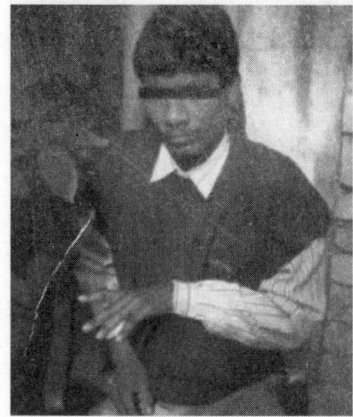

Mr. B. M. with vesicular dermatitis before treatment

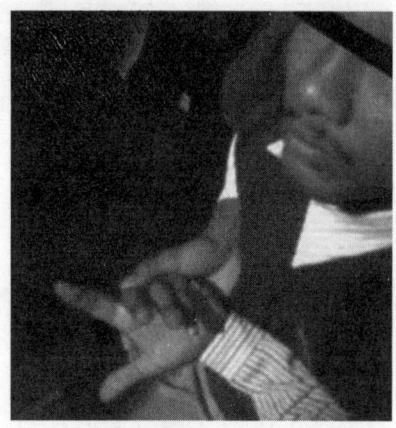

Before treatment

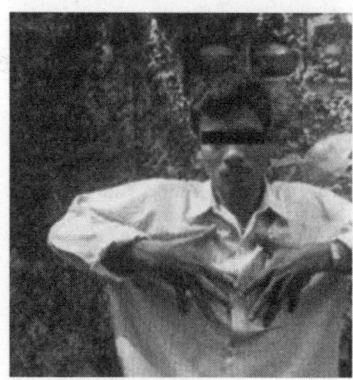

5 months after treatment

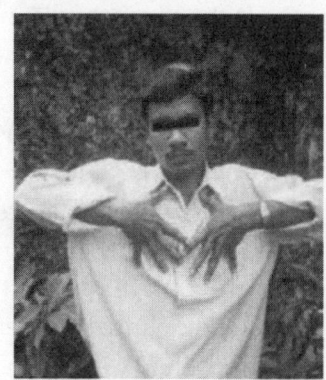

Vesicular Dermatitis, 16 months after treatment

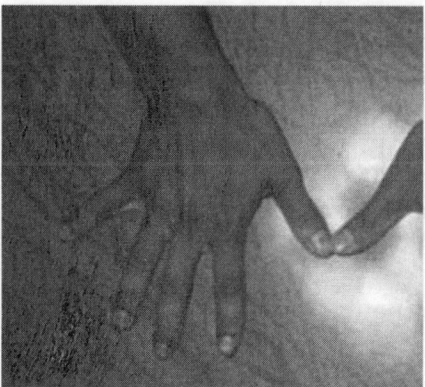

Vesicular Dermatitis, after treatment

11. A CASE OF FACIAL ACNE - MISS R.D.

Case No. D011

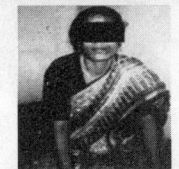

Miss R.D. before treatment

Presenting Complaints

- Acne: all over the face, shoulders; elevated, looks like large boils. Itchy, on scratching pus and fluid oozes.
- Patient is extremely depressed (+++), as she thinks this is awful and hates this appearance, the sight of her face, has tried allopathy (creams, lotions, shots), Ayurvedic (Naturopathy etc.) without any lasting improvement.
- Head: Nothing Abnormal Dectected (N.A.D).
- Eyes: O.K.
- Ears: White discharge from both ears. Type of discharge: thin and sticky.
- Nose: Occasional stoppage of nose.
- Mouth: Apthae in winter, bad odour in mouth, occasional salivation, drooling of saliva at night.
- Teeth: Gums swollen, pyorrhoea.
- Tongue: Thin, ulcer on tongue in winter.
- Throat: Pain in winter. Tonsils swell easily from exposure to cold.
- Lungs: Cough: moist, sticky phlegm comes out, breathing trouble present.
- Heart: Palpitation.
- Chest: Pain (occasional) in the left side, better by pressure, aggravation by respiratory movement.
- Abdomen: Nothing Abnormal Detected.
- Stomach: Appetite decreased.
- Sweat: Nil.
- Urine: N.A.D clear.
- Stool: Constipated. Mucus (occasional), offensive odour. Itching in rectum from pinworms (++), crawling in rectum at night.
- Upper Extremities: Occasional pain.
- Palms: Occasional sweat in summer.
- Skin Disease: Acne on face for the last 6 years.

Dermatological Diseases-Cured Cases

- Mental Symptoms: (a) Irritable temper, abusive (esp. to her brother). (b) Suicidal tendency, suspicious mood. (c) Depressed (+++). (d) Talkative, (e) Timid (++). (f) Desires to be neat and clean, desires company. (g) Fear of death. (h) Memory weak. (i) Weeping mood. (j) Patient cries when reprimanded. (k) Sympathetic. (l) Fear of ghosts, animals, cockroaches, lizards, literally all insects and animals, even ants!
- Exciting Cause of the Disease: Mental worry and fear. Abuse of homoeopathic and allopathic medicines.
- Present habit - tobacco chewing.
- History of accumulation of fluid inside chest. (Hydrothorax treated allopathically).
- History of Typhoid, skin disease (treated allopathically), Measles.
- Chilly patient, likes to sleep with closed doors and windows. Likes to bathe in summer, not in winter. Catches cold easily.
- Menses: Time - irregular (40 -50 days interval, sometimes even in 20 days) duration - 8 - 9 days. Character of flow - scanty bleeding. Flow more during 2nd day. Colour - blackish/dark. Odour – offensive. Pain - no pain.
- Leucorrhoea: Profuse white discharge, generally after menses, lasts for almost 15 days. Watery or sometimes thick and slippery. Slightly yellowish in colour.
- Desire of Foodstuffs: Hot pungent, fried food, bitter, potato, onion, fruits, warm food, cold drink, Ice cream.
- Aversion: Sweet +/-, sour, milk, vegetables, egg, fish, meat, spicy and fat food, cold food.
- Thirsty.
- Sleep: Sleep okay during the 1st part of the night, disturbed sleep in the late night.
- Dreams: Snakes, robbers, dead persons.
- Patient is unmarried.
- Family History: Father, mother and brother - have suffered from Tb.

CASE ANALYSIS, MIASMATIC DIAGNOSIS AND FINAL PRESCRIPTION

Miss R.D. was a young unmarried lady and she was extremely depressed by this long standing acne. In India, this had some social implications and was difficult to arrange her marriage.

Miasmatic Analysis

- Acne: all over the face, shoulders, recurrent: Tubercular
- Pus and fluid oozes: Syphilo-tubercular.
- Depressed (+++): Syphilitic or Syphilo-tubercular (continued or recurrent depression is syphilo-tubercular)
- Mouth: Apthae in winter, bad odour in mouth, occasional salivation, drooling of saliva at night: Syphilitic.
- Teeth: Pyorrhoea: Syphilitic.
- Tongue: Thin, ulcer on tongue in winter: Syphilitic.
- Throat: Tonsil swells easily from exposure to cold: Tubercular.
- Cough: sticky phlegm: Tubercular.
- Heart: Palpitation: Tubercular.
- Chest: Pains ameliorated by pressure: Sycotic.
- Rectum: Itching in rectum from pinworms: Tubercular.
- Stool: Constipation: Psora. Offensive: Psora – syphilio – tubercular.
- Mental Symptoms: (a) Irritable temper, abusive (esp. to her brother): Syco-tubercular.
  - Suicidal tendency: Syphilitic.
  - Talkative: Sycotic.
  - Timid: Psora.
  - Fear of death: Psora
  - Memory weak: Psora.
  - Fear of ghosts, animals, cockroaches, lizards literally all insects and animals, even ants: Psora-tubercular (though fears are generally psoric, but here fears everything, which can be reflected as complete destruction of mental stamina, confidence; thus Syphilitic miasm joins, therefore Psora-syphilitic = Tubercular miasm).
  - Desire to be neat and clean: Sycotic (over the top or excess).
  - Suspicious: Sycotic.
- Chilly patient, catches cold easily: Tubercular.
- Menses: Time – irregular, offensive: Syphilitic. Scanty: Psora.
- Leucorrhoea: After menses, yellow, watery: Tubercular.
- Desire of Foodstuff: Hot, pungent: Psora-tubercular; Cold drinks: Syphilitic; Potatoes: Tubercular;
- Aversion: Meat: Syphilo-sycotic; Cold food :Tubercular; Milk: Psora-sycotic.

- Disturbed sleep at night: Syphilitic.

It is a mixed miasmatic case with Tubercular preponderance.

Final Prescription Made on the Basis of

- Recurrent acne.
- Long lasting depression and discontentment: I took this as one of the background themes (mental essence) as the result of the physical manifestation of acne.
- Ears: Long lasting thin and sticky discharge.
- Throat: Tonsils swell easily from exposure to cold.
- Heart: Palpitation.
- Rectum: Itching in rectum from pin-worms. Crawling in rectum at night.
- Mental Symptoms: (a) Irritable temper, abusive (esp. to her brother). (b) Suicidal tendency, (c) Patient cries when reprimanded. (d) Fear of ghosts, animals, cockroaches, lizards, literally all insects and animals, even ants!
- Chilly patient, catches cold easily.
- Family history of tuberculosis.
- Appetite decreased.
- Sleep disturbed.

This is a tubercular case with strong elements of the other miasms. The miasmatic analysis of Tuberculinum is Psora +++, Sycosis +++, Syphilis ++, Tubercular +++ and therefore covers the case well.

Final Prescription

TUBERCULINUM, 200 C: 1 globule (No. 10 : poppy seed size) in sugar of milk sachet, asked the patient dissolve the powder in half or one litre of pure water and sip it slowly throughout the day, save a little at the bottom, top it up next morning, keep sipping throughout the next day. Generally I give instruction to my patient to dilute the medicated water (top it up with water) as many times as s/he likes. Continue like this for 10 days. Then 10 days of no medicine. Followed by another dose to be shaken and sipped for 10 days.

In cases where there is a history of Tuberculosis, a tubercular remedy should be prescribed with caution: starting with a high potency can re-establish walled off tubercular infection. In this case, however, the patient's vitality was very strong and this allowed me to begin with a potency of 200c.

Remedy Reaction

Patient improved dramatically and was cured within 9 months. A detailed prescription chart is unfortunately not available.

Authenticity of Cure

CD Reference: D011-FACIAL ACNE-RD

Dermatological Diseases-Cured Cases

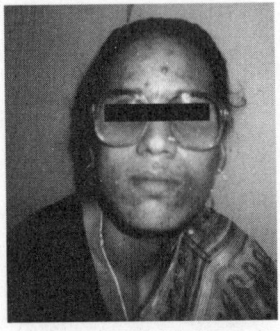

Photo of the patient Miss R.D. before treatment

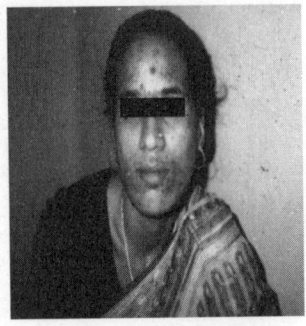

Photo of the patient Miss R.D. before treatment

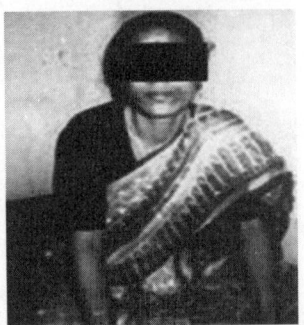

Photo of the patient before treatment

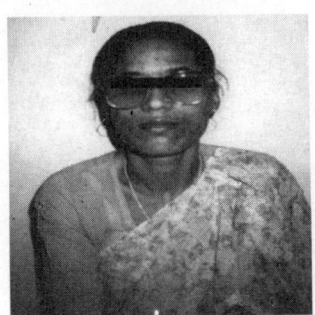

Photo of the patient before treatment

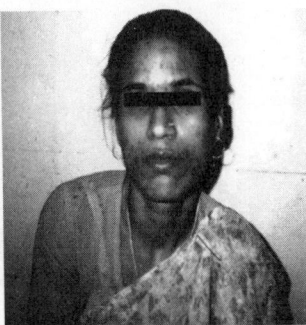

Photo of the patient after 6 months treatment

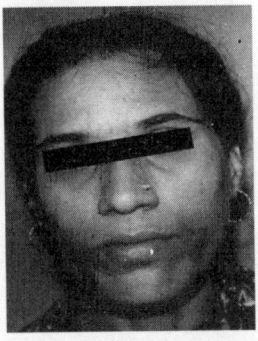

Photo of the patient after 9 months treatment

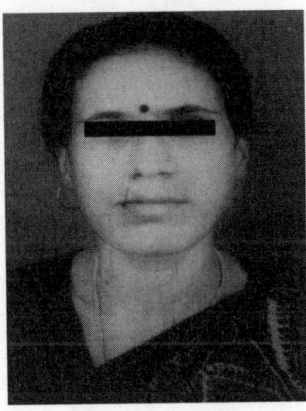

After Treatment

3 E.N.T. Diseases - Cured Cases
CHAPTER

1. A CASE OF CHRONIC SUPPURATIVE OTITIS MEDIA (C.S.O.M): MR. N.D.

Case No. ENT001

A 30 year-old man as on 4th September, 1991.

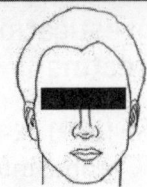

Photo of the patient, Mr. N.D.

Presenting Complaints

- Hardness of hearing in left ear. Hissing in ears. Weight/heavy feeling of left ear.
- Otorrhoea → Whitish, watery discharge → offensive discharge from left ear.
- Occasional itching. No pain. Discharge coming in the morning, burning pain inside the ear.
- History of mastoiditis with boils and ulceration behind the ear – 10 years back; surgically treated.
- Stool: Regular: no mucus in the stool.
- Urine: Okay.
- Appetite: Decreased.
- Occasional acidity, 2-3 hours after meals; aggravates after awakening → Sour taste in mouth.
- Thirst: Average. Chilly patient.
- Profuse perspiration in axilla, chest, back à bad smell to sweat.
- Heals: Okay.
- Sleep: good.

- Dreams: Nothing particular.
- Desires: Sweet++, salt+++, salty, vegetable and spinach; fish, egg+, warm food, cold drinks.
- Mind: Angry, talkative; desires company; sympathetic; cannot tolerate blood-letting. Memory: weak.
- Past History: Chickenpox.
- Family History: Father: Tumours (dermoid cysts). Mother: Heart complaints.
- Ear: Sore and tender > by heat.
- Aggravation from cold.
- Worse open air.
- Physical energy: Low.

Investigations Carried Out Before/After Dr. Banerjea's Treatment

18th Jul'91: X-ray of Mastoids: Left mastoid – Bony sclerosis and rarefaction = Chronic infective changes with cholesteatoma at left mastoid.

14th Jun'94: X-ray Left Mastoid: Left mastoid poorly pneumatized. Internal meatii of both sides appear normal.

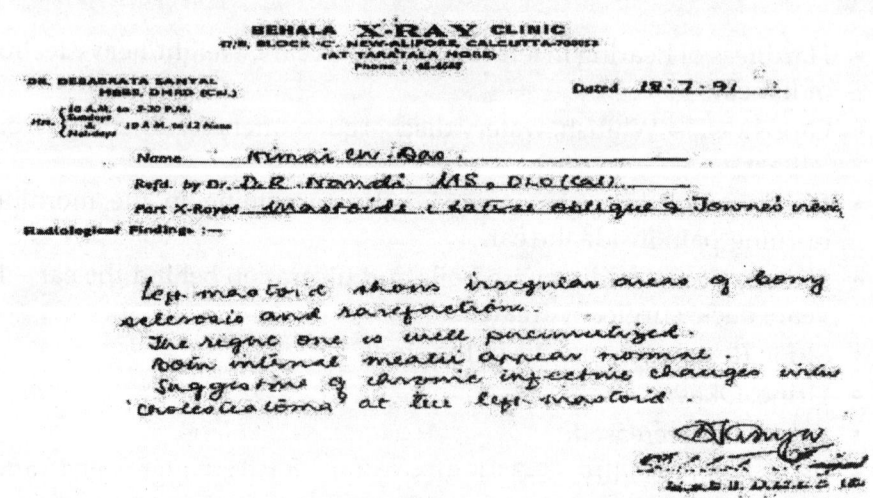

X-Ray report of Mr. N. D. before treatment

E.N.T. Diseases – Cured Cases

BEHALA X-RAY CLINIC
47/B, BLOCK 'C', NEW ALIPORE, CALCUTTA-700053
(AT TARATALA MORE)
Phone : 478-6667

DR. DEBABRATA SANYAL
MBBS, DMRD (Cal.)

Dated: 14.6.94

Name: Nimai Das
Refd. by Dr.: Subrata KK Banerjee NIMS (Cal).
Part X-Rayed: Left Mastoid Towne's view

Radiological Findings :—

The left mastoid is poorly pneumatized. Internal meatii of both sides appear normal.

DR. DEBABRATA SANYAL
MBBS, DMRD (CAL)

X-Ray report of Mr. N. D. after treatment

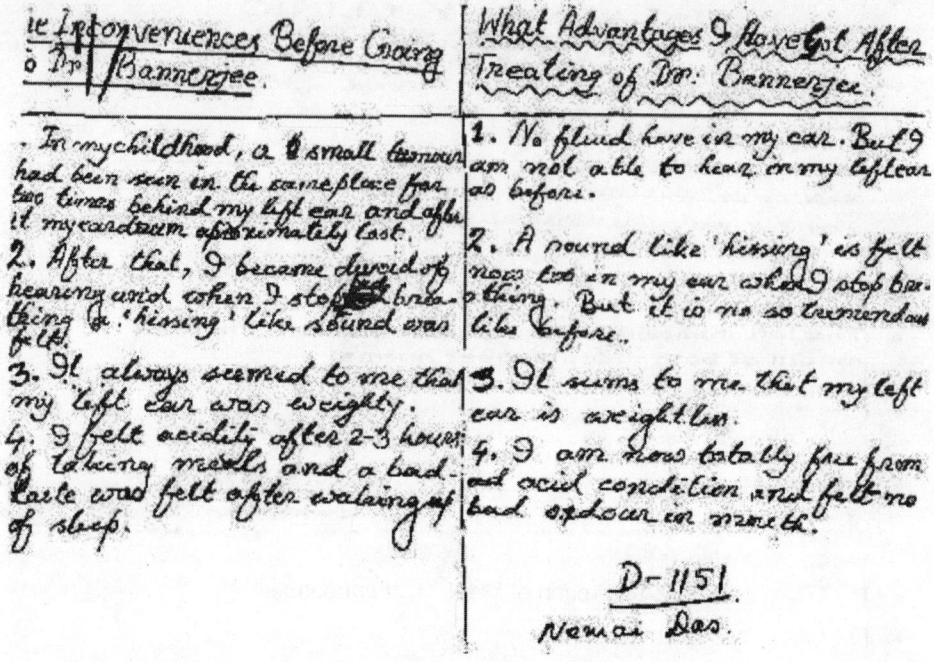

Patient's comments after treatment

CASE ANALYSIS, MIASMATIC DIAGNOSIS AND FINAL PRESCRIPTION

Chronic Suppurative Otitis Media is a long drawn out process and many children these days do suffer from it, the consultant offering them surgery. Here is another example where Homoeopathy can replace surgical intervention.

Miasmatic Analysis

- Otorrhoea: Syco-Syphilitic.
- Profuse perspiration: Sycosis.
- Burning pain, offensive discharge: Syphilitic.
- Itching in ear: Psora.
- Boils and ulceration behind ear: Syphilitic.
- Decreased appetite: Psora.
- Acidity and sour taste in mouth: Psora.

- Chilly patient: Psora.
- Desires: Sweet: Psora. Salt: Syco-tubercular. Warm food: Sycosis. Cold drinks: Syphilitic.
- Mind: (a) Talkative: Sycosis; cannot tolerate blood-letting: Psora. (b) Memory: weak: Psora.

Final Prescription Made on the Basis of

- Hardness of hearing in left ear.
- Otorrhoea → Whitish, watery discharge → offensive discharge from left ear.
- Capsicum has a "Marked tendency to suppuration in every inflammatory process" [Boericke].
- Inflammation of mastoid. Per Clarke, "Caps. is among the remedies of the front rank in stomatitis; in inflammation of the middle ear, with involvement of mastoid cells.....".
- Profuse perspiration in axilla, chest, back à bad smell in sweat.
- Desires: Sweet++, Salt+++, Salty.
- Mind: Angry, talkative; desire for company; sympathetic; cannot tolerate blood letting. Memory: weak.
- Sour taste in mouth (Clarke).
- Burning pain inside the ear with general chilliness. Clarke states that "The well-known burning effect of red pepper is a leading indication for its use: 'Burning pains' wherever occurring demand that Capsicum should have the first consideration, if there are no other determining symptoms in favour of another remedy."
- Chilly patient;
- Decreased appetite.
- Ear: Sore and tender > by heat.
- Aggravation from cold.
- Worse open air.
- Physical energy: Low.

The miasmatic breakdown of Capsicum is Psora ++, Sycosis +, Syphilis +, Tubercular ++.

Final Prescription

CAPSICUM, 1M: 1 globule in sugar of milk sachet dissolved in water and sipped over 10 days. Then 10 days of no medicine, followed by another dose to be shaken and sipped for 10 days.

I began treatment with the 1M potency of Capsicum as it was so clearly indicated and I could therefore begin with a high potency.

Remedy Reaction

The prescription of Capsicum was followed by prescriptions of Sulphur and Calcarea sulph. This is a chain of medicines, as Calcarea follows Sulphur well. In just over 3 years the patient noted that there was no longer fluid in his ears, however his hearing was still diminished in his left ear. The ear no longer felt weighty. Hissing was still noted in his ears when he stopped breathing, however this was much reduced. The acidity after eating and sour taste on wakening has disappeared.

Prescription Chart

Date	Prescription Done on the Basis of	Treatment
4th Sep'91	History of mastoiditis. Swelling and boil behind ear. Burning pain inside the ear.	Capsicum 1M, 2 doses.
9th Oct'91	Watch and wait for change.	Sac lac.
1st Nov'91	Watch and wait for change.	Sac lac.
18th Dec'91	No appreciable change.	Capsicum, 1M, 1 dose.
22nd Jan'92	Standstill, so went higher in potency.	Caps, 1M, 2 doses → 10M, 1 dose.
19th Feb'92	50–60% better.	Sac lac.
1st Apr'92		Sac lac.
6th May'92	Wait and watch. 60 % better but now at standstill.	Sac lac.
24th Jun'92	Went higher in potency as still standstill.	Capsicum 10M → 50 M.
29th Jul'92	Wait and watch.	Sac lac.
2nd Sep'92	60 % Better, but now standstill. Change in the plan of treatment, use of anti-.psoric remedy.	Sulphur 200C, 2 doses
21st Oct'92	Wait and watch.	Sac lac.
25th Nov'92	No further change; went higher in potency.	Sulphur, 10 M, 1 dose.
6th Jan'93	Doing much better. Wait and watch.	Sac lac.
10th Feb'93	Wait and watch.	Sac lac.

E.N.T. Diseases – Cured Cases

Date	Prescription Done on the Basis of	Treatment
17th Mar'93	75% better, but now standstill.	Sulphur, 10M, 1 dose.
7th Apr'93	Wait and watch	Sac lac.
7th Jul'93	75% better	Sac lac.
18th Aug'93	Standstill. Wait and watch.	Sac lac.
29th Sep'93	Change in the plan of treatment: Calcareas are the natural followers of Sulphur.	Calc. Sulph. 200, 2 doses.
5th Jan'94	No appreciable change.	Sac lac.
9th Feb'94	Wait and watch.	Sac lac.
9th Mar'94	Chronic Suppurative Otitis Media much better.	Sac lac.
20th Apr'94	Better, but standstill.	Sac lac.
18th May'94	Went higher in potency.	Calc. Sulph. 1M, 2 doses
27th Jun'94	Better. X-ray report shows normal internal meatii.	Sac lac.
20th Jul'94	Wait and watch.	Sac lac.
31st Aug'94	Doing much better. Wait and watch.	Sac lac.
26th Oct'94	Cured.	

Authenticity of Cure

CD Reference: ENT001-CHRONIC SUPPURATIVE OTITIS MEDIA-ND

2. A CASE OF RECURRENT EPISTAXIS (NOSE BLEEDING): MR. A.B.S.

Case No. ENT002

Age   : 22 year-old as on 28.11.1992.
Sex   : Male
Height : 5 ft. 3 inches
Weight : 41 kgs.

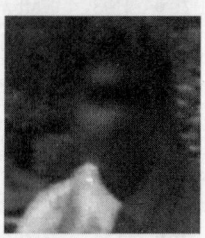
Photograph of Patient

Presenting Complaints

- Heavy bleeding from Nasal cavity. Epistaxis:- Duration 18 years. Causation → catches cold easily since childhood. Any mild injury or pressure on nose – during clearing process → generally bright red blood comes out through nose (20 – 25 drops of blood). > cold application on the part (nose).
- Thyroid gland little enlarged. Tonsillitis: frequent sore throat (+++). 4 – 5 times per year. Tendency of recurrent infection of tonsil with the tendency of catching a cold easily → settles in tonsils: recurrent worse during wet weather. Associated with fever (++).Tonsillitis:- Both side. Sudden inflammation of gland with pain < during change of weather. < during cough and cold infection. Duration – 2 years. Causation → Susceptibility to cold and intake of cold drinks.
- Constipation (Bowels are not clear).
- Amoebic dysentery (white). Occasional presence of blood in stool. Stool with blood (++), associated with pus and crampy pain abdomen. Constipation with Amoebic Dysentery. Duration → 1 year. Causation – No clear stool since child hood. Generally no stool for 2 days after that dysentery starts.
- Allergic condition (Allergy from time to time). Allergy (occasionally). Generally red moles appear with itching.
- Dry cough.
- Sore throat < morning, evening.
- Increase of Nasal Bleeding – in the morning and evening.
- Motion >. Epistaxis < winter.
- Increased in winter. But it occurs from time to time (any season).

- Bleeding is better by the shower with cold water and cold application.
- Bleeding increased during stress, anxiety.
- It increases when sleep is disturbed (aggravation from night watching).
- Both nostrils are occasionally blocked. Discharges occur: White phlegm.
- Throat: feels pain in both sides. Both glands are swollen.
- Dry cough at first → It turns moist thereafter.
- Abdomen:- Distension of abdomen. Whole abdomen. Eructation. Passing of flatus relieves the patient.
- Stomach:- Appetite decreased.
- Urine:- Normal.
- Stool:- Dark type. Ineffectual. Constipated. Dysentery (white). It seems stools are not cleared.
- Sweat of feet < winter.
- Skin Disease:- Outer layer of the skin of the fingers on both hands are coarse or rough. Exfoliation of skin of hands & feet < during winter.
- Mental Symptoms:- Mild. Extrovert. Patient very talkative. Desires to be neat and clean. Memory – active. Everything in a hurry. Very active. Extremities: Frequent pain in joints, especially knee and back. Aggravation during first course of motion, agg. during damp and wet weather; better from moving (continuous).
- Habit:- Smoking.
- Past Medical History:- Measles.
- Chilly patient.
- Likes cold, winter.
- Likes open air. Prefer to lie with doors and windows open.
- He likes to bath in winter/summer; catches cold easily though occasionally he is chilly.
- Food desires:- Sweet++; Sour+; Pungent and hot+; Meat++; Cold food++; Onion; Egg; Cold drinks; Ice Cream.
- Generally thirsty++
- Sleep:- Ideas crowd his mind.
- Family Medical History:- Father and mother alive. Asthma – Grandfather and Grandmother.
- Sneezing < after bathing. Dry cough. Duration → 2 years. Causation → Tonsillitis. Cough < during winter.

- Temperament:- Extrovert+++; Methodical+++; Organised+++; Positive (Optimistic)+++; Restless+++; Sympathetic+++; Greedy+++; Neat/clean+++; Sociable+++; Talkative+++; Angry+; Stubborn+; Suspicious+.
- Food Preferences:- Sweet+++; Spice+++; Meat+++; Fish+++; Chicken+++; Egg+++; Ice Cream+++; Sour+; Salt/Salty+; Savoury+; Green leafy+; Fat+; Cold food.

CASE ANALYSIS, MIASMATIC DIAGNOSIS AND FINAL PRESCRIPTION

Miasmatic Analysis

- Thyroid gland little enlarged: Sycosis.
- Tonsillitis: frequent sore throat: Tubercular.
- Tendency of recurrent infection of tonsil and tendency of catching a cold easily: Tubercular.
- Tonsils, recurrent worse during wet weather: Syco-Tubercular.
- Inflammation of gland with pain < during change of weather: Sycotic.
- Amoebic dysentery: Syphilitic.
- Occasional presence of blood in stool: Tubercular.
- Bleeding is better by the shower with cold water and cold application: Syphilitic.
- Bleeding increased during stress, anxiety: Psora-Tubercular.
- Mild: Psora; Extrovert: Syco-Tubercular. Patient very talkative: Sycotic. Desires to be neat and clean: Sycotic. Everything in a hurry: Sycotic. Very active: Sycotic.
- Extremities: Frequent pain in joints: Sycotic.
- Joint pains aggravation during damp and wet weather: Sycotic;
- Joint pains, better from moving (continuous): Sycotic.
- Haemorrhagic tendency: Tubercular.

Prescription Made on the Basis of

- Thyroid gland little enlarged. Tonsillitis: frequent sore throat (+++). 4 – 5 times per year. Tendency of recurrent infection of tonsil with the tendency of catching a cold easily → settles in tonsils: recurrent worse during wet weather. Associated with fever (++).Tonsillitis:-

Both side. Sudden inflammation of gland with pain < during change of weather. < during cough and cold infection. Duration – 2 years. Causation → Susceptibility to cold and intake of cold drinks.
- Amoebic dysentery (white). Occasional presence of blood in stool. Stool with blood (++), associated with pus and crampy pain in abdomen. Constipation with Amoebic Dysentery. Duration → 1 year. Causation – No clear stool since child hood. Generally no stool for 2 days after that dysentery starts.
- Bleeding is better by the shower with cold water and cold application.
- Bleeding increased during stress, anxiety.
- Mental Symptoms:- Mild. Extrovert. Patient very talkative. Desires to be neat and clean. Memory – active. Everything in a hurry. Very active. Extremities: Frequent pain in joints, especially knee and back. Aggravation during first course of motion, agg. during damp and wet weather; better from moving (continuous).
- Considering: Recurrent Throat infections, 4-5 times a year (where cold à settles and affects the throat) → Sore Throat.
- Constipation: Followed by dysentery with blood. Haemorrhagic tendency.
- Presence of triad: Rhus Tox type of joint pains + Mercury type of dysentery + Phosphorus type of haemorrhage and allergy.

Streptococcin has the miasmatic breakdown: Psora ++, Sycosis ++, Syphilis +, Tubercular +++.

Final Prescription and Remedy Reaction

I prescribed Streptococcin 200C to start with and in the course of time, gradually ascended up to 10M potency and the patient got totally better. Not only the nose bleeding of 18 years duration but also the sore throat, joint pains, allergy and dysentery all got better in about 16 months.

I finished the case with Tuberculinum 200C, thereafter 1M as a Miasmatic coverage and the presence of symptoms like (a) Tendency to catch cold easily, (b) Haemorrhagic diathesis, (c) Recurrence (+++) of nasal bleeding from childhood and also the recurrence of sore throat.

Authenticity of Cure

CD Reference: ENT002-RECURRENT EPISTAXIS NOSE BLEEDING-ABS

Cured Cases

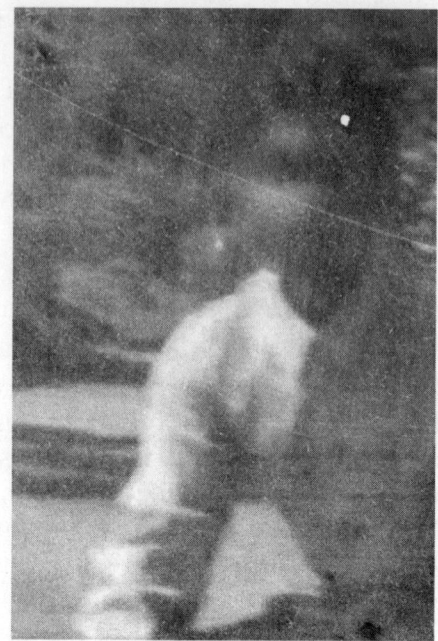

Photograph of Patient

c/o.
Recurrent Epistaxis.

Before the treatment of   After:
Dr. Banerjee
problems were:-
1) Bleeding from nose or nasal   1. Now
   cavity in anytime or any-   stopped
   season or Bleeding due to-   by
   mild hit, thrust or sneezing
   since childhood.

1. Tonsilitis - Enlargement of   2. Tonsil
   glands - Burning irritation   But feel
   of larynx due - Cold -   comfort
   Cut is unbearable.   weather
                                   sometime

1. Constipation.

Patient's comments 16 months after treatment

4 Endocrinological Disorders – Cured Cases

1. A CASE OF DIABETES MELLITUS   MR. M.M.

Case No. E001

Age : 55 years.
Height : 5 ft. 4 inches.
Weight : 64 Kgs.
Present & past occupation: Teacher.
Married.
Only son died six years back.

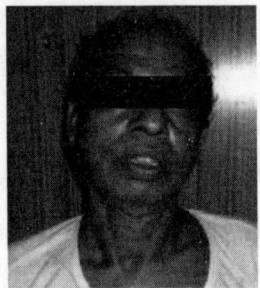

Photo of the patient,
Mr. M.L.M.

Presenting Complaints

- Weakness and drowsiness more towards evening, aggravated by movement, exertion
- Frequent urination.
- Burning after urination: urethra feels scalded.
- Disturbed sleep.
- Wormy irritation in anus.
- Headache occasionally in the evening. Shifting, piercing pain.
- Chilly patient.
- Head - (1) Hot feeling in vertex. (2) Occasional vertigo after day's work.
- Mouth - (1) Dryness of mouth; 2) Foetor oris.
- Teeth - Swelling of gums.
- Abdomen - Occasional gas & distension of abdomen.

- Stomach - Appetite: increased.
- Sweat - Profuse sweat, no odour.
- Urine - (a) Yellowish colour. Occasionally turbid. (b) 18-20 times per 24 hours. Frequent urination, and profuse. More at night. (c) No odour. (d) Burning after urination. (e) Discomfort and uneasiness in urethra after urination.
- Stool - Regular.
- Upper Extremities - Occasional stiffness of small joints aggravated severely during new moon and full moon.
- Joints - Painful stiffness of joints, was severe during 1985, a little better after allopathic treatment.
- Lower Extremities - Occasional weakness & trembling of the lower extremities towards evening, after a day's work. Stumbles.
- Male Genital Organs – History of masturbation during youth up to his 30's, power deficient since. Lax penis.
- Skin Disease - (1) Dandruff. (2) Barber's itch.

Mental Symptoms

Irritable & indifferent attitude. Depression. Likes to be alone, introvert type. Gradual weakness of memory. Weepy +. Works slowly. Fear of incurable diseases.

First Cause of Break Down of Health

Death of his son, 6 years of age: Never Been Well Since (N.B.W.S.)

Past History

History of masturbation during youth up to 30's.

Allopathic medicines used for the last 4 years without appreciable effect.

(i) History of measles in childhood; (ii) Malaria 2-3 times; (iii) Stiff joints (rheumatism), barbers' itch treated with cortisone group of medicines (since 1985-86); (iv) Diabetes; diagnosed 4 years previously. (v) Suffered from chicken pox in childhood.

Homoeopathic Generalities

Catches cold easily. Food desires: (i) Salty (+) (ii) Milk (+) (iii) Fruits (++) (iv) Chicken (+) (v) Cold food & drinks (+) (vi) Rich & spicy foods (++). Thirsty (+). Sleep - Disturbed.

Family History

History of skin disease and pleurisy with father.

Investigations Carried out before and During Dr. Banerjea's Treatment

8th Mar'90: Blood Sugar Post Prandial (BSPP): 228
20th Apr'90: Blood Sugar Post Prandial (BSPP): 171
20th Jun'90: Blood Sugar Post Prandial (BSPP): 95

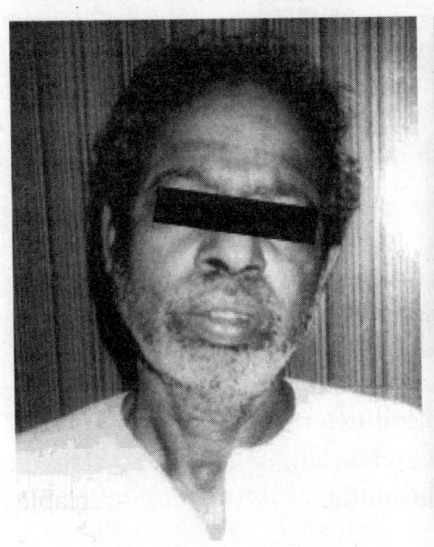

Mr. M.L.M., a case of Diabetes before treatment

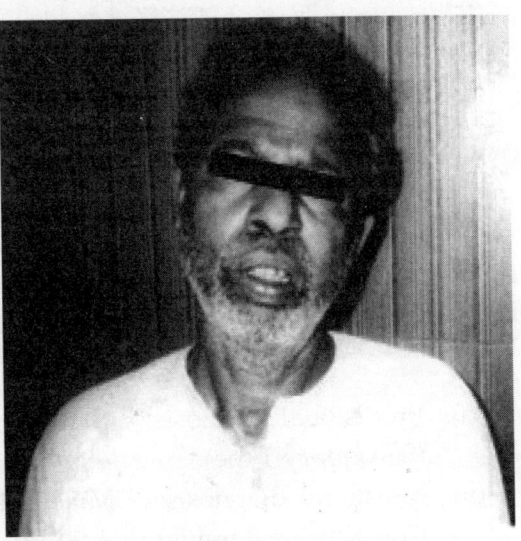

before treatment

Cured Cases

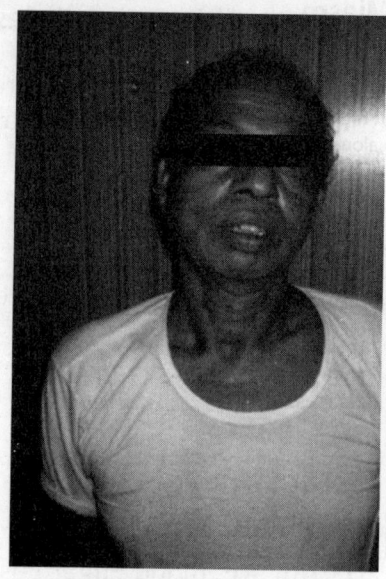

Smiling face after treatment

Blood reports, before treatment

CASE ANALYSIS, MIASMATIC DIAGNOSIS AND FINAL PRESCRIPTION

(i) Provisional diagnosis: Diabetes Mellitus (Secondary Type).
(ii) Miasmatic diagnosis: Mixed Miasmatic.
(iii) Constitutional remedy: Acid Phos.

Miasmatic Interpretation of Acid Phos Case

Psoric	Sycotic	Syphilitic	Tubercular
(1) Likes to be alone (Psora + Syphilis). (2) Weakness aggravated by exertion, movement. (3) Dandruff. (4) Fear of incurable diseases.	(1) Stiffness of joints. (2) Joint pains are also Sycotic painful stiffness. (3) Light physical exertion fatigues – patient stumbles (Syco-tubercular). (4) Barber's itch. (5) Gradual weakness of memory. (6) Profuse urine (Syco –Tubercular)	(1) Urethra feels scalded (irritation & burning of parts). (2) Depression & indifference. (3) Introvert.	(1) Wormy irritation, pinworms. (2) Foetor oris (Psoric + tubercular). (3) Diabetes is tubercular. (4) History of masturbation (++), with weakness of sexual organs. (5) History of pleurisy with father. (6) Weakness after micturition: Tubercular miasm. (7) Tubercular miasm: Urine loaded with phosphate, sugar, etc. always tubercular miasm. (8) Catches cold easily. (9) Polyuria, nocturnal. (10) Small joint stiffness aggravated at full and new moon.

Miasmatic Derivation from the Pathological Point of View

MIXED MIASMATIC: As it is a secondary type of diabetes mellitus (a result of some primary degenerative condition or the after effects of some strong drugs: here in this case prolonged cortisone-therapy). From the homoeopathic point of view, this secondary type of diabetes mellitus is caused by suppression of rheumatism by cortisone therapy → resulting diabetes mellitus.

Note: A dose of Causticum to end with, which will follow Acid Phos., as well as Sycotic coverage and deep acting from the psychic side too.

PROGNOSIS

As here in this case the primary degenerative condition, rheumatism, was suppressed and currently is not present at its peak → with the homoeopathic remedy the suppressed condition could flare up → if it does not reach its peak → the total status of the patient is favourable and curable.

Points Favouring The Choice of Acid Phos

- Weakness and drowsiness: the system has been exposed to the ravages of excesses & grief.
- Dryness of the mouth with polyurea (Clarke).

- Vertigo towards evening (Boericke).
- Profuse sweat (Clarke).
- Burning after urination (Boericke). Polyurea at night (Boericke).
- Great debility of the lower extremities & stumbles easily (Boericke).
- History of prolonged vital drainage: masturbation.
- Though always thinks of sexual enjoyment, but due to prolonged history of masturbation, the sexual power is deficient and the penis is lax.
- The legs tremble whilst walking and the hands are as difficult to control as the thoughts (Clarke).
- History of shock from the death of his son; since last 6 years. Effects of grief and mental shock (Boericke).

The miasmatic breakdown of Phos. acid is: Psora ++, Sycosis ++, Syphilis +, Tubercular +++.

Phosphoric Acid

(1) Apathetic, listless, absent mindedness, indifferent attitude. It has the indifference of Sepia + Apis.

(2) Mental debility first, later physical (--reverse Mur. acid)

(3) Initial indifference → mental prostration.
Phos. acid is coined as an anti-tubercular remedy: so if the symptoms are suppressed during the youth → by non-homoeopathic means → debilitated tubercular state. So therefore the ill-effects of prolonged masturbation, polyurea, chronic diarrhoea or the indifference arising from a typhoid state and thereby resulting in debility → if suppressed → the lungs are affected.

(4) Indigestion → undigested food particles with stool → yet canine hunger peculiarly uncommon → associated with chronic diarrhoea → empty all gone sensation (Anac., Chelid., Sep., Sulph., Phos., Zinc met.) → though eats well, but indigestion → so diarrhoea aggravates → so the emptiness aggravates → more hunger: alternately resulting profound apathetic, indifferent states → thin and debilitated. The specific gravity of urine in diabetes mellitus is 1010 or below (Dr.N.M. Chowdhury says high). Whey, milky urine: → weakness after urination → empty, all gone sensation in lungs (chest), abdomen & urinary bladder (like Phos.).

(5) There is also a post urination sensation of dryness in the entire skin → characterised by the sensation as if the white portion of the egg was applied to the skin and dried up. Remember, Phos. acid patient is capable of getting up from the bed to go to the toilet even in the

advanced stages of the disease, but due to profound melancholic mental prostration & indifferent apathetic attitude → he does not have the intention to get up → "let it go" feeling (attitude) → lies like a log. The essence here is that the exhaustion is less in comparison to his advanced physical status.

Dr. N.M. Chowdhury suggests, indifferent, listlessness & apathy (ILA) are the red-strand of the remedy.

Impotency is the natural sequence, but it is not the total and complete impotence of Selenium. The sensibility of the penis is still there, erections happen, but they are weak and inefficient.

To make matters worse, they are troubled with a constant desire to urinate. The urine passed is larger in quantity than usual and is intensely debilitating.

Tripod for the choice of Phos. Acid in diabetes:

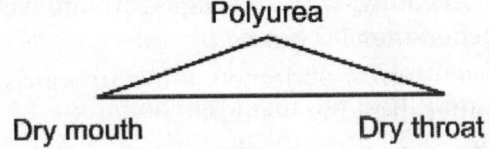

Prescription Chart

Date	Report after Last Medication	Prescription done on the basis of	Treatment
19th Mar'90			Acid Phos, 200 C: 2 doses.
23rd Apr'90			Sac Lac
23rd May'90	As a whole much better.		Sac Lac
25th Jun'90	Blood sugar normal.		Sac Lac

Authenticity of Cure

CD Reference: E001-DIABETES-MLM

2. A CASE OF HYPO-THYROIDISM: MR. S. C.

Case No. E002

Age : 55 years as on 14.8.99.
Sex : Male.
Height : 5'-3"
Weight: 62 kgs.

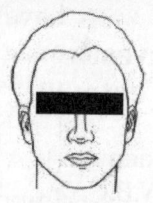

Photo of the patient, Mr. S.C.

Presenting Complaints

- Main problem: Diagnosed as hypo-thyroidism. Went to doctor because he was feeling weakness (+++), tired all the time and nervousness. Also gradually increasing body weight.
- Weakness after eating, with lots of gas formation especially in upper abdomen, better after 1-2 hours.
- Gas and distension of abdomen: wind upwards. Weak digestion. Discomfort after drinking water.
- Pain in buttock & calf muscles – aggravates after first motion, better rest.
- Stool not clear, 2-3 times; bad odour ++. Mucus ++. Occasionally ineffectual urging for stool. Previously treated by Dr. Banerjea for sciatic pain, took homoeopathic medicine from him & improved [History of: sciatic pain with feeling of numbness of the left leg: aggravates after waking from sleep; better from flexing the leg on abdomen: Gnaphalium 1M was given in 1995 and was better in 3 months].
- Talkative.
- Desire for company. Indifference. Pessimism.
- Gradual loss of memory.
- Fear of dogs/snakes/animals/thunderstorm/incurable diseases/accidents/failures.
- Had history of skin diseases in childhood treated allopathically.
- Chilly patient, but craves fresh open air.
- Catches cold easily.
- Desires: Salty +++, salt ++, sweet ++, pungent and hot; warm food.
- Bleeds easily and it does not stop easily.
- Thirst: Profuse (++).

Endocrinological Disorders – Cured Cases

- Sleep: Average.
- Sweat: Average.

Investigations Carried Out before/After Dr. Banerjea's Treatment

Haemoglobin 13.00 gm% Red Blood Corpuscles:- 4.6×10^6 White Blood Cell (W.B.C.) 9,000, Neutrophill 51; Lymphocyte 37, Monocyte1, Eosinophyl 1, Erythrocyte Sedimentation Rate – 32, Blood Sugar Post Prandial (BSPP) 86 mg%, Cholesterol 216.

2nd Aug'99: Urine: Albumin – Trace. Pus cell – 3-4 hpf

7th Aug'89: T3-0.6 (Normal 0.8-2.1) T4 2.8 (Normal 4.2-12.0); TSH 41.7 (Normal 0.2 – 5.0)

30th Apr'00: T3 1.2, T4 8.4, TSH 2.8 (Normal).

Blood report of Mr. S.C., a case of Hypothyroidism, before treatment

Blood report after 8 months of treatment

CASE ANALYSIS, MIASMATIC DIAGNOSIS AND FINAL PRESCRIPTION

Miasmatic Analysis

- Hypo-thyroidism: Psora.
- Weakness (+++) and tired: Psora.
- Nervousness: Psora.
- Increasing body weight: Sycosis.
- Lots of gas formation: Indigestion (lack of digestion) : Psora
- Weak digestion: Psora.
- Talkative: Sycosis.
- Indifference: Syphilo-tubercular.
- Pessimism: Syphilis.
- Gradual loss of memory: Psora.
- Fear of dogs/snakes/animals/thunder-storm/incurable diseases/accidents/failures: Psora.
- Chilly patient but craves fresh open air: Tubercular.
- Catches cold easily: Psora- tubercular.
- Desires: Salty +++, salt ++: Tubercular.
- Bleeds easily and it does not stop easily: Haemorrhagic diathesis: Tubercular.
- Carbo Vegetabilis has the miasmatic breakdown: Psora ++, Sycosis +, Syphilis ++, Tubercular +++.
- This is a mixed miasmatic case with Psora-Tubercular preponderance.

Final Prescription and Remedy Reaction

Please refer to prescription chart below for the reasons for the choice of remedy. 200 C potency was used to begin with as Carbo Vegetabilis is an inert substance in the crude form and therefore works more effectively in the higher potencies. Patient was much improved in just under a year, a final potency of 1M being used.

Prescription Chart

Date	Prescription done on the basis of Treatment	Treatment
14th Aug'99	Weakness (+++) and tired; Nervousness. Lots of gas formation especially upper abdomen. Gas and distension of abdomen: wind upwards. Weak digestion. Stool not clear, 2-3 times; bad odour ++. Mucus ++. Desire for company. Indifference; pessimism. Gradual loss of memory. Fear of Dogs Chilly patient, but craves fresh open air. Catches cold easily. Desire: Salty +++, Salt ++. Bleeds easily and it does not stop easily: haemorrhagic diathesis. Tuberculo-psoric preponderance. Miasmatic analysis of Carbo Veg: Psora ++, Sycosis +, Syphilis ++, Tubercular +++.	Carbo Veg. 200C, 2 doses.
11th Oct'99	Doing better	Sac lac.
1st Dec'99	60 kg. Doing better.	Sac lac.
2nd Feb'00	Stand still status. Occasional throbbing sensation on left side of the chest. Occasional gas formation in abdomen better by passing of flatus. Heaviness of body with difficulty In breathing, ameliorated by rest. Occasional cramping of calf muscles.	Carbo Veg 200C, 2 doses.
22nd Mar'00	Doing better: 50%, but then stand still status for last 15 days. Occasional gas formation in abdomen, ameliorated by passing of flatus Wind ascending, discomfort felt in chest, ameliorated by eructation.	Carbo Veg 1 M, 2 doses.
12th May'00	Doing better. Thyroid function normal (according to the pathological report of April 2000) Appetite – normal; Stool – Okay.	Sac lac.

Authenticity of Cure:

CD Reference: E002-HYPOTHYROIDISM-SC

3. A CASE OF DIABETES - MR. M.K.C.

Case No. E003

Age : 45 years as on 29th April 1995.
Height : 5 ft. 5½ inches
Weight : 59 kgs.

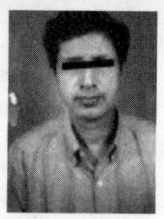

Photo of the patient,
Mr. M.K.C.

Presenting Complaints

- Main problem: Diabetes which he thinks may have started after typhoid, but there is no such correlation.
- Hot patient.
- Desires: Sweet++, pungent and hot+, meat++, warm food+.
- Changeability
- Warmth unbearableness
- Aggravation from warmth & warm room
- Amelioration from cold food, drinks and cold applications
- Sound sleep in the morning, wakes up unrefreshed
- Fanatic & religious
- Sympathetic (but gives to receive)
- Needs approval,
- Clingy, fanatical
- Consolation >
- Eye: Vision = +1.5
- Mental Symptoms: Mild. Weepy.
- Thirst: average
- Urination: profuse
- Sweat: average

Investigations Carried Out Before Dr. Banerjea's Treatment

22nd Jul'95: Post Prandial Blood Sugar (BSPP): 227 mg%
Diagnosis: Diabetes.

Endocrinological Disorders – Cured Cases

Blood sugar report, before treatment

Investigations Carried Out After Dr. Banerjea's Treatment

16th Oct'96: Blood Sugar Post Prandial (BSPP): 124 mg%.

Blood-sugar report, 18 months after treatment

CASE ANALYSIS, MIASMATIC DIAGNOSIS AND FINAL PRESCRIPTION

This case is another good example about how Classical Homoeopathy can take care of pathological conditions like diabetes; the blood sugar level became completely normal.

Miasmatic Analysis

- Main problem: Diabetes: Mixed miasmatic with syco-tubercular.
- Changeability: Tubercular.
- Fanatic & religious: Sycosis
- Needs approval: Psora (low confidence)
- Clingy: Psora (low confidence)
- Fanatical: Sycosis.
- Mild: Psora.
- Weepy: Sycosis.
- Desires warm food: Sycosis. Desires sweet: Psora.
- Amelioration from cold, aggravation warmth: Syphilis.

It is a mixed miasmatic case with Sycotic preponderance.

Final Prescription Made on the Basis of

- Main problem: Diabetes : covers the mixed miasmatic state.
- Changeability
- Warmth-unbearableness
- Aggravation from warmth & warm room
- Amelioration from cold food, drinks and cold applications
- Sound sleep in the morning, wakes up un-refreshed
- Fanatic & religious
- Sympathetic (but gives to receive)
- Needs approval,
- Clingy, Fanatical
- Consolation >
- Mental Symptoms: Mild. Weepy.

The miasmatic breakdown of Pulsatilla is: Psora ++, Sycosis +++, Syphilitic +, Tubercular ++.

Pulsatilla covers mixed miasmatic background with Sycotic preponderance as well.

Final Prescription

PULSATILLA, 200 C: 1 globule in sugar of milk sachet, dissolved in pure water and sipped slowly throughout the day, continuing for 10 days. Then 10 days of no medicine, followed by another dose to be shaken and sipped for 10 days.

Remedy Reaction

The case was begun with Pulsatilla 200, taking into account the patient's vitality and the totality of the symptoms. The patient dramatically improved and within a few months the blood sugar level came down to normal.

Prescription Chart

Date	Prescription Done on the basis of	Treatment
29th Jul'95	Calm, quiet, amiable, appearance. See above for further indications of Puls.	Pulsatilla 200C, 2 doses
20th Sep'95	Much better.	Sac lac.
17th Nov'95	Wait & Watch with Wisdom!	Sac lac.
5th Nov'96	Feels like stand still status.	Pulsatilla 200C 2 doses → followed by 1M, 1 dose
2nd Feb'96		Sac lac.
10th Mar'96	Much Better.	Sac lac.
25th Apr'96		Sac lac.
6th Jun'96		Pulsatilla 1M, 2 doses
3rd Jul'96	As a whole better re. diabetes	Sac lac.
2nd Aug'96		Sac lac.
27th Apr'96		Sac lac.
22nd Jun'96	Better Blood Pressure: 120/84. Stand still status.	Pulsatilla 10M, 2 doses
27th Jul'96	Better but now stand still status.	Pulsatilla 50M, 2 doses
24th Aug'96	Feels better. Asked to do repeat the blood sugar test.	Sac lac.
17th Oct'96	Report of 16th October, 1996: Blood sugar normal.	

Authenticity of Cure:

CD Reference: E003-DIABETES-MKC

4. A CASE OF DIABETES MELLITUS- MR. S.B.

Case No. E004

Age   : 71 years as on 23/12/95
Height : 5 ft. 11 inches
Weight : 64 kgs.

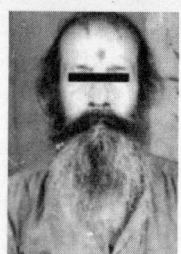

Photo of the patient, Mr. S.K.B.

Presenting Complaints

- Main problem: Diabetes.
- Burning left leg and sole, ameliorated by cold application.
- Hot flashes. Hot sensation on vertex.
- Sensation of contraction felt in the right side of the leg, aggravated by sitting; ameliorated from standing → since 2 months back.
- Occasional tingling of left hand, aggravated in cold water.
- Gas forms in abdomen, ameliorated by passing of flatus.
- Weakness++
- Stool: Regular; mucus (++) in stool.
- Urine: Okay.
- Appetite: Normal.
- Thirst: Average.
- Sweat on head.
- Heals Okay.
- Sound sleep.
- Desires: Sweet+++, bitter++, milk+, veg and spinach, fish, luke warm food, cold drinks.
- Mind: Mild; talkative; wants to be alone; patient gets angry when reprimanded; sympathetic; no fears; selfish; introvert.
- Intellectual interests, talks about God.
- Past history: Malaria; chickenpox.
- Family history: Diabetes.
- Hot patient.

Investigation Carried Out Before/After Dr. Banerjea's Treatment

6th Dec'95: C. T. Scan Brain :- NAD.

3rd Dec'95: Blood Sugar Post Prandial (PPBS): 196 mg%. Serum urea 25 mg%.

Endocrinological Disorders – Cured Cases

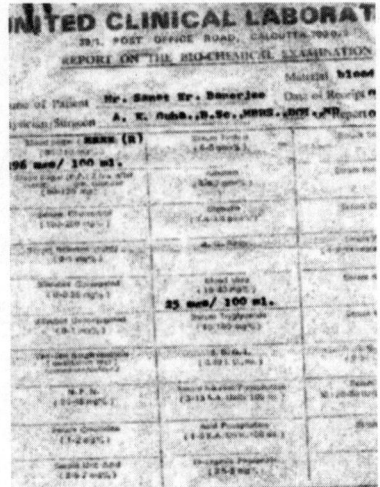

Blood-sugar report, before treatment

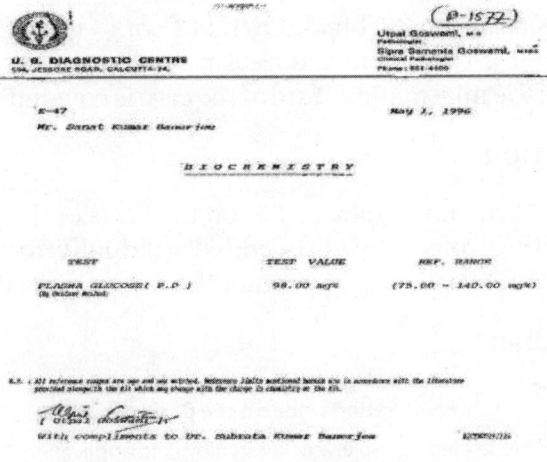

Blood-sugar report 5 months after treatment

1st May'96: Blood Sugar Post Prandial (BSPP): 98 mg%.

CASE ANALYSIS, MIASMATIC DIAGNOSIS AND FINAL PRESCRIPTION

Miasmatic Analysis

- Diabetes: Mixed miasmatic with Syco-tubercular.
- Burning in leg and sole, ameliorated by cold application: Syphilitic.
- Cramps in lower extremities: Tubercular.

- Tingling (neurological pains), aggravated by cold: Psora.
- Weakness: Tubercular.
- Mucus (++) in stool: Sycotic.
- Desires: Sweet+++: Psora; luke warm food: Sycotic; cold drinks: Syphilitic.
- Selfish: Sycotic; introvert: Syphilitic.

Final Prescription Made on the Basis of

- Burning pains, ameliorated by cold applications – Sulphur is a leading burner.
- Burning with hot flashes.
- Desires sweet.
- Selfish, introvert.
- Intellectual interests – philosophises about God.
- Appearance: Ragged philosopher.

Sulphur has a miasmatic breakdown of Psora +++, Sycosis ++, Syphilis +++, Tubercular +++. This is a mixed miasmatic case with a Syco-tubercular preponderance; the miasmatic nature of the case is covered well by Sulphur.

Remedy Reaction

The case was begun with Sulphur 200C on the basis of the patient's vitality and the presenting complaint. I ascended gradually to 50M during the period of just over 4 years at which point the patient was cured.

Prescription Chart

Date	Prescription Done on the Basis of	Treatment
23rd Dec'95	Burning left leg and sole, ameliorated by cold application. Hot flashes. Hot sensation on vertex. Weakness++ Stool: Regular; mucus (++) in stool. Urine → Okay. Appetite → Normal. Thirst → Average. Sweat on head. Heals Okay. Sound sleep. Desire: Sweet+++, Milk+. Mind: Mild; talkative; wants to be alone; Patient gets angry when reprimanded; Selfish, introvert. Intellectual interests, talks about God. BP: 118/76	Sulphur, 200C, 2 doses

Endocrinological Disorders – Cured Cases

Date	Prescription Done on the Basis of	Treatment
22nd Jan'96	BP: 136/80 Better.	Sac lac.
21st Feb'96	Nose cold; left nose. Burning left sole aggravates at night. Stool: not clear.	Sac lac.
9th Apr'96	Standstill status. Thirst average. Sound sleep. Appetite: good. Right sided sciatica, aggravates from sitting.	Sac lac.
1st Jun'96	Burning left leg and sole. Gas++. BP: 132/80. PPBS 98% - normal.	Sac lac.
25th Jun'96	BP: 132/76. Standstill status. Repeat.	Sulphur 200C, 2 doses.
24th Jul'96	Wait & watch.	Sac lac.
13th Sep'96	Darting pain from shoulder to foot (left) aggravated by cold. Pimples on buttocks aggravated from sitting. Burning on sole (left) ameliorated by cold water. Hot feeling in vertex. Patient cannot sit for a long time, after sitting 25/30 minutes tingling sensation in right knee joint. Wait & watch.	Sac lac.
14th Oct'96	No change. Hot flushes on vertex++, ameliorated by cold water. Thirst++, Sleep+, Sweat+, Lethergy+.	Sulphur, 1M, 2 doses
3rd Dec'96	As a whole feels better. Burning on left leg a little better but still present; aggravates from touch and ameliorated by cold water. Hot flushes on head. Gas in lower abdomen. Thirst little, Appetite+, Sleep+.	Sac lac.
18th Jan'97	Doing better. Burning on sole was better now, stand still. Gas+ ameliorated by passing flatus. Hoarseness of voice + tough sputum comes out from throat. Constant clearing of the throat. Thirst+ Appetite+ sleep+. Sensation of stoppage of breathing aggravated in supine position. Wait & watch.	Sac lac.
18th Mar'97	BP: 140/80. Burning on soles (both). aggravated evening and at night. Hoarseness of voice, aggravated by fanning. Tingling sensation left half of the body aggravated from touching of clothes. Itching of left nostril. Thirst little, Appetite+, Sleepless. Feels like 1M is not holding. Go higher.	Sulphur, 10M 2 doses
9th May'97	BP: 130/74. Had spicy food outside.	Sac lac
28th Jun'97	BP: 130/90. No change. Lump on left buttock + aggravates from pressure. Burning on soles standstill. Hoarseness ameliorated by hawking. All the complaints are aggravated in the left half of the body.	Sulphur, 10M, 2 doses
27th Jul'97	BP: 140/80. Doing better. Burning on left leg better. Lump on left buttock standstill. Hot flushes on head ameliorated by cold water.	Sac lac.
12th Aug'97	BP: 130/80. Doing better. Hot flushes better. Hoarseness little better but still there, ameliorated by expulsion of phlegm. Thick, whitish mucus. Stool normal, thirst less, Appetite+, Sleep+, Sweat+.	Sac lac.

Date	Prescription Done on the Basis of	Treatment
26th Sep'97	Doing better. Burning on soles was better but now came back. Burning in left side of thigh. Hoarseness standstill. Swelling of left foot aggravates during evening and morning. Stool normal.	Sulphur, 50M, 2 doses
26th Nov'97	Doing better.	Sac lac.
2nd Jan'98	Now boils on buttock aggravated from sitting on hard substances, ameliorated by walking. Hoarseness ameliorated by constant hawking. Heat on vertex ameliorated by cold applications. Stye on left eye. Stool normal. BP: 150/90. Weight: 65.5 kgs.	Sac lac.
13th Feb'98	Boils standstill. Burning (left) side of the body. Hot flushes on chest and back.	Sulphur, CM, 2 doses
2nd Apr'98	BP: 150/80. Burning in leg little better. Hot flush present but better. Occassional swelling.	Sac lac.
21st May'98	BP: 166/90. Weight: 66 kgs. Gas better. Hot feeling and burning: better. Burning vertex: better. Dry mouth with sticky phlegm in throat.	Sac lac.
1st Jun'98	Burning in the right knee to leg. Hot feeling chest and back. Swelling of the right foot. Oedema in leg. Hot feeling in feet.	Sac lac
19th Jun'98	Burning left leg and hot vertex. Better after last medication.	Sac lac
10th Jul'98	Wait & watch.	Sac lac
14th Aug'98	BP: 150/88. Weight: 66 kgs. Burning + and hot feeling of the body – slightly present. Hot vertex. Burning of knee and left foot, more left sided, aggravated at night. Husky voice. Gas. Stool: Constipation. 50% better.	Sac lac
15th Sep'98	All other complaints are ameliorated but burning+++ in legs.	Sac lac.
23rd Nov'98	Voice – No improvement. Hot sensation throughout the body all the time: came back 30%. Dryness of mouth when sleeping. Hot vertex.	Sulphur CM, 2 doses
2nd Jan'99	BP: 170/96. Standstill.	Sac lac.
14th Apr'99	BP: 150/90. Weight: 67.5 kgs. Gas and distension better. Burning better.	Sac lac
3rd Jun'99	BP: 138/78. Weight: 67 kgs.	Sac lac
17th Jun'99	All symptoms aggravated after taking last medicine, burning with hot sensation in chest (left). Burning in left leg ameliorated during morning. Voice husky. Standstill status. Hot sensation in vertex - standstill. Pain on right side of the back, aggravates from inspiration.	Sulphur CM, 2 doses
23rd Jul'99	BP: 146/80. Weight: 68 kgs. Doing better. Burning in chest – decreased. Occasional burning left leg, aggravated when bowels do not get clear. Swelling of both legs - better. Occasional discomfort feeling. Appetite: Ok, Thirst: scanty. Mucus in stool.	Sac lac.

Date	Prescription Done on the Basis of	Treatment
14th Sep'99	Much better.	Sac lac.
20th Sep'99	Doing better.	Sac lac.
23rd Nov'99	Doing much better. Told the patient to repeat the blood report and will finish the case soon.	Sac lac.
29th Dec'99	Better	Sac lac.
11th Feb'00	Better.	CURED. NO PRESCRIPTION.

Authenticity of Cure

CD Reference: E004-DIABETES-SKB

5. A CASE OF DIABETES - MR M.M.

Case No. E005

Age : 50 years as on 1/8/97
Height : 5 ft.
Weight : 50 kgs.

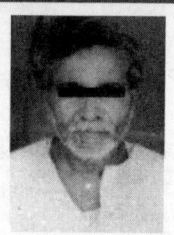

Photo of the patient, Md. M.

Presenting Complaints

- Main complaint: Diabetes.
- Knee pain (left) aggravated in the morning.
- Cold affects glands, especially nasal polyps get swollen if he gets a cold.
- Catches cold easily, but aggravated in warm room and indoors. Desires: fresh open air.
- Occasional pain in fingers, ameliorated by pressure.
- Now, pain on both soles – for the last month, aggravated after waking; aggravated during 1st motion, ameliorated by continued motion.
- Cyst (dermoid) on abdomen.
- Stool: Constipated.
- Urine: Ok.
- Appetite: Normal.
- Thirst: Normal.
- Hot patient.
- Profuse sweating.
- Sleep: good.
- Desire: Sweet +++, Sour ++, Salty++, Pungent+, Bitter, Vegetables and Spinach, Chicken, Cold food, Cold drinks.
- Mind: Mild, silent habit, desire for company, sympathetic.
- List maker: fear of forgetting.

Investigations Carried Out Before/After Dr. Banerjea's Treatment

21st **Jun'96:** Blood Sugar Post Prandial (BSPP) – 400 mg%
6th **Aug'96:** Blood Sugar Post Prandial (BSPP) – 257 mg%

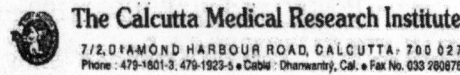

Blood-sugar report, before treatment

Blood-sugar report, 8 months after treatment

1st Mar'97: Blood Sugar Post Prandial (BSPP) – 200 mg%
25th Jul'97: Blood Sugar Post Prandial (BSPP) 198 mg%.
18th Aug'97: Blood Sugar Post Prandial (BSPP) 160 mg%.
15th Nov'97: Blood Sugar Post Prandial (BSPP) 175 mg%.
1st Apr'98: Blood Sugar Post Prandial (BSPP) 120 mg%.

CASE ANALYSIS, MIASMATIC DIAGNOSIS AND FINAL PRESCRIPTION

Miasmatic Analysis

- Diabetes: Mixed miasmatic.
- Knee pain: Joint pains: Sycotic.
- Cold affects glands: Scrofulous diathesis: Tubercular.
- Nasal polyps get swollen if he gets a cold: Tubercular.
- Catches cold easily: Psora-tubercular.
- Catches cold easily but desires fresh open air: Tubercular.
- Cyst on abdomen: Sycosis.
- Stool: Constipated: Psora.
- Profuse sweating: Sycosis.
- Mind: Mild: Psora.
- List maker: Sycosis.
- Fear of forgetting: Psora.
- Desires sweet (Psora), Sour (Psora-syphilitic), Cold food and cold drinks (syphilitic).
- This is a mixed miasmatic case with Syco-psoric preponderance.

Final Prescription Made on the Basis of

- Symptoms and features of Calcarea and Tubercular miasm in a hot patient.
- Catches cold easily but desires fresh air; aggravation in a warm room.
- Cold affects glands - this is a very important symptom for Calc. Iod.
- Desires cold food.
- Desires sweet and sour.
- Constipated.
- List maker – fear of forgetting.

The miasmatic breakdown of Calc. Iod. Is Psora ++, Sycotic +++, Syphilitic +, Tubercular +++.

Calcarea Iod also covers the case miasmatically.

Remedy Reaction

This case was started with Calc. Iod. 200 on the basis of patient's vitality. The patient was cured in just under a year without a higher potency being required.

Prescription Chart

Date	Prescription Done on the Basis of	Treatment
1st Aug'97	BP: 140/86. Cold affects glands, especially nasal polyps get swollen if he gets a cold. Catches cold easily but aggravated in warm room and indoors. Desires: fresh open air. Cyst on abdomen. Stool: Constipated. Hot patient. Profuse sweating. Desires: Sweet +++, Sour ++, Salty++, Cold food. Mind: Mild, silent habit, desire for company. List maker: fear of forgetting. Syco-psoric preponderance.	Calc.Iod, 200C, 2 doses
20th Aug'97	Feels better now. Blood sugar: better. normal. Dermoid cyst on body: present. Asked patient to gradually wean off the conventional anti-diabetic drugs and to keep a balance of the sugar level, gave Gymnema Q.	Sac lac. Gymnema Q (10 drops in half a cup of luke warm water, twice daily X 6 weeks).
29th Sep'97	Feels better now. Occasional vertigo (at noon). Dermoid cyst present, but better (on abdominal wall). Asked patient to gradually wean off the conventional anti-diabetic drugs and to continue Gymnema Q.	Sac lac. Gymnema Q.
17th Nov'97	Standstill status.	Calc. Iod. 200C, 2 doses Gymnema Q.
22nd Dec'97	Pains reduced. Sugar standstill. Wait and watch.	Sac lac.
6th Dec'98	BP: 160/100. Weight: 55 kgs. As a whole much better. Reduced Gymnema to 5 drops twice daily. Stopped conventional anti-diabetic.	Sac lac Gymnema Q: 5 drops twice daily for 6 weeks.
3rd Apr'98	Much better. Wait & watch. Blood sugar normal.	Sac lac.
29th May'98	Much better. Wait & watch.	Sac lac.

Date	Prescription Done on the Basis of	Treatment
17th Jul'98	BP: 118/76. Now feels better. Cyst on abdomen better, but present. Stool: clear.	Sac lac.
20th Aug'98	Much better. Wait & watch.	Sac lac.
26th Sep'98	Much better: physically & mentally.	Sac lac.
21st Nov'98	BP: 150/90. Weight: 54 kgs. Better. Diabetes cured.	Sac lac.

Authenticity of Cure

CD Reference: E005-DIABETES MELLITUS-MD.M

6. A CASE OF HYPOTHYROIDISM – MRS M.G.

Case No. E006

Age : 46 years as on 25.9.93.
Sex : Female
Height : 5' - ½"
Weight : 70 kg.

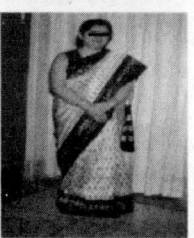

Photo of the patient
Mrs. M.G.

Presenting Complaints

- Hypothyroidism since 1989 – swelling of feet, loss of memory, tiredness. Previously there was loss of appetite, tongue: thick & flabby. Taking Eltroxin 2 tablets once daily.
- Piles – No bleeding at the moment. Occasional constipation. Bearing down sensation of rectum if constipation is severe. Occasional bloody stool. Stool: offensive.
- Spondylitis in both hips & neck. Doing exercises. Occasional reeling of head.
- High blood pressure. Pressure charts: on 2.8.93 – 148/90; 11.8.93 – 120/78; 21.8.93 – 140/82. For pressure: not taking any allopathic medicine.
- Acidity, gas – sour mouth.
- Catches cold easily and in most of the cases it turns to fever. Sensitive to heat as well as cold: < by heat, < by cold.
- Occasional weakness of arms, cannot hold anything for a long time. Bone pains << night.
- Perspiration profuse and offensive – throughout the body, not only head.
- Vision is alright at the moment.
- Nose – Rhinitis: sneezing.
- Coated thick tongue, not very clear.
- Sour taste. Saliva: profuse (+++).
- Palpitation sometimes after heavy work.
- Uneasy sensation in the middle of the chest.
- Gas – yes, passing of flatus relieves.
- Hunger – normal.

- Bad odour from sweating. Profuse sweat.
- History of B-coli infection a few times in the last 2 years. Now drinks lots of water.
- Stool – colour yellow – no bad odour but constipated ++.
- Bloody stool when there is problem of piles.
- 2 miscarriages – RH Negative – sexual desire – absent.
- Menstruation started at the age of 12 yrs. Pain before menses – much less. 27 or
- 28 day cycle, regular. Stays for 4 days – blackish red –clotted.
- Leucorrhoea < night.
- Piles: present. Started 18 years ago. Sometimes creates a problem.
- Small reddish eruption on both legs, no burning and itching. Occasionally gets pussy.
- Slow and sluggish. Lack of self confidence. Weepy.
- History of skin disease –amelioration when moist, ulcer – amelioration by homoeopathic treatment.
- Very easily catches cold.
- Talks in sleep.
- Disturbed sleep – deep sleep during the later part of the night.
- Married – one child: girl – 22 years. Very attached.
- Family history: Mother died of hypertension. Father died due to kidney failure.
- Food desires: Sweet, salty. Aversion: None.
- Thirst: Profuse (+++).

Investigations Carried Out Before/After Dr. Banerjea's Treatment

1st Nov'89: T3 – 1.8 (Normal 0.8 – 1.6); T4 – 7.2 (Normal – 5.0 – 11.5); TSH – 9.2 (Normal = 0.5 – 4.0).

13th Jun'95: T3 – 0.85 (Normal); T4 – 6.2 (Normal); TSH – 2.56 (Normal).

26th Feb'96: T3 = 1.25 (Normal = 0.8 – 1.8); T4 = 8.40 (Normal = 3.5 – 11.7); TSH = 3.6 (Normal = 0.2 – 3.8).

Endocrinological Disorders – Cured Cases

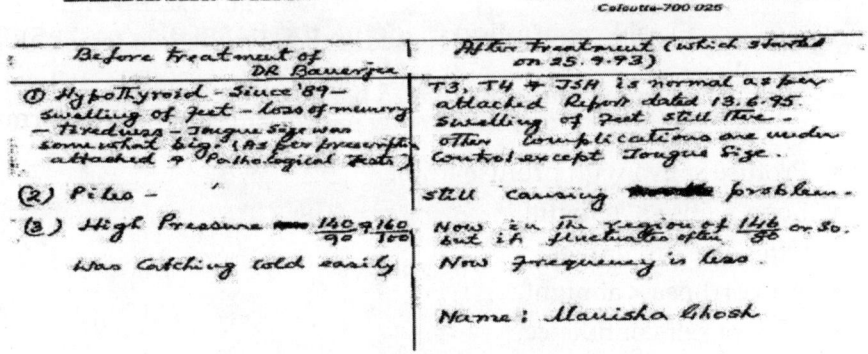

Blood report, before treatment

Blood report, 21 months after treatment

Comments of the patient, before and after treatment

CASE ANALYSIS, MIASMATIC DIAGNOSIS AND FINAL PRESCRIPTION

Miasmatic Analysis

- Hypothyroidism: Psora.
- Appetite poor: Psora.
- Constipation: Psora.
- Occasional bloody stool: Tubercular; Haemorrhoids: Sycotic.
- Stool: offensive: Syphilis.
- High blood pressure: Sycosis.
- Acidity, gas: Psora.
- Catches cold easily: Psora –tubercular.
- Occasional weakness of arms: Tubercular.
- Bone pains << night: Syphilis.
- Perspiration profuse and offensive: Syco-syphilitic.
- Saliva: profuse (+++): Sycosis.
- Sexual desire – absent: Psora.
- Menses: clotted: Tubercular.
- Leucorrhoea < night: Syphilitic.
- Pussy eruptions: Syphilitic.
- Lack of self confidence: Syphilo-sycotic.
- Weepy: Sycosis.
- Very easily catches cold: Psora-tubercular.
- Talks in sleep: Psora.

It is a mixed miasmatic case with Syphilo-Sycotic preponderance.

Final Prescription Made on the Basis of

- Human thermometer: sensitive to heat as well as cold: < by heat, < by cold.
- Profuse saliva with profuse thirst.
- Bone pains << at night.
- Offensive discharges.
- Leucorrhoea < at night.
- Lack of self confidence.
- Weakness of extremities (hands).
- Coated thick tongue.

The miasmatic analysis of Mercurius is: Psora +++, Sycosis ++, Syphilis +++, Tubercular+++.

Mercurius covers the case miasmatically as well.

Remedy Reaction

This case was started with Mercurius Sol. 200 and finished with 10M. The initial potency of 200 was chosen because it was an endocrine problem, which is helped well by that potency, and on the basis of the patient's vitality. Tiredness and memory loss of the patient improved, as well.

Prescription Chart

Date	Prescription Done on the Basis of Treatment	Treatment
25th Sep'93	Loss of memory, tiredness. Occasional bloody stool. Stool: offensive. Catches cold easily. Sensitive to heat as well as cold: < by heat, < by cold.	Mercurius Sol. 200 C, 2 doses.
	Occasional weakness of arms, cannot hold anything for a long time. Bone pains << night.	
	Perspiration – profuse and offensive smell, throughout the body.	
	Coated thick tongue, not very clear.	
	Saliva: profuse (+++). Bad odour from sweating. Profuse sweat.	
	2 miscarriages – RH Negative – sexual desire –absent. Leucorrhoea < night.	
	Small reddish eruption on both legs, no burning itching. Occasionally gets pussy.	
	Slow and sluggish. Lack of self-confidence. Weepy. Very easily catches cold.	
	Talks in sleep. Disturbed sleep – deep sleep in the later part of the night.	
20th Nov'93	Doing a little better.	Sac lac.
	Skin eruptions better	
	Pain along the tibia: bone pains: a little better. Pitting oedema: a little better.	
	Occasional left maxillary tenderness.	
18th Dec'93	Doing a little better.	Sac lac.
	Skin eruption better.	
5th Mar'94	Blood pressure: 150/100	Sac lac.
	Pain (left) leg lower end of tibia; pitting oedema aggravates at night. Wait & watch.	

Date	Prescription Done on the Basis of Treatment	Treatment
9th Apr'94	Pitting pedal oedema. Moist, flabby tongue with imprint of teeth. Macroglossia. Repeat as there is no further improvement. Stand still status.	Merc Sol. 200C, 2 doses.
14th May'94	Doing better: pitting oedema; brown spots on the cheeks; puffiness of eyes.	Sac Lac
25th Jun'94	Had fever- took allopathic medicine. Feels all symptoms are worse since. Pitting oedema++; puffiness of eyes; lumbago. Periods – alternate months: scanty.	Merc Sol. 1M, 2 doses.
23rd Jul'94	Stand still. Wait & watch.	Sac lac.
27th Aug'94	B.P.: 160/90; Weight: 72 kg No further change. Feeling Okay.	Sac lac.
22nd Oct'94	Doing better: Cramps in the legs >; pitting oedema >; brown spots >.	Sac lac
3rd Dec'94	73 kg. As a whole Okay, but blood pressure high; didn't want to take allopathic medication, so gave Crataegus Q. B.P.: 160/100	Sac lac Crataegus Q.
14th Jan'95	B.P.: 140/95..better. 71.5 kg.	Sac lac.
25th Feb'95	As a whole better; B.P: 150/86 Thirst – average 73 kg.	Sac lac.
29th Apr'95	As a whole better B.P.: 140/90 72 kg.	Sac lac
17th Jun'95	Oedema aggravates pre-menstrually. B.P.: 134/90. 73 kg. Eltroxin has been reduced from 2 tabs daily to now: ½ tab T3, T4 and TSH reports normal. Tiredness and memory loss of the patient got better, as well.	Merc Sol 1M, 2 doses.
5th Aug'95	Swelling of leg aggravated during menses. Tiredness and memory are under control. Spots – stand still now. Stool – Okay. B.P.: 146/80 73 kg.	Sac lac.

Date	Prescription Done on the Basis of Treatment	Treatment
12th Sep'95	Stand still status.	Sac lac.
21st Oct'95	Wait & watch	Sac lac.
9th Dec'95	As a whole better B.P.: 140/90. 73.5 kg.	Sac lac.
20th Jan'96	Stand still status.	Sac lac.
2nd Mar'96	No appreciable change.	Sac lac.
27th Apr'96	As a whole Okay. 75 kg. Piles better.	Sac lac.
22nd Jun'96	B.P.: 160/86	Sac lac.
10th Aug'96	B.P.: 156/84 75 kg. Stand still status.	Sac lac.
1st Oct'96	Red spots on both cheeks & legs +: feels like coming back. Stand still status.	Merc Sol 10 M, 2 doses.
30th Nov'96	Occasional right knee pain, aggravates at night. Otherwise Okay. B.P.: 160/90. 76 kg.	Sac lac.
18th Jan'97	Feeling much better. Thyroid better. Stopped conventional medication.	Sac lac.
29th Mar'97	Much better	Sac lac

Authenticity of Cure:

CD Reference: E006-HYPOTHYROIDISM-MG

7. A CASE OF HYPO-THYROIDISM: MISS R.M.

Case No. E007

Age : 28 as on 27.11.99.
Sex : Female
Height : 150 cms/5'-1"
Weight : 66 kgs.

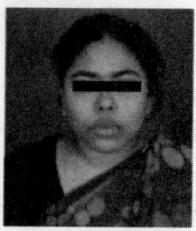

Photo of the patient, Miss R.M.

Presenting Complaints

- Main problem: Hypo-thyroidism. Premature greying of hair and hair falling. Tingling sensation in hands. Sleeplessness.
- Weight gain.
- Severe breathing problems.
- No energy to do any work, always feels tired. Weak physically. General exhaustion.
- Eruptions on face. Black patches on face, extremities and back part of the body.
- Constipation with piles a problem.
- Pain in throat, swelling of throat during talking.
- Cough is dry, teasing, and constant (++). Tendency to catch cold.
- Appetite: normal.
- Menses: started at 11 years. Severe stomach pain on the first day.
- Delayed at times. Painful periods with nausea. Quantity – Profuse.
- Associated symptoms with menses: Nausea & coldness of palms and feet.
- Obstinate.
- Desires to be neat & clean/she desire company. Restless.
- Memory active. Needs excitement. Superstitious. Dissatisfied → easily bored.
- Having involuntarily sighing. Consolation aggravates.
- Patient is intensely sympathetic. Does everything in a hurry.
- Fearless.
- Suffered from chickenpox once.
- Chilly patient +++. Very susceptible to cold. Takes cold easily, but likes open fresh air.
- Generally thirsty.
- Sleep: disturbed.

Endocrinological Disorders – Cured Cases

- Unmarried.
- Father & Mother are both alive.
- Food desires.

Investigations Carried Out Before/After Dr. Banerjea's Treatment

17th Apr'99: T3 1.12 (Normal), T4 5.8 (Normal), TSH 5.19 (Normal 0.2 – 3.8)
14th Jun'00: FNAC left Breast lump :- simple cyst.
28th Nov'00: T3 1.61, T4 6.97, TSH: 2.67 (Normal)

Blood report, before treatment

Blood report, 19 months after treatment

Comments of the patient after treatment

CASE ANALYSIS, MIASMATIC DIAGNOSIS AND FINAL PRESCRIPTION

Miasmatic Analysis

- Hypo-thyroidism: Psora.
- Premature greying of hair: Sycosis.
- Tingling sensation in hands: Psora.
- Sleeplessness: Lack: Psora.
- No energy to do any work, always feels tired: Psora.
- Weak physically: Psora.
- Black patches on face, extremities & back part of the body: Hyper-pigmentation: Sycosis.
- Constipation: Psora.
- Swelling of throat: Syco-tubercular.
- Cough is dry, teasing, and constant (++): Psora-Tubercular.
- Tendency to catch cold: Psora-Tubercular.
- Menses: Quantity – Profuse: Tubercular. Nausea during: Tubercular.
- Obstinate: Tubercular.
- Mental restlessness: Sycosis.
- Needs excitement: Dissatisfied: Tubercular.
- Dissatisfied → easily bored: Tubercular.
- Patient is intensely sympathetic: Sycosis.
- Does everything in a hurry: Sycosis.
- Fearless: Tubercular.
- Chilly patient +++. Very susceptible to cold. Takes cold easily, but likes open fresh air: Tubercular.

It is a mixed miasmatic case with Psora-Tubercular preponderance.

Points In Favour Of Remedy Selection

- Takes cold easily, but likes open fresh air.
- Dissatisfied and easily bored, obstinate, restless.
- Does everything in a hurry: restless and hyperactive.
- Needs excitement.
- Sensitive.

- General exhaustion – weakness, no energy to do any work.
- Hard dry cough.
- Poor sleep.
- Miasmatic analysis of Tuberculinum is: Psora +++, Sycosis +++, Syphilis ++, Tubercular +++.

Tuberculinum covers the case miasmatically as well.

Remedy Reaction

I started the case with Tuberculinum 30C; a low potency being used because of the patient's lowered vitality and general weakness. I finished the case with the 200C potency after one year's treatment.

Prescription Chart

Date	Prescription Done on the Basis of Treatment	Treatment
27th Nov'99	Chilly patient +++. Very susceptible to cold. Takes cold easily, but likes open fresh air. Tendency to catch cold. No energy to do any work, always feels tired. Weak physically. General exhaustion. Black patches on face, extremities & back part of the body. Pain in throat, swelling of throat during talking. Severe breathing problems. Cough is dry, teasing, and constant (++). Delayed at times. Painful periods with nausea. Quantity – Profuse. Obstinate. Restless. Memory active. Needs excitement. Fearless. Superstitious. Dissatisfied → easily bored. Tubercular preponderance.	Tuberculinum, 30C, 2 doses.
29th Jan'00	Repeated attacks of cough and cold, but feels like the teasing cough is a little better or stand still.	Sac lac.
18th Mar'00	Feeling much better.	Sac lac.
13th May'00	Cough is back. Stand still status.	Tuberculinum, 30C, 1 dose.
1st Jul'00	Blood pressure: 106/70 62 kg Lump on left breast, FNAC done: NAD. Eruption on forehead. As a whole better.	Sac lac.
29th Aug'00	Breast lump stand still or better. Throat was better, now standstill.	Tuberculinum, 200C, 1 dose.

Date	Prescription Done on the Basis of Treatment	Treatment
17th Oct'00	Wait and watch. Breast lump better.	Sac lac.
28th Nov'00	64 kg. TSH returned to normal. Breathing considerably better and constipation improved. No pain in throat.	CURED.

Authenticity of Cure:

CD Reference: E007-HYPOTHYROIDISM-RM

Endocrinological Disorders – Cured Cases

8. A CASE OF DIABETES – MRS. A.D.

Case No. E008

Age : 48 years as on 30/5/97

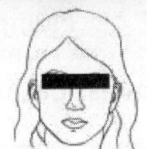

Photo of the patient, Mrs. A.D.

Presenting Complaints

- Muscular pain from waist to leg (mostly left) felt at night.
- Main complaint: Diabetes.
- Warts and moles: all over the body.
- Stool: loose generally.
- Acidity aggravates during the evening.
- Catches cold easily. Dust allergy – produces sneezing.
- Hypertension present. Occasional neck pain present.
- Headache aggravated by heat. Sunlight disagrees.
- Chilly patient.
- Sweat: more on back. Sweat only on covered parts of the body when she sleeps, stops when she wakes.
- Craving: Sour++, pungent and hot++, salty+, bitter+. Thirst: Less than normal.
- Aversion: Vegetables.
- Head: Heat and burning on vertex when blood pressure increased due to tension.
- Mouth: Occasional aphthous ulcers.
- Heart: Palpitation++ due to tension.
- Abdomen: Distension of whole abdomen, passing flatus.
- Appetite: Decreased.
- Stool: Regular.
- Lumbago: Aggravates after exertion.
- Menstrual cycle stopped at the age of 35 years.
- Mental: Mild. Desire to be neat and clean - fussy (++). Weeping mood. Cannot tolerate blood letting.
- Non Flexible: Fears of being exposed.
- Closed and rigid.
- Conceals feelings; Secret obsession about money.
- Fears: Ghosts, darkness.
- History of Typhoid, Malaria and accident (falling injury).

- Sleep: Okay.
- Urine: Normal.
- Plumpy abdomen can go in the final Rx.

Investigations Carried Out After Dr. Banerjea's Treatment

25th Jun'97: Electro Cardio Gram (ECG): WNL (within normal limit).

18th Sep'97: Blood Sugar Post Prandial (BSPP):- 242 mg%. Haemoglobin 11.2 White Blood Cell (W.B.C.) 7, 100 Neutrophill 50 Lymphocyte 47 Monocyte, Eosinophyl 2

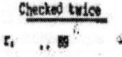

Blood sugar report of Mrs. A. D., during treatment

Blood sugar report of Mrs. A. D., 2 months after treatment

Cholesterol 218 mg%. Triglyceride 171 mg%.

19th Nov'97:   Blood Sugar Post Prandial (BSPP) – 112mg%.

CASE ANALYSIS, MIASMATIC DIAGNOSIS AND FINAL PRESCRIPTION

Miasmatic Analysis

- Muscular pain at night : Syphilis.
- Diabetes: Mixed miasmatic.
- Warts and moles: Sycosis.
- Stool : loose: Sycosis (constipation is psoric, dysentery is syphilitic)
- Acidity: Psora.
- Headache aggravated by heat: Syphilitic.
- Catches cold easily: Psora.
- Dust allergy: Psora-Tubercular.
- Hypertension: Sycosis.
- Mouth: aphthous ulcers: Syphilis.
- Desires sour: Psora-syphilitic. Pungent and hot: Sycotic.
- Palpitation: Tubercular.
- Distention of abdomen from gas: Psora.
- Desire to be neat and clean: fussy: Sycosis.
- Cannot tolerate blood letting – Psora.
- Weeping mood: Sycosis.
- Non Flexible: Syco-syphilis.
- Closed and rigid: Syco-syphilis.
- Conceals feelings: Sycosis.
- Secret obsession about money: Sycosis.
- Fears: Ghosts, darkness: Psora.

It is a mixed miasmatic case with Sycotic preponderance.

Final Prescription Made on the Basis of

- Warts and moles all over body.
- Sweat only on covered parts of the body when she sleeps, stops when she wakes. These are PQRS symptoms of Thuja.
- Conceals feelings, secret obsessions about money: Thuja guards and conceals – "Ducks and Hides" and has secret obsessions.

- Fixed ideas about health and hygiene.
- Emotional sensitiveness – weeping mood.
- Closed and rigid opinions.
- Non flexible – fears of being exposed.

The miasmatic analysis of Thuja is: Psora ++, Sycosis +++, Syphilis ++, Tubercular ++.

Thuja covers the case miasmatically as well.

Remedy Reaction

This case was started with Thuja 200 based on the diagnoses of diabetes and the patient's vitality. I ascended in potency to Thuja 10M and the patient was cured of her symptoms in less than 2 years.

Prescription Chart

Date	Prescription Done on the Basis of	Treatment
30th May'97	Muscular pain from waist to leg (mostly left); Warts and moles: all over the body. Catches cold easily. Hypertension. Occasional neck pain. Chilly patient. Sweat: more on back. Sweat only on covered parts of the body when she sleeps, stops when she wakes (PQRS). Craving: Salty+; Aversion: Vegetables. Mental: Desire to be neat and clean - fussy (++). Weeping mood. Non flexible: Fears of being exposed. Closed and rigid. Conceals feelings; Secret obsession about money.	Thuja, 200C, doses2
30th Jun'97	BP: 144/110. Doing a little better.	Sac lac.
6th Aug'97	BP: 160/100. Pain on left thigh aggravates at night. Pain and numb feeling on left hand. Occasional pain on left lower abdomen.	Sac lac.
22nd Sep'97	BP: 206/100. As BP got worse, so dropped a potency. Also diagnosed with high blood sugar (Blood report given above).	Thuja, 30C, 2 doses → 200C, 1 dose.
22nd Oct'97	BP: 174/94. Weight: 46 kgs. Occasional pain.	Sac lac.
5th Dec'97	BP: 170/108. Weight: 45 kgs. Feels better. Now pain in lower abdomen (occasional) only. Falling of hair. PPBS of 19/11/97 normal.	Sac lac.
30th Jan'98	BP: 166/90. Weight: 46 kgs. PPBS normal.	Sac lac.
30th Mar'98	BP: 162/90.	Sac lac.
15th May'98	BP: 136/90.	Sac lac.

Date	Prescription Done on the Basis of	Treatment
10th Jul'98	BP: 180/100. Waited for nine months!! Has been better. Pain in knee to heel aggravates when sitting on the floor.	Thuja, 1M, 2 doses.
14th Aug'98	BP: 146/100. Weight: 49 kgs.	Sac lac.
16th Sep'98	Doing better.	Sac lac.
16th Oct'98	BP: 156/100. Weight: 48 kgs. Acidity aggravates in evening. Appetite less. Pain in calf muscle aggravates when in sitting position. Thirst: More. Pain in the heel better. Emotionally better.	Sac lac.
27th Nov'98	Weight: 50 kgs. Dust allergy. Sneezing + and coryza followed by cough. Dry cough aggravated for last month. Catches cold easily. Knee pain ameliorated.	Thuja 10M, 1 dose
10th Feb'99	Better Blood sugar controlled.	Sac lac

Authenticity of Cure

CD Reference: E008-DIABETES MELLITUS-AD

9. A CASE OF HYPERTHYROIDISM: MRS. I.B.

Case No. E009

Age   : 33 years as on 8.7.96
Sex   : Female
Height : 5'-3"
Weight : 69 kgs.

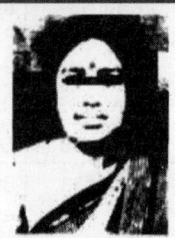
Photo of the patient, MRS. I.B.

Presenting Complaints

- Main problem: Hyperthyroidism.
- Small cervical polyp.
- Acute acidity.
- Palpitation, weakness (especially in morning) and sweating: 1st observed in 1985-86.
- Aforesaid problems are often associated with nausea & vomiting.
- Breathing trouble and restlessness with dry cough.
- Muscles: feels weakness and doesn't like the flabbiness.
- Puffiness and oedema.
- Pre-menstrual irritability. Periods are regular & Okay.
- Stool: Regular; no mucus.
- Urine: Okay.
- Appetite - Normal
- Thirst - Normal
- Chilly Patient ++; catches cold easily. Hates: Rainy weather.
- Profuse perspiration → No bad odour.
- Heals: In normal time: Okay.
- Sleep: Okay.
- Desire: Sweet +++; salty ++; salt +; bitter; veg. + & spinach.
- Fish ++; Luke warm food; cold drinks.
- Mind: Angry ++; Obstinate; talkative ++; desire for company; Gets angry when reprimanded; Sympathetic;
- Weepy mood; consolation aggravates.
- Fear of darkness; accident.
- Irritable < least opposition.
- Irritable +++, before menses.

- Depressed (especially on waking)
- Mentioned in the history about maladjustment with husband and stress (+++) thereby (2 years after marriage; around 1984 –85 and problem could have been triggered by that).
- Past History: Measles –
- Family History: Father died of cerebral thrombosis. Mother – Diabetes.

Investigations Carried Out Before/After Dr. Banerjea's Treatment

3rd Jul'95: T3 0.9 (Normal: 0.79 – 1.73) T4 7.2 (Normal: 5.2 – 12.7) TSH 10.2.

29th Apr'96: Haemoglobin 11.0 gm%. White Blood Cell (W.B.C.) 11,800, Neutrophil 69, Lymphocyte 26, Monocyte 6, Eosinophyl 5, Basophil 6.

18th Oct'96: T3 1.46 mg T4 9.12 TSH 3.67. Cholesterol 181, Triglycerides 117 mg%, Haemoglobin – 11.7 gm%.

26th Jul'97: T3 – 1.44, T4 – 13.6, TSH – 0.14 (Normal).

6th Dec'97: T3 1.16, (Normal) T4 10.8 (Normal), TSH-2.71 (Normal)

8th Apr'99: T3 1.14 (Normal), T4 10.3 (Normal), TSH 2.52 (Normal)

21st Dec'00: T3 0.96, T4 9.5, TSH – 3.41 (Normal), Blood Sugar Fasting (BSF):- 87 mg%, Blood Sugar Post Prandial (BSPP) 90 mg%.

CASE ANALYSIS, MIASMATIC DIAGNOSIS AND FINAL PRESCRIPTION

- Miasmatic Analysis:
- Hyperthyroidism: Sycosis.
- Small cervical polyp: Sycosis.
- Acute acidity: Psora.
- Palpitation: Tubercular.
- Weakness: Psora.
- Sweating: Sycosis.
- Dry cough: Psora.
- Muscles: feels weakness: Psora.

Blood report of Mrs. I. B. before treatment

Blood report of Mrs. I. B. 6 months after treatment

Calcutta

Respected
Dr. S. Banerjea

In response of your letter dt 12.10.96, I furnish below the report of progress as I feel after undergoing your kind treatment along with the copies of prescriptions of alopathy treatments :—

Before treatment of Dr. Banerjea i.e. during alopathy treatment	After & during continuation of Dr. Banerjea's treatment
1) Weakness (better) specially during morning and after urinal release. Acute acidity.	
2) Breathing trouble, restlessness, nespenging accompanying cough and shaking of whole body.	All these complains subsides subject to continuation of Dr. Banerjea's medicines.
3) Unwillingness of undertaking any work	
4) Unnecessary fear, anger, and angry huizyness.	

Humble submission for your kind requirement.

Thanking you,

yours obedient
Indrani Banerjee.
(MRS. INDRANI BANERJEE)

THYROTOXICOSIS

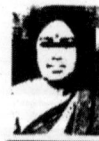

Patient's comments after treatment

- Flabbiness: Lack of tone: Psora.
- Puffiness & oedema: Sycosis.
- Pre-menstrual irritability: Hormonal: Sycosis.
- Hates: Rainy weather: Sycosis.
- Profuse perspiration → Sycosis.
- Angry ++: Sycosis.
- Obstinate: Tubercular.
- Talkative ++: Sycosis.
- Fear of darkness; accident: Psora.
- Irritable +++, before menses: Syco-Tubercular.
- Depressed (especially on waking): Psora- syphilis.
- Family History: Father died of cerebral thrombosis. Mother – Diabetes: Syco- tubercular background.
- It is a mixed miasmatic case with Syco-Psoric preponderance.

Points in Favour of Remedy Selection

- Main problem: Hyperthyroidism
- Small cervical polyp.
- Palpitation, weakness and sweating: 1st observed in 1985-86.
- Aforesaid problems are often associated with nausea & vomiting: In Thyroidinum: nausea and vomiting is a concomitant.
- Muscles: feels weakness & doesn't like the flabbiness.
- Puffiness & oedema.
- Pre-menstrual irritability.
- Chilly Patient++; catches cold easily. Hates: Rainy weather.
- Desire: Sweet +++; salty ++; salt +.
- Mind: Angry ++; obstinate; talkative ++;
- Weepy mood;
- Irritable < least opposition;
- Irritable +++, before menses;
- Depressed (especially on waking).
- Mentioned in the history about maladjustment with husband and stress (+++) thereby (2 years after marriage; around 1984 – 85 and problem could have been triggered by that). This (maladjustment) is a very important causative factor for Thyroidinum.
- Mixed miasmatic with Sycotic preponderance.

- The miasmatic analysis of Thyroidinum is: Psora ++, Sycosis +++, Syphilis ++, Tubercular +++.
- Thyroidinum covers the case miasmatically as well.

Final Prescription

Thyroidinum 200 C, a good potency for endocrine disorders, was initially prescribed. I finished the case with Thyroidinum 10M.

Prescription Chart

Date	Prescription Done on the Basis of	Treatment
8th Jul'96	B.P. – 110/70. Polyp. TSH – High. Desire Sweet. Catches cold easily.	Thyroid, 200C/2
3rd Aug'96	Acidity. Gas formed in upper abdomen by eructation. Burning and load feeling in throat. Weakness during acidity. Hot patient. Desire – Fish, Bread, Salt, Hot food. Aversion – Bitter. Appetite – poor, Sleep and dream – Normal, dreams of daily business. Thirst – For large quantity of cold water at long interval. Sweat uncovered part, uneasy feeling. Due to acidity – Allopathic medicine.	PL5 SOS – Carbo Veg
14th Sep'96	Weight – 69 kgs. Acidity was > No other problem.	PL5
12th Oct'96	Acidity and Debility++. Exhausted feeling after passing stool early in the morning. Dry tongue thirst++. Sleep and dreams of dead person. Sweat+. TSH level came from 102 to 3.67 (N).	PL5
22nd Nov'96		Thyroid, 200C/2

Authenticity of cure:

CD Reference: E009-HYPER THYROIDISM-IB

10. A CASE OF HYPERTHYROIDISM: (49 YEAR OLD MALE)

Case No. E010

MR. B. K. M.

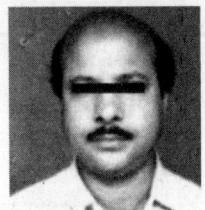

Photo of the patient
Mr. B.K.M.

Presenting Complaints

- Acidity, nauseatic tendency while tooth brushing in the morning. Loss of appetite, tasteless mouth. For last 3 weeks. Acidity < vomiting. Sneezing, uneasiness of throat, heaviness of head for air condition atmosphere, stoppage of left nose. Head – Heat on vertex, Perspiration on head. Bald head.
- Abdomen – No problem.
- Stomach – Appetite decreased.
- Sweat – Average, more on upper part, with odour.
- Stool – One time daily, clear.
- M.G.O. (Male Genital Organs) – Sexual desire less.
- Anus – No problem.
- Skin – No problem.
- Typhoid – at 8 years old – Allopathic. Measles – at childhood. Pox. Gastric troubles for 3 years.
- Patient thinks for last three, four years (since age 45-46) he is suffering with weakness, started putting on weight, loss of appetite, catches cold easily etc.
- Obese ++
- Patient is Chilly.
- Likes – Sweet +++, Egg, Warm food.
- Thirst – Thirsty.
- Sleep – Sound sleep.
- Mental- Feels withdrawn and disconnected with family. Mild, occasional desire for company. Memory - Active.
- Patient is married.

Investigations

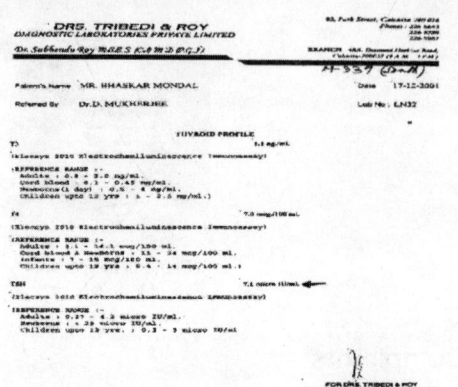

Blood report, before treatment

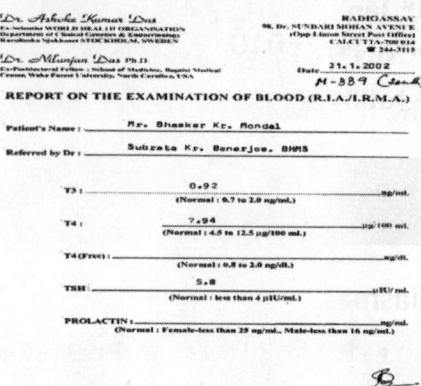

Blood report, 1 month after treatment

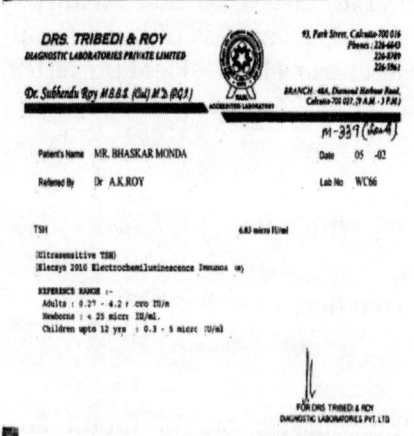

Blood report, 9 months after treatment

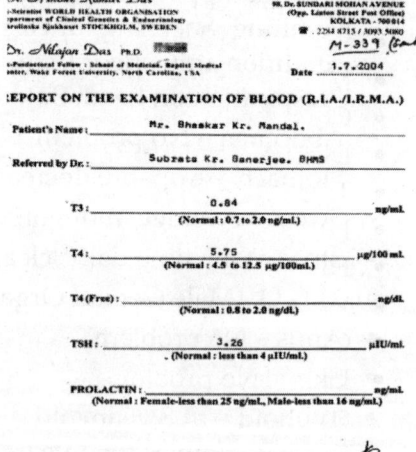

Blood report, 27 months after treatment

Before Treatment of Dr. S. K. Banerjee	After Treatment of Dr. S. K. Banerjee
1 Sudden weight gain	1 Weight almost stable
2 There had been hoarse voice	2 Now recovered
3 Sexual capability reduced considerably	3 Sexual capability regained

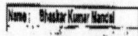

Comments of the patient, before and after treatment

17th Dec'01:	T_3 – 1.1, T_4 – 7.0, TSH – 7.1
31st Jan'02:	T_3 – 0.92, T_4 – 7.94, TSH – 5.8
5th Nov'02:	TSH – 6.03
1st Jul'04:	T_3 – 0.84, T_4 – 5.75, TSH – 3.26 (Normal)

CASE ANALYSIS, MIASMATIC DIAGNOSIS AND FINAL PRESCRIPTION

Miasmatic Analysis

- Hyperthyroidism: Sycotic.
- Acidity, nausea, vomiting: Psora.
- Loss of appetite: Psora.
- Heaviness of head: Sycotic.
- Sexual desire less: Psora.
- Mind – mild: Psora. Desire for company: Psora.
- Chilly++: Psora.
- Desire sweet: Psora. Warm food: Sycotic. Spicy: Psora.
- Thirsty: Sycotic.
- Hoarseness – Psora-Sycotic.
- Easily catches cold: psora-Tubercular.
- Weakness: Psora.
- Obesity: Sycosis.
- Patient thinks for last three, four years (since age 45-46) he is suffering with weakness, started putting on weight, loss of appetite, catches cold easily etc: related to imbalance of hormone: Sycosis.

It is a mixed miasmatic case with Syco-Psoric preponderance.

Final Prescription Made on the Basis of

- Hyperthyroidism which is sycotic.
- Obese++.
- Hoarseness.
- Nausea and vomiting, acidity.
- Chilly patient++. Easily catches cold.
- Sweet +++.
- Loss of appetite. Patient thinks for last three, four years (since age 45-46) he is suffering with weakness, started putting on weight, loss of appetite, catches cold easily etc: I interpreted that hormonal

imbalance during the change of life (middle age crisis in men), which Thyroidinum takes care of it.

The miasmatic breakdown of Thyroidinum is Psora ++, Sycosis +++L, Syphilis ++, Tubercular +++, C+++.

Thyroidinum covers the case miasmatically as well.

Prescription Chart

Date	Prescription Done on the Basis of	Treatment
29th Dec'01	Blood pressure: 126/80. 72 kgs. Getting obese++. TSH – high 7.1. Desire – Sweet+, Spicy++, Fish. Stool – Regular, Chilly++.	Thyroidinum, 200C, 2 doses.
9th Feb'02	140/85. 71 kgs. Wait and watch.	Sac lac.
6th Apr'02	125/80. As a whole >. Wait and watch.	Sac lac
1st Jun'02	130/85, 70 kgs.	Sac lac.
20th Jul'02	130/80. 71 kgs. As a whole doing >. Heaviness of voice during high pitch notations or singing. Wait and watch.	Sac lac. Given some Phytolacca Q for gurgling.
5th Oct'02	120/80. 72 kgs. As a whole > occ. congestion in throat.	Sac lac.
16th Nov'02	120/84. 69.5 kgs. Desire – Sweet. Appears to be standstill	repeat Thyroidinum 200C, 2 doses.
15th Feb'03	124/80. 70 kgs. As a whole doing >. Occ. Acidity + Sour eructation. Wait and watch.	Sac lac.
10th May'03	124/80. 72 kgs. As a whole >.	Sac lac.
July'03	126/80. 70 kgs. As a whole doing >.	Sac lac.
20th Sep'03	140/80. 70 kgs. Pain in left knee. < ascending. Pain Occ. in right elbow. Felt 200C is not holding, so went for next potency.	Thyroidinum, 1M, 2 doses.
13th Dec'03	140/80. Pain in left knee >. Right elbow pain >. As a whole doing >.	Sac lac.
7th Feb'04	122/80. Wait and watch.	Sac lac.
24th Apr'04	126/80. 72 kgs. >.	Sac lac. As the patient is doing much better, therefore asked him to repeat the blood investigation.
10th Jul'04	128/80. 72 kgs. As a whole doing >. TSH normal. Stopped treatment.	

Authenticity of Cure

CD Reference: E010-HYPER THYROIDISM-BKM

11. A CASE OF DIABETES: MR. J.K.S.

Case No. E011

Age   : 37 years-old as on 06.03.1989.
Sex   : Male

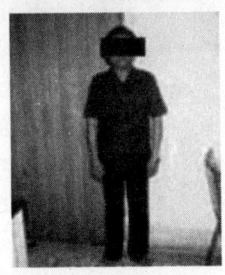

Patient Mr. J. K. S.

Presenting Complaints

- Patient has been diagnosed with high blood sugar and does not like, to take allopathic medicines.
- Burning while passing urine. Hot urine.
- 7 – 8 months: have been diagnosed with high blood sugar.
- Weakness and Vertigo++.
- Stomach:- Occasional discomfort. Burning (++) when the stomach is empty. Better by cold drink.
- Sweat:- Profuse sweating (+++) all over the body. Offensive (++) smell.
- Urine:- Strong smelling.
- Stool:- Loose; Not clear; Hot feeling; No mucus.
- Male Genital Organs:- Spermatorrhoea for 2 years.
- Mental Symptoms:- Angry. Suicidal tendency. Very talkative. Fear of death. Memory – medium. Sympathetic. Forgetful (++). Indolence, does not have energy, to get up and do things; procrastinates and leave lots of things undone. Also does not take care of his clothes etc., leaves them untidy.
- Habit of smoking: regular 10 – 12 cigarettes per day. Occasionally drinks wine.
- H/O Skin disease → 16 years ago → allopathic treat → Weakness developed
- Suffered from Chicken pox in past.
- Hot patient.
- Likes Bitter++, Vegetables, Chicken, Warm food, Bread, Milk, Egg++. Desire: Sweet (++), Sour (+).
- Generally thirsty.
- Sleep:- Sound (O.K.).

- Great weakness, semen expels out within ½ minute during coitus; semen – very much thin. Began – 2 years, ago; semen passing during micturition, and stool;
- Burning micturition began – 2 years ago – hot urine; strong smelling. Frequent micturition, not clear.
- All complaints arise after Diabetes. Stool not clear, ineffectual desire, scanty, semi-solid, or hard. Hot, offensive smelling:
- Dim vision after Diabetes. Itching of whole body – when Diabetes increases, aversion to eat.

Investigations Carried Out Before/After Dr. Banerjea's Treatment

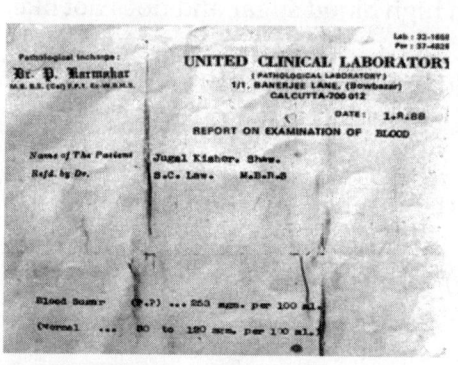

Blood Sugar report before treatment

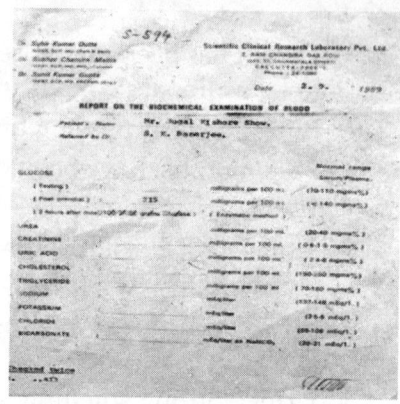

Blood Sugar report 7 months after treatment

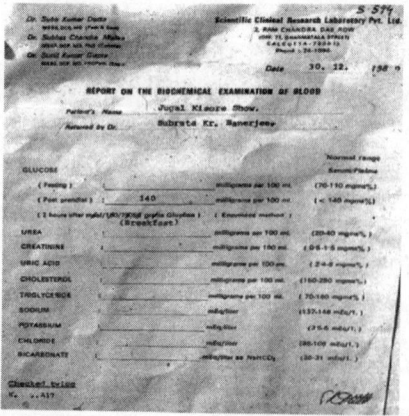

Normal Blood Sugar report, 10 months after treatment

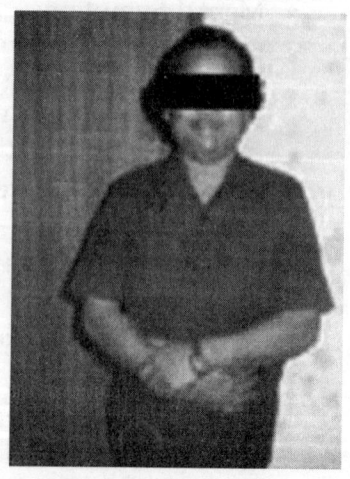

Patient Mr. J. K. S.

23rd Nov'87: Blood Sugar Post Prandial (BSPP): 260.
1st Aug'88: Blood Sugar Post Prandial (BSPP): 253.
28th Sep'88: Blood Sugar Post Prandial (BSPP): 220
29th Dec'88: Blood Sugar Post Prandial (BSPP): 140 (Normal)
19th Jan'89: Urine:- Epithelial cells 3 – 6 HPF. Pus Cells 6 – 8 HPF, Red Blood Corpuscles occasionally. Albumin: Trace.
2nd Sep'89: Blood Sugar Post Prandial (BSPP): 215.
10th Dec'89: Blood Sugar Post Prandial (BSPP): 140 (Normal).
30th Dec'89: Urine: Albumin: Trace, Pus Cell 1-2 HPF. Blood Sugar Post Prandial (BSPP): 140.

CASE ANALYSIS, MIASMATIC DIAGNOSIS AND FINAL PRESCRIPTION

- Miasmatic Analysis:
- Burning while passing urine: Syphilitic.
- Stomach:- Burning (++) when the stomach is empty. Better by cold drink: Syphilitic.
- Sweat:- Profuse sweating (+++) all over the body: Sycotic. Offensive (++) smell: Syphilitic.
- Suicidal tendency: Syphilitic. Very talkative: Sycotic. Fear of death: Psora. Forgetful (++): Psora-Syphilitic. Indolence: does not have the energy to get up and do things: Psora. Procrastinates and leaves lots of things undone: Psora. Also does not take care of his clothes etc., leave them untidy: Psora.
- H/O Skin disease → 16 years ago → allopathic treat → Weakness developed: Psora-Tubercular.
- Great weakness, semen expels out within ½ minute during coitus: Psora.
- Semen passing during micturition, and stool: Sycotic.

Prescription Made on the basis of

- Burning while passing urine. Hot urine.
- Stomach:- Occasional discomfort. Burning (++) when the stomach is empty. Better by cold drink.

- Sweat:- Profuse sweating (+++) all over the body. Offensive (++) smell.
- Mental Symptoms:- Angry. Suicidal tendency. Very talkative. Fear of death. Memory – medium. Sympathetic. Forgetful (++). Indolence, does not have the energy to get up and do things; procrastinates and leaves lots of things undone. Also does not take care of his clothes etc., leave them untidy.
- H/O Skin disease → 16 years ago → allopathic treat → Weakness developed
- Hot patient.
- Likes Bitter++, Vegetables, Chicken, Warm food, Bread, Milk, Egg++. Desire: Sweet (++), Sour (+).
- Great weakness, semen expels out within ½ minute during coitus; semen – very much thin. Began – 2 years, ago; semen passing during micturition, and stool;
- Burning micturition began – 2 years ago – hot urine; strong smelling. Frequent micturition, not clear.

The miasmatic breakdown of Sulphur is: Psora L+++, Sycotic++, Syphilitic+++, Tubercular+++

Final Prescription and Remedy Reaction

SULPHUR 30C, 2 doses.

Prescription Chart

I started the case in February, 1988 with Sulphur 30C. Gradually I went up to Sulphur 1M and in December, 1989 the blood sugar report was normal. Patient did follow-up till end of 1989 to make sure that the blood sugar remained stable and normal.

Authenticity of Cure

CD Reference: E011-DIABETES-JKS

Chapter 5

Gastro-Intestinal (G.I.) Diseases - Cured Cases

1. A CASE OF SALIVARY DUCT CALCULUS: MR. L.D.

Case No. GA001

Age   : 34 years at 4th February, 1989
Height : 5 ft. 4 inches
Weight : 62 kgs.

Photo of the patient, Mr. L.D.

Presenting Complaints

- Stone in salivary duct (as diagnosed by radiographic X-Ray plate): two and half months back, it was diagnosed radiologically and the patient refused to undergo surgery (operation).
- Sudden pain in the lower jaw (left side) with swelling. Excruciating pain (+++) while eating.
- Extreme dryness of mouth.
- Extreme weakness (+++) after the pain, especially after eating. Can't stand then with profuse drenching sweat, which often follows nervous trembling and scared feeling; he cannot eat food (as eating = pain) and so he is scared.
- Pale and anaemic; due to lack of quantitative intake of food.
- Occasional swelling of face with puffiness & bloated appearance.
- Aggravation in the evening and night.
- Better by rest.
- Aggravation by jar.
- Tremendous aggravation by eating & chewing (+++).
- Head: Occasional frontal headache in the evening & night, better in the morning.

- Tongue: Coated when indigestion takes place.
- Throat: Occasional throat pain (left sided), better by warm gurgling. Congested & dry feeling of the fauces, more on the left side.
- Heart: Occasional palpitation during excruciating lower left mandibular pain, while eating.
- Abdomen: Distension of abdomen with gas. Belching relieves. Occasional right sided abdominal colic, which is better by warm milk.
- Sweat: Profuse drenching perspiration during and after eating. No smell.
- Urine: Increased flow. Occasional burning of the urethra.
- Stool: Regular. No mucus.
- Lower Extremities: Occasional pain in the knees.
- Skin Disease: Fungal infection in the webs (especially in feet). Itching which follows oozing of sticky offensive fluid. Cracks in the webs. Itching aggravated at night & after removing the socks.
- Mental Symptoms: A constant grumbler. Melancholic. Memory weak. Fear of eating.
- Suffered from: History of jaundice (hepatitis) in the year 1978.
- Chilly person (+++).
- Extremely sensitive to cold: catches cold readily.
- Desire Foods: Sweet+++, sour+, pungent & hot+, salt+, milk+, meat+, rich & spicy++, fat food+, cold drinks+.
- Thirst+++ for cold drinks+++.
- Father died of diabetes.

Investigations Carried Out Before/After Dr. Banerjea's Treatment

23rd Nov'88: X-ray left salivary duct: Remark:- Small radio-opaque stone near the terminal end of left submandibular salivary duct.

18th Aug'89: X-ray left lower jaw: Remark: - No evidence of any radio-opaque calculus in the submandibular salivary duct.

Gastro-Intestinal (G.I.) Diseases – Cured Cases

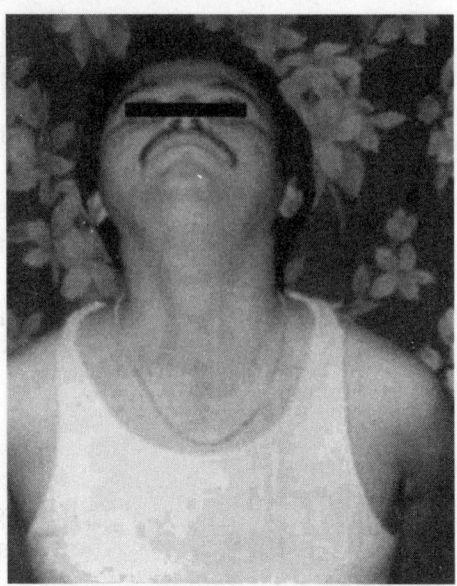

Mr. L.D., Salivary Duct Calculi, before treatment of Dr. Banerjea.

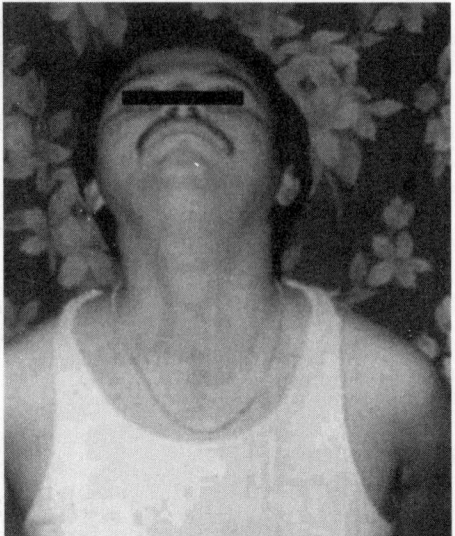

X-Ray report, before treatment

Small radio opaque stone near the terminal end of left submandibular salivery duct is shown.

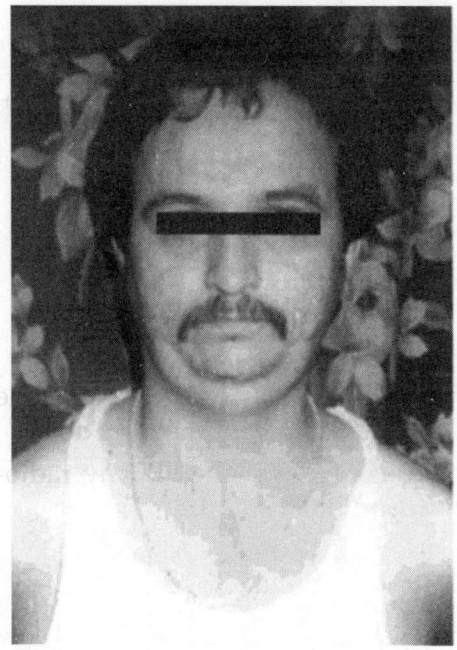

After 6 months of treatment

X-Ray report after treatment

No evidence of any radio opaque calculus in the submandibular salivery duct.

CASE ANALYSIS, MIASMATIC DIAGNOSIS AND FINAL PRESCRIPTION

Miasmatic Analysis

- Salivary duct calculus: Sycosis.
- Dryness of mouth: Psora.
- Profuse sweat: Sycosis.
- Fear of eating: Psora.
- Pains followed by weakness: Tubercular.
- Swelling and puffiness: Sycotic.
- Pale and anaemic, lack of intake of food: Psora.
- Aggravation at night: Syphilis.
- Frontal headaches: Sycosis.
- Head pain ameliorated in morning, aggravated at night: Syphilis.
- Throat pain better by warm gargling, dry feeling of fauces: Psora.
- Distension of abdomen with gas: Psora.
- Abdominal colic, better by warm milk: Sycosis.
- Increased flow of urine: Sycosis; burning of urethra: Syphilis.
- Joint pains: Sycosis.
- Fungal infection: Syphilitic.
- Itching of skin with sticky offensive fluid: Psora-Syphilitic.
- Cracks in webs: Psora-Syphilitic.
- Itching aggravated at night: Syphilitic.
- Mental: Melancholic –Syphilitic, weakness of memory: Psora.
- Jaundice: Sycosis.
- Chilly person: Psora.
- Extremely sensitive to cold: catches cold readily: Psora – Tubercular.
- Desires sweet: Psora, sour: Psora-syphilitic, pungent and hot: Sycotic, Spicy: Psora, fat food: Psora-tubercular, cold drinks: Syphilitic.

Reasons for Prescriptions

(1) Thuja

- Chilly patient but desire for cold drinks.
- Occasional frontal headache.
- Profuse sweat.

Gastro–Intestinal (G.I.) Diseases – Cured Cases

- Increased flow of urine (excess=sycotic).
- Extreme weakness; anaemic.
- Extremely sensitive to cold.
- Location: Lower jaw (Left side); Throat- pain in the left side; Congested dry feeling of fauces: more on the left side: left sided affinity.
- Loss of memory, forgetful.
- Sycotic preponderance. Incordination (salivary duct calculi; joint pains).
- Miasmatic breakdown of Thuja is Psora ++, Sycosis +++, Syphilis ++, Tubercular ++.

(2) Thyroidinum

- Grumbling.
- Melancholy and irritable.
- Weakness of memory.
- Puffiness and oedema: oedema of the face.
- Desires sweet (+++).
- Thirst for cold water (+++).
- Dryness of the mouth & throat.
- Pain more on the left side.
- Chilliness < cold.
- Weakness (+++) and anaemia with trembling.
- Easily catches cold.
- Mixed miasmatic with strong sycotic and tubercular preponderance (Psora ++, Sycotic +++, Syphilitic ++, Tubercular +++).

Physical Make-up

Thyroidinum acts best on anaemic, obese persons – a state of puffiness and obesity is a keynote. Conditions which point towards it are a loss of balance in the human economy due to strain, during some particular period of development; due to climatic variations or due to some other mental and emotional factors. The want of metabolic, nervous or vascular adjustment: or a combination of some or all of them.

Remedy Reactions

This case was started with Thuja 30C, this potency was chosen based on the low vitality of the patient. The remedy was changed to Thyroidinum

200C after insufficient reaction to the Thuja prescription and the case was finished with Thyroidinum 10 M after 19 months of treatment.

Prescription Chart

Date	Prescription Done on the Basis of	Treatment
4th Feb'89	Chilly. Desires cold food. Aversion vegetables: hydrogenoid. Sycotic preponderance & inco-ordination.	Thuja, 30 C: 2 doses
11th Mar'89	No change. Pain & dryness increased. Felt Thuja is not touching the case, changed in the plan of treatment.	Thuja, 200 C: 2 doses.
8th Apr'89	No change. Excruciating (+++) pain after eating. Change in the plan of treatment.	Thyroidinum, 200 C: 2 doses.
10th Jun'89	No appreciable change, but no worse. Stand still.	Thyroidinum, 200 C: 2 doses
15th Jul'89	Stand still. Increase potency: sarcodes act better in highest potencies.	Thyroidinum, 10m: 2 doses
19th Aug'89	Feeling much better. Pain reduced totally. Dryness has disappeared. Weakness, appetite: all improved. Stone has disappeared (radiologically verified 18.8.89).	Sac lac.
21st Oct'89	Everyway better. Fungal infection is also better.	No medicine
2nd Sep'90	Called back the patient to repeat the X-ray though complaining of no symptoms. X-ray done on 11th September, 1990: No stone. Cured.	No medicine

Authenticity of Cure

CD Reference: GA001-SALIVARY DUCT CALCULI-LD

2. A CASE OF DUODENAL ULCER - MR M.M.

Case No. GA002

Age : 52 years as on 23rd September, 1988.
Sex : Male
Height : 5 ft.6 inches.

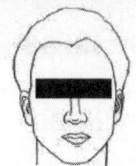
Photo of the patient, Mr. M.M.

Presenting Complaints

- Had History of irregular diet.
- Pain in epigastric region; aggravated on empty stomach, ameliorated after eating.
- Aching pain.
- Wind in abdomen, better by passing of flatus and by eructation.
- Acidity aggravated in the afternoon.
- Sour taste in mouth = plug like sensation in throat.
- Heaviness of abdomen aggravated in afternoon.
- Heartburn aggravation towards afternoon, evening.
- Hunger, but can't eat much followed by pain around the navel region.
- Ameliorated before & after voiding of stool.
- Burning of anus.
- Stool: Regular: Semi-solid stool. White mucus in stool.
- Urine: Frequent urination; burning sensation in urethra after micturition.
- Appetite: Decreased
- Thirst: Average.
- Chilly patient
- Sweat all over the body.
- Heals ok.
- Sleep: Good.
- Desires: Bitter (++), vegetables, fish, warm food
- Mind: Mild; Silent – habit; Wants to be alone; Cannot tolerate blood letting. Mental worry. No confidence. Plans everything ahead.
- Past History - Nothing particular.
- Family History – Father – rheumatism.

Investigations Carried Out Before/After Dr. Banerjea's Treatment

13th Jul'88: Barium meal X-ray stomach & duodenum: Remark:- Chronic duodenal ulcer.

1st Nov'89: Barium meal X-ray Stomach & duodenum: Remark:- Nothing Abnormal Detected.

Barium meal report of Mr. M. M, Duodenal ulcer, before treatment of Dr. Banerjea

Barium meal report after 14 months of treatment

Gastro-Intestinal (G.I.) Diseases – Cured Cases

CASE ANALYSIS, MIASMATIC DIAGNOSIS AND FINAL PRESCRIPTION

Miasmatic Analysis

- Distention of abdomen from gas: Psora.
- Aching pains: Psora.
- Acidity: Psora.
- Sour taste in mouth: Psora.
- Plug-like sensation in throat: Syco-Psoric.
- Heaviness of abdomen with occasional distention: Psora.
- Heartburn: Psora.
- Hunger – satisfied easily: Psora.
- Burning of anus – Syphilitic.
- Stool with mucus: Sycotic.
- Urine: Frequent urination: Sycosis; burning sensation in urethra after micturition: Syphilis.
- Poor appetite: Psora.
- Desire: warm food: Sycosis.
- Mind: Mild; Silent – habit: Psora; wants to be alone: Psora- syphilitic; cannot tolerate blood letting: Psora; mental worry: Psora; No confidence: Psora; Plans everything ahead: Sycotic.

It's a mixed miasmatic case with Psora-Sycotic preponderance.

Reasons for Prescription

- Pain in epigastric region = aggravated in empty stomach
- Ameliorated after eating.
- Sour taste in mouth = plug like sensation in throat; Acidity agg. in the afternoon.
- Heaviness of abdomen aggravated in afternoon.
- Heartburn: aggravation towards afternoon, evening.
- Hunger, but can't eat much, followed by pain.
- Chilly patient
- Desire: Warm food

Mind: Mild; Silent – habit; Wants to be alone; Cannot tolerate blood letting. Mental worry. No confidence. Plans everything ahead.

The miasmatic analysis of Lycopodium is Psora +++, Sycosis +++, Syphilis ++, Tubercular +++.

Lycopodium covers the case miasmatically as well.

Final Prescription and Remedy Reaction

The case was started with Lycopodium 200 C, a good potency for gastrointestinal complaints and taking into account the energy of the patient. Unfortunately a detailed prescription chart is not available for this particular case, however the patient was cured of his duodenal ulcer in just over a year, as shown by the Barium meal X-rays.

In my experience, Lycopodium which is prepared from "moss", which survived on the face of the planet for millions of years; therefore according to the Doctrine of Signature, Lycopodium is one of our longest acting medicine, meaning after a dose of Lycopodium, you can safely and surely wait for a very long time. I have waited even over 2 years after one single dose of Lycopodium 200 C and saw the patient was still improving under the action of the original dose.

Authenticity of Cure

CD Reference: GA002-DUODENAL ULCER-MM

Gastro-Intestinal (G.I.) Diseases – Cured Cases

3. A CASE OF CHOLELITHIASIS (GALL BLADDER STONE) : MR. S.S.

Case No. GA003

26 year-old unmarried male.

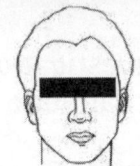

Photo of the patient, Mr. S.S.

Presenting Complaints

- Severe pain felt in abdomen on 21st February 1991 night and vomiting occurred the next morning.
- Then jaundice set in.
- This accompanied with fever 103°F for 6 days.
- Vomiting occurred occasionally after food.
- Went to Dr. Chakraborty – Suspected stone in gall bladder.
- USG abdomen report → A chain of gall stones detected; advised to go for surgery; but the patient declined.
- He decided to try homoeopathy, and came to me for treatment.
- Urine: Natural colour, 7 to 8 times.
- Skin Disease: Dry rash on finger. Itchy.
- History of ringworm in groin applied B.Tex ointment.
- Irritable temper.
- Silent habit.
- Absent minded, loner, introvert.
- Desire to be neat and clean. Courteous, self disciplined.
- Does everything in a hurry.
- Very active.
- Fear of dogs and ghosts.
- Suffered with Chickenpox at 20 years of age.
- Suffered with measles at the age of 2 years.
- Catches cold easily.
- Hot patient.
- Desires: Sweet++, salty+, bitter+, milk+, potato+, vegetables and spinach+, fish+, meat/chicken++, egg+, rich, spicy and fat food+; cold food++, cold drinks+, ice cream+.
- Thirsty.

- Appetite: Large, but cannot eat much.
- Bowels: More towards constipation.
- Sleep: Average.

Investigations Carried Out Before/After Dr. Banerjea's Treatment

5th Mar'91: Ultra Sonography upper abdomen:- Remark:- Cholecystitis and calculi seen in gall bladder and associated pancreatitis.

24th Feb'93: Ultra Sonography Upper abdomen. Remark:- Gall Bladder lumen is clear. NAD (Nothing Abnormal is Detected).

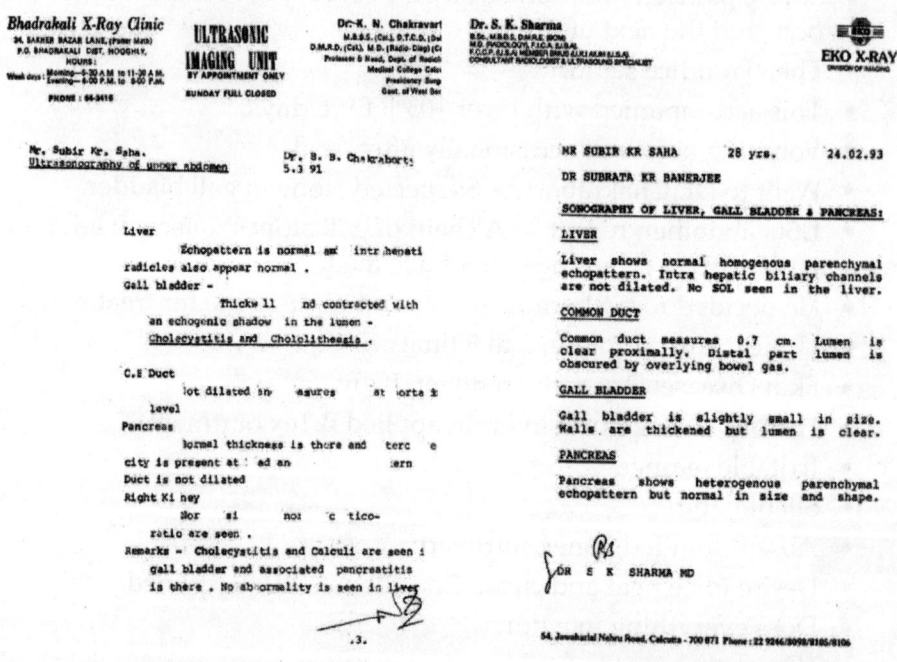

Sonography report of Mr. S.S., Cholecystitis and Calculi, before treatment of Dr. Banerjea

Sonographic report, after 23 months of treatment

CASE ANALYSIS, MIASMATIC DIAGNOSIS AND FINAL PRESCRIPTION

Cholelithiasis is a very common ailment with which a patient comes to a Homoeopath! I say very clearly to my patients at the outset as follows:-

- It is a surgical problem but Homoeopathy can cure about 50% to 60% of these cases.

- I will generally treat for about a year and do a repeat ultra-sonogram. If I find that the stones are either reducing in their size or have broken into pieces, then the Homoeopathic prognosis is good.
- If there is no change during this period, as revealed in the follow-up ultra-sonogram then I advise the patient to go for surgery.
- During the treatment I ensure diet restriction e.g. fat free diet (as far as possible and practicable).

Miasmatic Analysis

- Suffering from jaundice: Sycotic.
- USG abdomen report → Gall stones: Sycotic.
- Skin Disease: Skin disease on finger. Dry, itchy: Psora.
- History of Ringworm: Tubercular.
- Irritable temper: Sycotic.
- Silent habit: Psora.
- Absent minded: Sycotic;
- Loner, introvert: Psora-Syphilitic.
- Does everything in a hurry: Sycotic.
- Very active: Sycotic.
- Fear of dogs and ghost: Psora-Tubercular.
- Catches cold easily: Tubercular.
- Desires: Sweet: Psora.
- Mixed miasmatic case with Sycotic preponderance.

Final Prescription Made on the Basis of

- Suffering from jaundice; so liver is the weakest area here through which body manifests its symptoms. I give quite a bit of emphasis on weakest link in the body and sphere of action of the corresponding medicine. In Lycopodium, as we know, the liver is one of the main spheres of action.
- USG abdomen report → A chain of gall stones detected. Lycopodium being a Tri-miasmatic medicine and also having preponderant action on gastro-biliary apparatus, will cover this area.
- Skin disease on finger. Dry itchy.
- History of Ringworm in groin, suppressed by ointments.
- Irritable temper.
- Silent habit.

- Absent minded.
- Catches cold easily.
- Desire: Sweet++.
- Large appetite but cannot eat much.
- Loner, introvert, courteous, self-disciplined.

The miasmatic analysis of Lycopodium is Psora +++, Sycosis +++, Syphilis ++, Tubercular +++.

Lycopodium covers the case miasmatically as well.

Final Prescription and Remedy Reaction

I started the case with **LYCOPODIUM, 200 C** on 27th March'91. I waited for 3 months and in this period the jaundice got better and the pain was under control with much milder attacks; but vomiting after slightest food continued. I repeated 200 C, but with the second dose of 200 C there was no further improvement; so I decided to go for 1M of Lycopodium. With 1M, vomiting came under control and the patient felt much relieved by it. Pain was much milder and much less frequent. I waited for 2 months and then repeated 1M another time. But felt a standstill status, and then went to 10M and with this dose the mental symptoms significantly improved, including the feeling of 'loner'. The skin rash also cleared and the pain was totally absent. I asked the patient to repeat the Ultra sonography and the result was very positive, all the stones had gone! Patient was completely cured of his gall stones in about 23 months, avoiding surgery.

Authenticity of Cure

CD Reference: GA003-CHOLECYSTITIS WITH CHOLELITHIASIS-SS

Gastro-Intestinal (G.I.) Diseases – Cured Cases

4. A CASE OF PEPTIC ULCER: MRS R.C.

Case No. GA004

Age   : 30 years as on 24th March, 1993
Weight : 57 kgs.

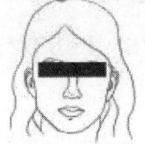

Photo of the patient, Mrs. R.C.

Presenting Complaints

- Stool: Regular but stool not clear. Frequent ineffectual urging.
- Discomfort felt in lower abdomen.
- Better by passing gas.
- Hard stool. Constipation;
- Required to strain during defecation.
- Stool with white mucus. Occasional pricking pain in upper abdomen.
- Loss of appetite.
- Acidity. More towards evening.
- Eructation, aggravated in the evening.
- Liver: sensitive to touch
- Indigestion: gas +++
- Debility, aggravation in the morning
- Backache: occipital to T12, pain aggravated by cold.
- Chilly patient.
- Desire: Egg+++, meat, sweet+, bitter, salty++, veg, warm food.
- Aversion: Sour, pungent, cold food.
- Thirst: Thirstless.
- Sleep: Sound sleep.
- Appetite: Decreased.
- Urine: Clear.
- Sweat: Average.
- Menses: Regular.
- Duration about 4 days.
- Mind: Indignation over trifles. Demanding (lacks confidence); very careful (++); safe person. Unable to decide (feels small)
- Past History: Measles, chickenpox.
- Family History: Mother – Rheumatism.

Investigations Carried Out Before/After Dr. Banerjea's Treatment

26th Feb'92: Barium meal stomach and Duodenum: Remark:- (1) Post bulbar peptic ulcer of duodenum; (2) Active duodenal ulcer; (3) Ascaris lumbricoides in small intestine.

2nd Jun'93: Gastroscopy:- Remark:- Stomach – Normal. Duodenum – Normal.

25th Jun'93: Faeces: Mucus + Occult Blood Test – ve, pus cell – occasional veg cell ++.

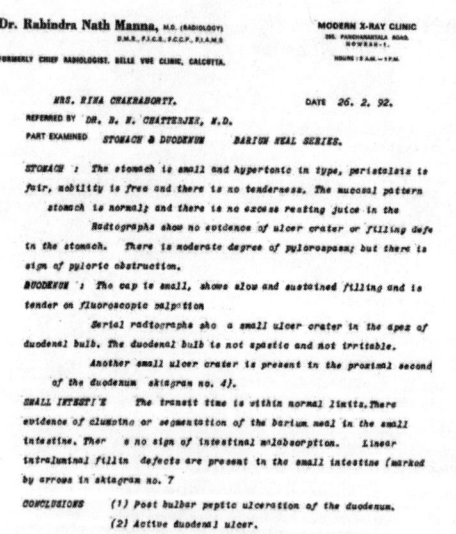

Barium meal report of Mrs. R.C., Peptic Ulcer, before treatment of Dr. Banerjea

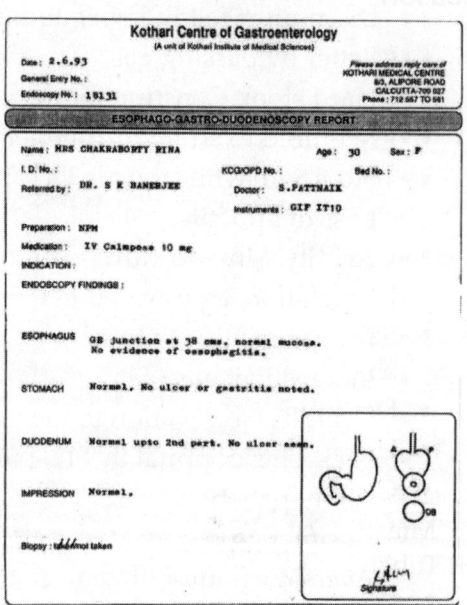

Oesophago-Gastro-Duodenoscopy report 3 months after treatment

CASE ANALYSIS, MIASMATIC DIAGNOSIS AND FINAL PRESCRIPTION

Miasmatic Analysis

- Constipation. Hard stool: Psora.
- Ineffectual urging for stool: Psora.
- Pricking pains: Sycotic.

- Distention of abdomen: Psora.
- Stool with mucus: Sycotic.
- Loss of appetite: Psora.
- Acidity: Psora.
- Aggravation from cold: Psora.
- Aversion to cold food: Psora.
- Mind: Lack of confidence: Psora-syphilitic.
- Very careful, safe person: Sycotic.

It's a mixed miasmatic case with Psora-Sycotic preponderance.

Reasons To Support The Prescription

- Constipation.
- Acidity, more towards evening.
- Eructations aggravate in evening.
- Temperament: Demanding (lacks confidence); safe person; very careful (++).
- Liver: sensitive to touch
- Physical → lethargy. Rectum → constipation
- Stomach → indigestion → gas +++. Discomfort felt in the lower abdomen.
- Debility aggravation in the morning
- Unable to decide (feels small).
- Chilly patient.

Miasmatic analysis of Lycopodium is Psora +++, Sycosis +++, Syphilis ++, Tubercular +++.

Lycopodium covers the case miasmatically as well.

Final Prescription and Remedy Reaction

LYCOPODIUM 200 C. The case was started with the 200C potency on the basis of the patient's vitality and also the digestive disorder being treated, which responds well to that potency. The patient improved in just over a year time as shown by the gastroscopy reports. Unfortunately a detailed prescription chart is not available for this case.

Authenticity of Cure:

CD Reference: GA004-PEPTIC ULCER-RC

5. A CASE OF HEPATOMEGALY: MR.R.M.

Case No. GA005

Age   : 25+ years as on 6th February, 1998.
Sex   : Male.
Height : 175 cm.
Weight : 60 kg.

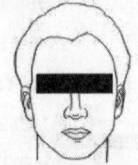
Photo of the patient, Mr. R.M.

Presenting Complaints

- Pain in upper right abdomen. Duration – 1 year. Causation – Jaundice. Pain aggravates on empty stomach, aggravation 3 hours after taking meal. Stitching pain with burning sensation on the part. Burning pain in the abdomen better cold food.
- Feels appetite in morning only, after taking something no appetite for the rest of the day.
- Duration -1 year. Causation - never been well since jaundice.
- Sleep -sound, but no freshness of mind and body in morning. Burning sensation in eyes, aggravates in morning.
- Stool – not clear → More in morning (quantity). Gradual loss of weight day by day.
- Pain in scapular region on both sides. Pain aggravates after loaded stomach and empty stomach also. Duration -2 years. Causation - gas.
- Desire open air. Desire cold food.
- Chilly patient.
- Mentally calm, amiable. Mild, timid; silent habit. Weeping mood.
- Fears failure
- Food desires:- Sweet++, Meat, Egg, Cold food++.
- Thirst: Less.
- Abdomen: Gas pains more on the right side; changeable or migratory in location.

Investigation Carried Out Before/After Dr. Banerjea's Treatment

27th Mar'98: Ultra Sonography upper abdomen:- Remark:- Hepatomegaly.

17th Sep' 98: Serum Bilirubin: 0.78 mg%.

2nd Apr'99: Ultra Sonography upper abdomen:- Remark:- Nothing Abnormal Detected.

Sonographic report of Mr. R.M., Hepatomegaly, before treatment of Dr. Banerjea

Sonographic report after 14 months after treatment

CASE ANALYSIS, MIASMATIC DIAGNOSIS AND FINAL PRESCRIPTION

Miasmatic Analysis

- Causation jaundice: Sycosis.
- Stitching pain: Sycosis; Burning sensation: Syphilitic.
- Pain aggravates on empty stomach, aggravation 3 hours after taking meal: Psora.
- Empty feeling in the morning: Psora; lack of appetite rest of day: Psora.
- Burning sensation in eyes: Psora-syphilitic.

- Unrefreshing sleep: Syphilitic.
- Hepatomegaly (enlargement of liver): Sycotic.

It's a mixed miasmatic Syco-Psoric case.

Reasons for Prescription

- Stitching pains. Gas pains more on the right side; changeable or migratory in location.
- Unrefreshing sleep – wakes unrefreshed.
- Burning sensation in eyes.
- Mentally calm and amiable.
- Want of appetite.
- Desire - Cold food (++); Desire open air. Chilly patient.
- Weeping mood.
- Occasional burning pain in the abdomen better cold food.

Miasmatic breakdown of Pulsatilla is Psora ++, Sycosis +++, Syphilis +, Tubercular ++.

Pulsatilla covers the case miasmatically as well.

Remedy Reaction

This case was started with Pulsatilla 1M, the potency chosen on the basis of totality and the vitality of the patient. The case was finished with Pulsatilla 50M after just over a year's treatment.

Prescription Chart

Date	Report After Last Medicine/Prescription Done on the Basis of	Treatment
6th Feb'98	BP: 136/80 Desires - cold food, open air, calm, amiable.	Pulsatilla, 1M, 2 doses.
8th Apr'98	Better. Wait & watch. U.S.G. report – Liver enlarged (27/3/98).	Sac lac.
27th May'98	Was better 60.5 kg. Now stand still.	Pulsatilla 1M, 2 doses.
15th Jul'98	Heaviness of abdomen Gas ++	Pulsatilla 10M, 2 doses.

Gastro-Intestinal (G.I.) Diseases – Cured Cases

Date	Report After Last Medicine/Prescription Done on the Basis of	Treatment
19th Aug'98	Pain in upper abdomen better. Appetite – Nil. Acidity + gas = Rare. Stool – constipated, not clear. Thirst – normal. Sleep – normal Heavy sensation in right side of abdomen Malaise & weakness – profound. Burning abdomen aggravated on an empty stomach, ameliorated by cold food, cold drinks. Desire for cold water, cold food.	Sac lac.
23rd Sep'98	Pain in upper abdomen better, but slightly present. Pain on back (both sides). Acidity + gas aggravates after meal. Stool – clear, generally hard. Thirst – normal. Appetite – improved. Sleep – sound. Weakness aggravates in morning Occasional burning sensation in abdomen. Feels slightly better.	Sac lac.
28th Oct'98		Sac lac.
2nd Dec'98	Pain in right upper abdomen better. Back pain – ameliorated, pain on waist more. Pain aggravates if stool not clear. Gas aggravates 3 hours after meal. Stool – semi-solid – one a day. Thirst – normal. Appetite – less, occasional acidity. Sleep – sound.	Sac lac.
27th Jan'99	Pain in liver region better. Occasional acidity aggravated in afternoon. Stool – clear but Mucussy (occasional) Thirst – normal. Appetite – normal. Occasional burning at side of abdomen to back and sensation of heat in abdominal cavity. Slightly better after taking medicine. Pain, aggravates after exertion, acidity slightly relieved, but there is distension of abdomen.	Pulsatilla 10M, 1 dose.

Date	Report After Last Medicine/Prescription Done on the Basis of	Treatment
17th Mar'99	Stool – not clear – one in morning. Distension of abdomen due to accumulation of gas. Gas aggravates 3 hours after meal aggravates easily in morning, afternoon. Pain in epigastric region aggravates in afternoon. Thirst – normal. Desires – sweet. Sleep – Okay.	Sac lac.

7th Apr'99	Pain in abdomen ameliorated but occasional trifling pain is there.
	Occasional pain in back due to gas, aggravates in morning, ameliorates after stool. Flatus ameliorates.
	Burning in eyes.
	Stool - normal if takes bread.
	    - light yellow + acidic after taking rice.
	    - USG report: Better: Hepatomegaly Cured.
		Pulsatilla 50M, 2 doses.

Authenticity of Cure

CD Reference: GA005-HEPATOMEGALY-RM

Gastro–Intestinal (G.I.) Diseases – Cured Cases

6. A CASE OF FATTY LIVER: MR. C.M.

Case No. GA006

Age   : 32 on 2nd April, 1998.
Sex   : Male
Weight : 42.5kg.

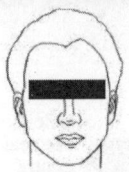

Photo of the patient, Mr. C.M.

Presenting Complaints

- Uneasy feeling left upper abdomen.
- Occasional mild pain - aggravates in afternoon aggravates when stool not clear.
- Had history of habit of taking rich, spicy food.
- Patient Never Been Well Since suffering Typhoid fever.
- Stool: Regular; not clear; occasional blackish colour; mucus in stool.
- Occasional distension of abdomen, better passing flatus.
- Urine: Okay.
- Gradual loss of body weight.
- Weakness ++.
- Appetite average.
- Thirsty.
- Sweating: Upper part of the body (+++).
- Sleep – good.
- Desire: Sweet +; salty; bitter ++; veg. & spinach;
- Luke warm food; cold drinks.
- Aversion to sour, pungent.
- Mind: Mild; silent habit; wants to be alone; fear of death.
- Occasional pain in backbone:- aggravated by jerking and from rest. Aggravated by lying. Touch aggravates. - ameliorated from motion.
- Thermal: Chilly Patient (++).

Investigations Carried Out After Dr. Banerjea's Treatment

13th Apr'98: Ultra Sonography upper abdomen: Remark:- Slightly enlarged size of liver with fatty changes in liver.

20th May'98: Total Protein: 7.8 gm%. Albumin 4.5, Globulin 3.3, Total Bilirubin 0.9.

Direct Bilirubin 0.5. SGPT 28, SGOT 26. Alkaline + Phosphate – 3.6

19th May'00: Ultra Sonography whole abdomen:- Remark:- Nothing Abnormal Detected.

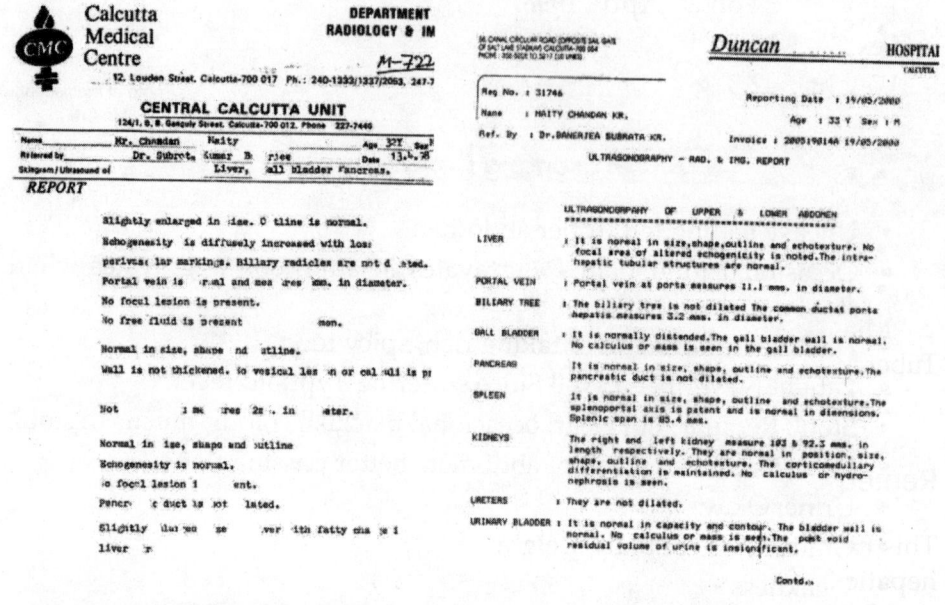

Sonographic report of Mr.C.M., Enlarged liver with fatty changes, before treatment

Sonographic report 24 months after treatment

CASE ANALYSIS, MIASMATIC DIAGNOSIS AND FINAL PRESCRIPTION

Miasmatic Analysis

- Stool: Occasional blackish colour: Syphilis; mucus in stool: Sycosis.
- Occasional distension of abdomen, better passing flatus: Psora.
- Weakness ++: Tubercular.
- Desire: Sweet: Psora; Salty: Syco-tubercular; Luke warm food: Sycosis; Cold drinks: Syphilis.
- Mind: Mild; silent habit: Psora; wants to be alone: Psora; fear of death: Psora.
- Occasional pain in backbone: - aggravated by movement: Syphilis; ameliorated by lying: Psora.

It is a mixed miasmatic case and as there is preponderance of Psora and Syphilis therefore Tubercular component is present in the surface.

Reasoning for Prescription

- Sweating on upper part of body accompanied by weakness and backache. Clarke says that "when there is a combination of "sweat, backache and weakness," the three, according to Farrington, constitute a grand characteristic."
- Occasional pain in backbone: - aggravated by jerking and from rest. Aggravated by lying. Touch aggravates. - ameliorated from motion.
- Fear of death (incurable diseases).
- Desire for sweets. Bloating and gastric disorders.

Miasmatic breakdown of Kali carb. is Psora++, Sycosis ++, Syphilis +, Tubercular +++.

Kali Carb covers the Psora-Tubercular aspect of the case.

Remedy Reaction

This case was started with Kali carb. 200C, which is a good potency in hepatic complaints of this nature and gastro-intestinal problems. The case was finished after just over 24 months of treatment.

I started the case with Typhoidinum to remove any block. If there is a clear aetiology or never been well since (NBWS), I prescribe the corresponding nosodes or the related medicine which is capable of clearing such block either in the beginning or as an intercurrent during the course of treatment. If there is a clear totality for a polychrest at the beginning, I will obviously prescribe the polychrest. In my experience there might be 60% - 80% improvement with the polychrest in ascending potencies and thereafter there will be a standstill status. At that stage you need to prescribe as an intercurrent to remove the block, e.g., Typhodinum for NBWS Typhoid; Streptococcin for NBWS Streptococcal infection; Morbillinum for NBWS Measles; Carcinosin for NBWS Diabetes; Meningococcinum for NBWS Meningitis; Influenzinum for NBWS Influenza; Pertussin for NBWS Whooping cough; Pneumococcin for NBWS Pneumonia etc.

After removing the block with Typhoidinum I prescribed Kali Carb on the basis of the totality of symptoms.

Prescription Chart

Date	Report after Last Medicine	Prescription Done on the Basis of Treatment
2nd Apr'98	42.5 kg. Never been well since Typhoid. To remove the bad effects of Typhoid fever.	Typhoidinum. 200, 2 doses in water. 1M, 1 dose in water.
16th May'98	No appreciable change. The ravages of the typhoid: to remove. X-ray report reveals Slightly enlarged size of liver with fatty changes in liver.	Typhoidinum. 1M, 2 doses in water. 10 M, 1 dose in water.
27th Jun'98	No appreciable change. Change in the plan of treatment.	Kali carb., 200, 2 doses in water.
15th Jul'98	43.5 kg. Weight gain. Slight improvement in feelings Thirst ++. Heaviness at side of abdomen aggravates 4 p.m. – 8 p.m. Burning in abdomen occasionally, Stool: Semi-solid, 2/3 times/day. Better 1st 15 days of last medicine taking. Now aggravated. Stool is not clear. Ineffectual desire.	Sac lac.
17th Aug'98	Fever started and after that every 3-4 days alternate fever came. Last fever arose 14th Aug'98, 15th Aug'98, and 16th Aug'98. Fever comes with chill and every time stays at 1030 F with profuse perspiration. Fever with great violence and with acute vertex headache. Last month this fever paroxysm was coming from every 2/3 days alternately. Weakness, fever comes from 2-3 p.m. Duration 3 hr. Chill – Fever – Perspiration. Thirst - ++. Stool with pinworms. Asked the patient to wait till the fever went and then take the medicine.	Kali carb. 1M, 2 doses
22nd Oct'98	Doing better	Sac Lac
5th Mar'99	Patient came back after 6 months, as was absolutely fine; no pain; no discomfort.	Sac Lac
6th Sep'99	Was better but now slight discomfort in abdomen	Kali Carbonica 10M, 1 dose
12th Mar'00	Patient came back again after 6 months, as was absolutely fine.	Sac Lac
22nd May'00	Came back with USG Report. Cured.	

Authenticity of Cure

CD Reference: GA006-FATTY CHANGE IN LIVER-CM

7. A CASE OF CHOLELITHIASIS: MRS. R.K.

Case No. GA007

28 year-old lady as on 27th June, 1994
Height – 5 feet 4 inches.

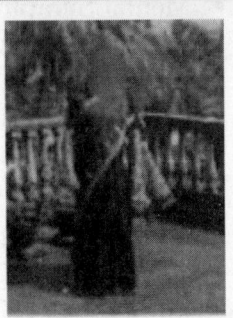

Photo of the patient, Mrs. R.K.

Presenting Complaints

- Pain in left hypochondrium and right iliac fossa.
- Aggravates after eating (especially taking fried and sour foods). Better by Allopathic medicine.
- Acidity → Sour taste in mouth.
- Wind formation in upper abdomen. Aggravates on empty stomach. Better by passing flatus.
- History of pain in abdomen → 4 months back → Pain comes suddenly. Better by taking allopathic tablets.
- Previous treatment – allopathy.
- Slight whitish tongue.
- Throat pain aggravates on taking cold, ameliorated by gurgling.
- Profuse sweating on face and back. No bad odour.
- Urine: Occasionally yellow in colour.
- Stool: Regular occasional loose stool. No mucus in stool.
- Menses: Time: regular. Colour: pale. Duration: 4 days.
- Vertigo: Better by lying down.
- Abdominal gas++. No eructation.
- Desire for company.
- Does everything in a hurry.
- Patient cries when reprimanded.
- Fear: Darkness, Snakes.
- Desire: Sour++, pungent and hot+, salty+++, potato+, vegetables and spinach+, fish++, egg+, rich spicy and fat food+, warm food+, cold drinks+
- Aversion to bitter.

- Thirsty.
- Mental Symptoms: Calm and quiet. Talkative. Anxious (++) about the disease and especially for surgery (doctor advised to do so). Sluggish, aversion to work or any exertion.
- Thermal: Chilly patient.
- ECC (Easily Catches Cold): Loves fresh air but catches cold easily.
- Sleep: average.
- Appetite: Good.

Investigations Carried Out Before/After Dr. Banerjea's Treatment

21st Jun'94: Ultra Sonography upper abdomen: Remark:- Gall Bladder with multiple calculi – cholelithiasis. Others normal. Clinical findings: - Cholelithiasis.

3rd May'95: Ultra Sonography upper abdomen: Remark: - Gall Bladder: - neither calculus shadow nor any intrinsic lesion noted. Liver – Enlarged in size (16.9 cm).

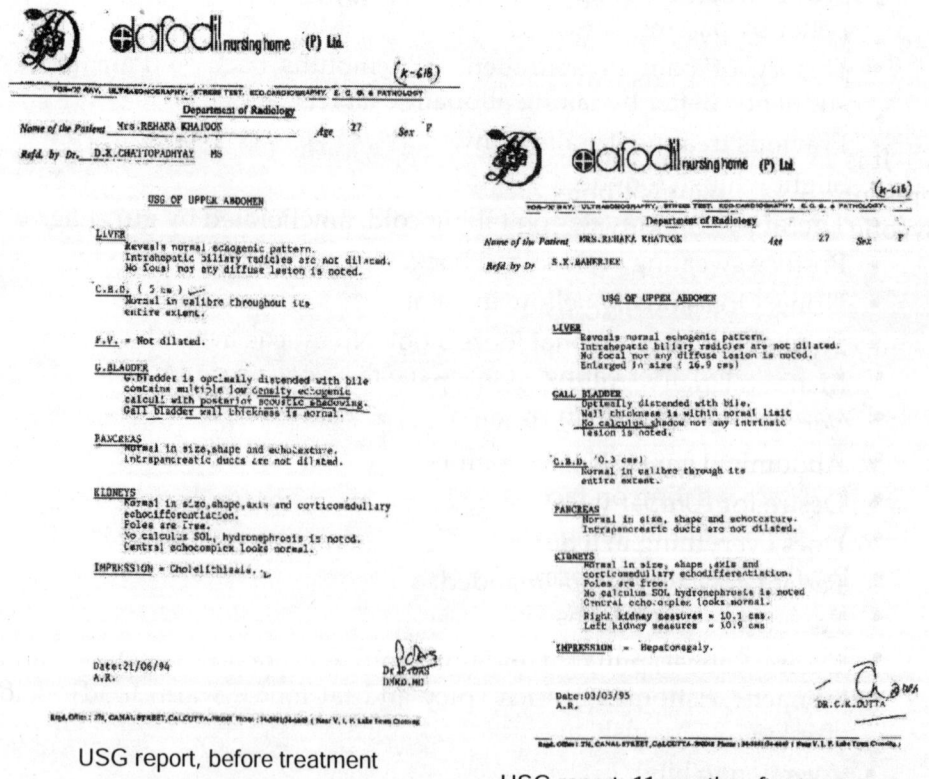

USG report, before treatment

USG report, 11 months after treatment

Gastro–Intestinal (G.I.) Diseases – Cured Cases

CASE ANALYSIS, MIASMATIC DIAGNOSIS AND FINAL PRESCRIPTION

This case is another example about how homoeopathy can cure even an apparently surgical problem, like Cholelithiasis (stone in the gall bladder). The concerned patient was not interested in undergoing surgery, therefore, she came to me to be treated homoeopathically and our beautiful art and science had the desired effect!

Miasmatic Analysis

- Acidity → Sour taste in mouth: Psora.
- Wind formation in upper abdomen: Psora.
- Vertigo: Better by lying down: Psora.
- Profuse sweating: Sycosis.
- Tongue, white coating: Tubercular.
- Desires: Salty: Syco-tubercular. Sour: Psora-syphilitic.
- Does everything in a hurry: Sycosis.
- Fear: Darkness, Snakes: Psora.
- Mind: (a) Calm and quiet: Psora. (b) Talkative: Sycosis. (c) Anxious: Psora. (d) Sluggish, aversion to work or any exertion: Psora.
- Cholelithiasis: Stone in the Gall Bladder: Sycosis.

It is a mixed miasmatic case with Psora-Sycotic preponderance. As the presenting complaint is Cholelithiasis therefore the formation of stone is a sycotic manifestation for which sycotic miasm is present in the surface.

Final Prescription Made on the Basis of

- Aggravation after eating.
- Acidity → Sour taste in mouth.
- Throat pain aggravates on taking cold, ameliorated by gurgling.
- Profuse sweating on face and back. No bad odour.
- Vertigo: Better by lying down.
- Patient cries when reprimanded.
- Fears: darkness, snakes.
- Desires: Sour++, salty+++, potato+, egg+, cold drinks+
- Mental Symptoms: (a) Calm and quiet. (b) Anxious(++) about the disease. (c) Sluggish, aversion to work or any exertion.

- Chilly patient but desires fresh open air and consequently catches cold easily.
- Syco-Psoric Case.

The miasmatic analysis of Calc Carb. is Psora +++, Sycosis +++, Syphilis ++, Tubercular +++.

Calcarea Carb covers the case miasmatically as well.

Final Prescription

CALCAREA CARB, 1 M/2: 1 globule (No. 10 : poppy seed size) in sugar of milk sachet, asked the patient to dissolve the powder in half or one litre of pure water and sip it slowly throughout the day, save a little at the bottom, top it up next morning, keep sipping throughout the next day. Generally I give instruction to my patient to dilute the medicated water (top it up with water) as many times as s/he likes. Continue like this for 7 days. Then 7 days without medicine. Followed by another dose to be shaken and sipped for 7 days.

Remedy Reaction

I started this case with Calc. Carb. 1M on the basis of the clear totality and the patient's vitality. The patient improved and in less than a year, the follow-up Sonography report was normal. So, in this case of gall bladder stone, Homoeopathy was capable of breaking the stone and clearing it up; which has been proved and confirmed by the follow-up Ultra-Sonography.

Prescription Chart

Date	Prescription Done on the Basis of	Treatment
27th Jun'94	Considering the appearance and reasoning for prescription has already been given above.	Calc Carb, 1M, 2 doses. For Emergency S.O.S: Cholesterinum 6, 3 doses
19th Jul'94	Was better. Burning oesophagitis. Sensation of something crawling upwards. Appetite: Improved. Pain in abdomen better. Nausea.	Sac lac.

Gastro–Intestinal (G.I.) Diseases – Cured Cases

Date	Prescription Done on the Basis of	Treatment
30th Aug'94	Pain in abdomen better Burning oesophagitis better, Appetite increased. Stool regular. Thirst ++. Nausea better. Sourness in the throat started after injury by a fish bone. Tonsils inflamed.	Sac lac.
25th Oct'94	Pain in upper (L) abdomen. Acidity heartburn. Flatulence. Frequent urination. Yellowish. Giddiness. Weak. Profuse sweat over entire body.	Calc.Carb., 1M, 2 doses.
15th Nov'94	Doing better dry cough aggravates in dry, cold wind, in morning, running nose at night.	Sac lac.
20th Dec'94	Coryza – watery aggravates in morning; thin, scanty whitish expectoration aggravates in morning.	Sac lac.
31st Jan'95		Sac lac.
27th Feb'95	Pain in right iliac region ameliorated after stool, heaviness of the lower abdomen.	Sac lac
11th Apr'95	Gall stone colic. Constipated stool, regular, not clear, fruitless urging occasionally. Offensive. Intolerance of heat. Urine – clear. Appetite – good. Intense thirst. Desires – Fish, egg, sour, pungent; aversion to bitter. Profuse sweat on whole body.	Calc Carb 10 M, 2 doses.
12th May'95	Gall Bladder colic. Wind aggravates after eating; hepatomegaly. USG: no calculi in gall bladder (3rd May'95).	Sac lac.
16th Jun'95		Sac lac.
2nd Aug'95	Now okay.	Sac lac.
6th Sep'95	Urine frequent, yellowish, no odour. Occasional Vertigo. Profuse sweat. Alopecia. Stool clean menses – clear.	Sac lac.
7th Oct'95	Vertigo suddenly, No gall stone colic. Urine frequent, slightly yellow. Menses 2 days, scanty, Gas better passing of flatus, by belching rolling of wind, stool regular, appetite good. Thirst normal. Profuse sweating from head to foot.	Sac lac.
5th Dec'95	Indigestion better. Gas stitches in abdomen (occasional).	Sac lac.
16th Jan'96	Occasional loose motion. Pain in lower abdomen ameliorated after urination. Urine frequent yellowish. Appetite good. Thirst normal. Stool clear.	Sac lac
27th Feb'96	Great liability to take cold.	Sac lac.

Date	Prescription Done on the Basis of	Treatment
16th Apr'96	Itching in various parts of body. Bleeds on scratching. Took allopathic medicine. Gas → chest pain, stool clear. Thick yellow, tenacious coryza sweat+++ Desires – egg, hot patient.	Sac lac.
22nd Jul'96	Pain in epigastrium. Gas rumbling. Appetite □.	Calc Carb, 50 M/1
10th Aug'96	Now patient is okay, no pain. Acidity aggravates after eating, ameliorates drinking water. Thirst++, Appetite+, Sleep+. Sweat profuse.	Sac lac.
30th Sep'96	Now acidity aggravates after eating, ameliorated by eructation. Sour eructation. No other problems.	Sac lac.
30th Oct'96	Patient feels better. Now gas and acidity aggravate half an hour after eating. Ameliorated by antacid. Stool normal. Thirst+, Appetite+, Sleep+.	Calc. Carb, 50M, 1 dose.
10th Dec'96	Was better now aggravated. Moving sensation in upper part of abdomen (L+), loss of appetite. Common cold + stoppage of nose. Thirst+, sleep+	Calc Carb, CM, 2 doses
11th Feb'97	Patient as a whole feels better occasional gas in whole abdomen aggravated morning ameliorated drinking water. Thirst++, Appetite+, Sleep+, Stool normal.	Sac lac.
16th Apr'97	Had pain in lower abdomen around the waist and patient took allopathic medicine. Heaviness in bladder, frequent urging to urinate. Excessive sweating from waist to feet (running down). Rumbling in abdomen, loose stool alternates with hard stool. Thirst+ Appetite, Sleep+, Sweat+.	Sac lac.

Authenticity of Cure

CD Reference: GA007-CHOLELITHIASIS-RK

8. A CASE OF CHOLECYSTITIS WITH THICKENED WALL OF GALL BLADDER : MISS B.C.

Case No. GA008

20 year-old girl (as on 27th March, 1998)
Height: 5 ft. 1½ inches

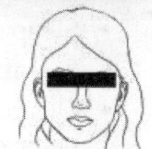

Photo of the patient, Miss. B.C.

Presenting Complaints

- Acidity and gas in abdomen, duration – 7 months. Causation – Had an attack of Jaundice in May 1996. → abdominal complaints started after that. Gas aggravates at night – 7 p.m.
- Acidity → obstruction felt in throat.
- Gas ameliorates after taking antacid.
- Indigestion aggravated by spicy and oily food.
- Pain in left lower abdomen.
- Generally constipated, but occasional diarrhoea, especially after long time of constipation. Stool: Not clear; hard stool; bad odour; no mucus.
- Duration – since childhood (constipation).
- Headache caused by excessive accumulation of gas. Also due to formation of gas → breathing trouble.
- Sick headache (with vomiting). Duration – 2 years. Causation – Mental work. Heat of sun, after board work, studies.
- Vertigo aggravated by accumulation of gas.
- Heavy sensation in abdomen and chest. Rumbling sound in abdomen.
- Pain around umbilicus.
- Backache aggravated by rest.
- Blocking sensation in throat, aggravated by gas.
- Catches cold easily. Duration – since childhood. Occasional dry cough with irritation in throat.
- Worm infestation (pinworms).
- In July, 1995 – Appendicectomy was done.
- Urine: Okay.
- Menses: Okay. Started at 11 years of age, now less. Delayed menses (5 – 6 days). Leucorrhoea: Slight white discharge.
- Appetite: Poor.

- Thirsty.
- Chilly Patient++.
- Heals: Okay.
- Sleep – good.
- Sweat: More on palms, armpits.
- Desire: Pungent+++, salty++, salt++, sour+, vegetable and spinach, eggs, cold food, cold drinks.
- Aversion to sweet, bitter.
- Mind: Mild, talkative, absent minded; desires company; patient cries when reprimanded; sympathetic; weepy mood.
- Fears: Ghosts; cockroaches++, thunderstorm.
- Skin: Allergy aggravates after taking brinjal (aubergine). Aggravated after taking flesh of tortoise.
- Past history of diseases: suffered before : Measles, jaundice, appendicitis.
- A case of Cholecystitis with thick walled gall bladder.

Investigations Carried Out Before/After Dr. Banerjea's Treatment

31st Dec'97: Ultra Sonography whole abdomen:- Remark:- Thick walled contracted gall bladder, no calculi.

30th Jan'99: Ultra Sonography Abdomen: Remark:- Normal wall thickness, no sonographically detected abnormality noted.

CASE ANALYSIS, MIASMATIC DIAGNOSIS AND FINAL PRESCRIPTION

This case is another good example of how Classical Homoeopathy can take care of some of the pathological changes and here the thickened gall bladder has been reversed to normal.

Miasmatic Analysis

- Acidity: Psora.
- Constipated: Psora.
- Vertigo aggravated by accumulation of gas: Psora.
- Headache with sun: Psora.

Gastro-Intestinal (G.I.) Diseases – Cured Cases

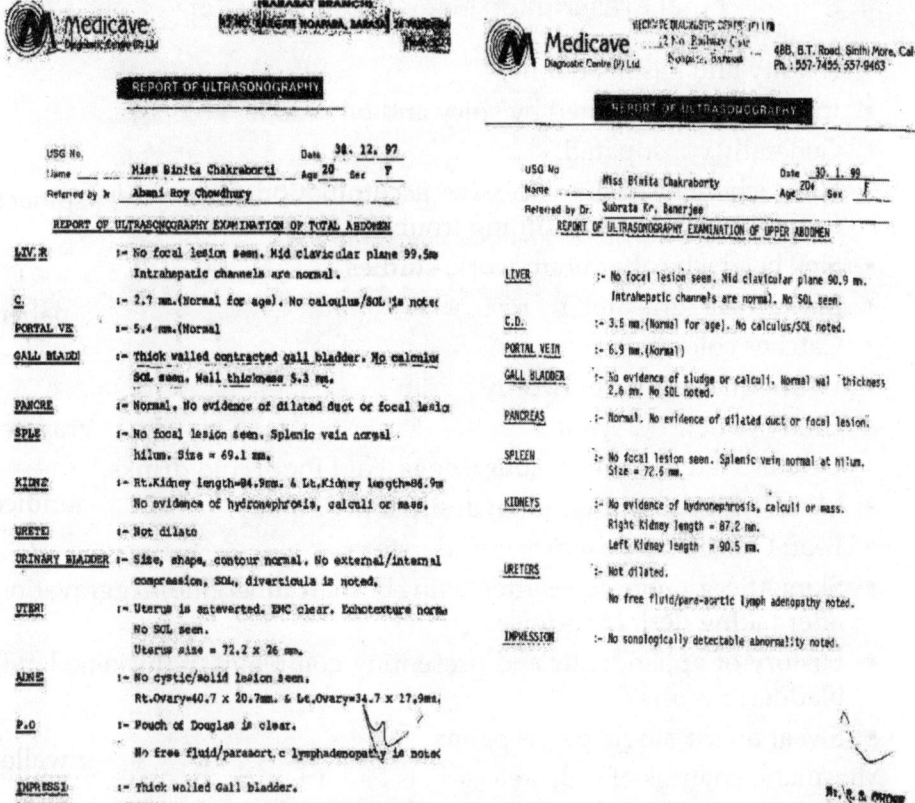

Sonography report of Miss B.C., before treatment.

Sonography report 10 months after treatment.

- Heavy sensation in abdomen and chest: Psora.
- Catches cold easily: Psora-Tubercular.
- Occasional dry cough with irritation in throat: Psora-Tubercular.
- Worm infestation (Pinworms): Tubercular.
- Appetite poor: Psora.
- Desires: Pungent: Sycosis; Salty ++, Salt ++: Syco-Tubercular.
- Mind: (a) Talkative: Sycosis. (b) Absent minded: Sycosis. (c) Weepy mood: Psora-Sycotic.
- Fear: Ghosts, cockroaches++, and thunderstorm : Psora.
- Skin: Allergy: Tubercular.

This is a mixed miasmatic case with Psora-Sycotic preponderance. Thickening of the wall of the gall bladder is Sycotic as excess deposition therefore Sycotic miasm is in the surface.

Final Prescription Made on the Basis of

- Acidity and gas in abdomen
- Indigestion aggravated by spicy and oily food.
- Generally constipated.
- Headache caused by excessive accumulation of gas. Also due to formation of gas → breathing trouble.
- Sick headache after brain work, studies.
- Backache aggravated by rest.
- Catches cold easily.
- Worm infestation (pinworms).
- Chilly Patient++.
- Desires: Salty++, salt++, sour+, eggs, cold food, cold drinks.
- Mind: Mild, absent minded; desire for company;
- Fear: Ghost; cockroach++, thunderstorm.
- Skin: Allergy aggravates after taking brinjal (aubergine). Aggravation after taking flesh of tortoise.
- History of appendicitis and presenting complaint of thickened gall bladder: Sycosis.
- Sweat on the single parts--palms.

Miasmatic analysis of Calcarea carb. is Psora +++, Sycosis +++, Syphilis ++, Tubercular +++.

Calcarea Carb is a Tri-Miasmatic medicine and accordingly it will cover the case miasmatically as well.

Final Prescription

CALCAREA CARB, 200C, 2 doses: 1 globule in sugar of milk sachet dissolved in pure water and sipped for 10 days. Then 10 days of no medicine, followed by another dose to be shaken and sipped for 10 days.

Remedy Reaction

This case was started with Calc. Carb 200C (based on the condition being treated and the good vitality of the patient) and finished with 50M; the patient improved and in just over a years time. The follow-up sonography report was normal. So, in this case of gall bladder thickening, Homoeopathy was capable of acting on the pathological gall bladder and bringing that back to normal, which has been proved and confirmed by the follow-up ultra-sonography

Prescription Chart

Date	Prescription Done on the Basis of	Treatment
27th Mar'98	Reasoning outlined above.	Calc. carb, 200C, 2 doses.
22nd May'98		Sac lac.
10th Jul'98	Eructation, gas, acidity. Pain in neck.	Calc carb, 200C, 2 doses.
14th Aug'98	Presenting complaints: (1) Stool not clear; (2) Eructation ameliorates; (3) Acidity, (4) Headache occasional burning abdomen.	Sac lac.
18th Sep'98		Sac lac.
28th Oct'98	Dropped a potency to go deeper and "clear the soil", 200 not acting sufficiently.	Calc. carb., 30C, 2 doses → 200/1
9th Dec'98	Gas +. Acidity better. Heavy sensation in head. Stool – one a day not clear. Thirst – Medium. Appetite – Normal. Sleep – sound.	Sac lac.
1st Feb'99	Gas and acidity aggravate, stool → constipated. Pain in head as before with heaviness in sleep → sound. Ultrasonography of abdomen done on 30th Jan'99: No abnormality noted.	Calc carb, 1M, 1 dose.
5th Apr'99	Gas +. Acidity was aggravated last menstrual period → scanty. Onions, weakness aggravated. Appetite less. Stool – almost regular but occasionally disturbed. USG (30/1/99) normal.	Sac lac.
4th Jun'99	Constipation was ameliorated, now aggravates. Stool – two or three day's interval. Pain in right upper abdomen aggravates 15 days. Thirst – More. Appetite – Normal. Gas +. Acidity was better now aggravates 1 month. Scanty – Menstruation → 30 day interval, leucorrhoea aggravates slightly.	Calc carb., 1 M, 2 doses.
24th Jul'99	Standstill	Calc. carb, 10 M, 2 doses.
14th Aug'99	Gas, acidity++. Stool – irregular, not clear 2 – 3 days interval; hard stool; sour smell. Headache – pain on forehead. Aggravates with journey - ameliorates after sleep.	Sac lac.

Date	Prescription Done on the Basis of	Treatment
11th Oct'99	Gas and acidity – slightly aggravated. Stool – not clear; 3 – 4 days interval. Headache ameliorated. Urine – okay. Menses: contractions felt in lower abdomen during periods. History of cold – sneezing+. Pain on extremities better by massage. Had History of exposure to cold. → cold since then. Appetite – average. Sleep – okay. Thirsty.	Sac lac.
2nd Dec'99	Was better, but again aggravates 7 – 8 days back. Gas + taking irregular food. Ameliorated by passing of flatus. Stool – clear. Leucorrhoea – before periods; thick; occasional contractions of lower abdomen. Memory – weak; Appetite – normal; Thirst – okay; Sleep: good.	Calc. carb., 50M, 2 doses.
3rd Feb'00	Weight : 49 kgs. Gas and acidity ameliorated. Stool – not clear; hard stool; constipation. Leucorrhoea aggravated before periods, thick. Anorexia; Thirst – average. Sleep – okay. Heaviness of abdomen. ameliorated by passing of flatus. History of cold with coryza → took Belladonna. Blood mixed with phlegm.	Sac lac.
27th Mar'00	Weight: 50 kgs. B.P.: 120/66. Was better but again aggravated. Occasional gas forms in abdomen. Acidity → obstruction felt in throat. Heaviness of head. Occasional eructation. Stool: irregular. Not clear; Appetite – less. Thirst – normal. Sleep – good.	Calc carb., 50M, 2 doses.
17th May'00	Weight: 51 kgs. Was better but again aggravated 3 – 4 days back. Gas + ameliorated by passing of flatus. Appetite – average. Sleep – okay. Stool – not clear; occasional mucus. Constant headache → mild pain on forehead and occipital region – since 1 week back.	Sac lac.
14th Jul'00	Had History of taking irregular food. Gas++ ameliorated by passing of flatus. Occasional pain right lower abdomen -- ameliorated passing of stool. Occasional acidity – plug like obstruction in throat. Ameliorated by drinking warm water. Stool: not clear; soft; no mucus. Headache better. Sleepless. Appetite: Poor.	Sac lac.
12th Sep'00	Occasional pain in right knee joints aggravated when going from sitting to standing. Stool: not clear. Acidity aggravates taking dahl (red lentil); bread, onion. History of cold --. Appetite: normal; Thirst: normal; Sleep: okay.	Sac lac.
28th Sep'00	Gas and acidity better. Stool: Regular; mucussy stool. Frontal headache ameliorated after sleep. Menses → scanty bleeding, stays 2½ days. Appetite – normal. Sleep good.	Sac lac.

Authenticity of Cure

CD Reference: GA008-CHOLECCYSTITIS WITH THICK WALL GALL BLADDER-BC

9. A CASE OF DUODENAL ULCER: MRS R.C.

Case No. GA009

Age   : 40 years as on 23rd May, 1992
Height : 5 ft. 1 inch
Weight : 43 kgs.

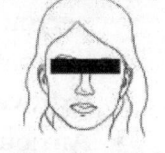
Photo of the patient, Mrs. R.C.

Presenting Complaints

- Patient complaints of an ulcer in the region of duodenum.
- Acid vomiting and regular acidity.
- Formation of gas regularly throughout the day and night.
- Leucorrhoea:
- Aggravates before and after menses.
- After micturition with backache.
- Discharge – scanty, thin white discharge. Occasional thin watery discharge.
- Menses: Time: Early, Duration about 7 days, Discharge: Bright red and black clots. No pain.
- Bearing down sensation.
- Piles.
- Slight swelling and itching of rectum improved after taking medicine.
- Weakness with palpitation, aggravation from hard work.
- Burning pains.
- Acute pain below the knee on both legs regularly.
- Allergy aggravates in winter season (appears once a year on body). Urticaria.
- Chilly patient.
- Desires: Fish+++, meat+, egg++, sweet+, salt++ (takes extra salt), bitter+++, veg, cold food+++, potato, fried+++.
- Aversion: pungent, warm food.
- Thirst: Average.
- Sleep: Disturbed sleep (during first part of night), sleeplessness.
- Appetite: Average.
- Stool: Regular. Occasionally not clear. Soft stool. Ineffectual urging. History of occasional dysentery.
- Urine: clear.

- Sweat: Profuse perspiration throughout the body, aggravates in summer. Offensive odour.
- Mind: Angry, irritable, talkative, desire for company, memory weak, nervous, sensitive, restless.
- Sympathetic.
- Extrovert, outgoing, dynamic, expressive.
- Anxious and sensitive, company >
- Fears: Disease & death, thunder.
- Startles easily.
- Past History: Typhoid, skin disease, mumps, chicken pox.
- Family History: Mother – Rheumatism and plies.

Investigations Carried Out Before/After Dr. Banerjea's Treatment

21st Oct'89: Barium meal – Stomach, duodenum: Remark:- Result strongly suggestive of an ulcer or erosion in the region of the duodenal bulb.

26th Feb'92: Barium meal – Stomach, duodenum: Remark:- Post bulbar peptic ulceration of duodenum. Active duodenal ulcer.

5th Jan'93: Barium meal – Stomach duodenum: Remark:- Oesophagus, stomach normal. Duodenum shows evidence of duodenitis.

CASE ANALYSIS, MIASMATIC DIAGNOSIS AND FINAL PRESCRIPTION

Miasmatic Analysis

- Leucorrhoea: Aggravates before and after menses: Tubercular.
- Scanty: Psora.
- Occasionally watery discharge: Tubercular.
- Menses: Discharge: Bright red and black clots: Tubercular.
- Piles with itching of rectum: Psora – sycotic.
- Occasional acidity: Psora.
- Urticaria: Tubercular.
- Desires: Salt++ (takes extra salt), cold food+++: Syco-tubercular.
- Ineffectual urging for stool: Psora.
- History of occasional dysentery: Syphilis.

Gastro-Intestinal (G.I.) Diseases – Cured Cases

MANISHA X-RAY CLINIC
P-10B, C. I. T. ROAD, CALCUTTA-700 014
FACILITIES FOR PORTABLE X-RAY AVAILABLE

Mrs. Rina Chatterjee
35 Years
Date: 21.10.89

Part Examined: Barium meal of stomach & duodenum
Ref. by Dr.: B. BHATTACHARJEE

STOMACH
It is normally sited.
Its tone, peristalsis and mucosal pattern are normal.
No ulcer crater nor any filling defect is shown.
Gastric emptying rate is normal.

DUODENUM
Mild coarsening of the mucosa is present.
Duodenal bulb and post bulbar region are spastic.
The width of the C-loop is normal.

CONCLUSION
Changes strongly suggestive of an ulcer or erosion in the region of the duodenal bulb are present though no ulcer could be demonstrated.

EKO DIAGNOSTIC
54, Jawaharlal Nehru Road,
Calcutta-700071
Ph. 22-9240/8098/8106/8106

Mrs. REENA CHATTERJEE   40 yrs.   05.01.93
Dr SUBRATA KR BANERJEA

RADIOLOGICAL EXAMINATION OF UPPER GASTRO INTESTINAL TRACT BY BARIUM MEAL AND DOUBLE CONTRAST STUDY :

OESOPHAGOGRAM
Passage of barium is unobstructed through the oesophagus. Oesophagus is normal in course and calibre. No evidence of hiatus hernia when examined in Trendelenburg's position.

STOMACH
Stomach is normal in size and shape. Both curvatures are smooth and no evidence of gastric ulcer. Pyloric end is contracting and relaxing well.

DUODENUM
Duodenal cap is normal in size and shape but shows coarse mucosal pattern – duodenitis. 'C' loop is not widened.

IMPRESSION
Oesophagus and stomach are normal. Duodenum shows evidence of duodenitis.

Barium meal, report of Mrs. R.C., before treatment.   Barium meal report, 8 months after treatment.

A DETAILS HISTORY REPORTS OF A CASE OF A PATIENT
NAME SMT. RINA CHATTERJEE.

Conditions of the Patient before the treatment of Homoeopathy under Dr.S.K. Banerjia. Perood: 10/89 to 7/92	Condition of the Patient after the treatment of Dr.S.K.Banerjia. Period : 5/92 to 1/93
1. Acid Vommitting	1. Not Present.
2. Regular Acidity	2. Feeling occasionally.
3. Ulcer in the region of duodenal bulb present	3. Duodenum shows evidence of duodenitis as on 05.01.93.
4. Formation of Gas heavily through out the day and night	4. Present to some extent.
5. Sleeplessness night	5. Now normal.
6. Dysentry through out the life.	6. Not present.
7. Soft stool nature through out the life	7. Still present.
8. Deep Black spot on both the side of nose.	8. Existing but gradually becoming fade.
9. Acute pain below the knee on both the legs regularly	9. Occasionally appearing.
10. Elergy appearing once in every year on the body.	10. Accordingly Elergy appeared during the year 1993 on 22.01.93.

Name : Smt. Rina Chatterjee.
Age : 40 years.

Patient's comments after treatment

- Sweat: Profuse perspiration throughout the body: Sycosis. Offensive odour: Syphilis.
- Mind: Irritable: Syco-psoric; Talkative: Sycosis; Memory weak: Psora; Restless (mentally): Psora.
- Extrovert: Sycosis.
- Anxious: Psora.
- Fears: Disease & death, thunder: Psora.

It is a mixed miasmatic case with Psora-Syphilo-Tubercular preponderance. As Tubercular miasm is a combination of Psora and Syphilis, therefore presence of Tubercular miasm will always include the presence Syphilitic miasm in the background.

Reasoning for Final Prescription

- Desires: Salt.
- Thirsty. Chilly patient.
- Desire: – Salt++ (takes extra salt), cold food+++.
- Fears thunder.
- Haemorrhagic. Last menstrual period: 10 days earlier, bleeding of menses continues.
- Burning/Pain.
- Nervous, sensitive, restless.
- Sympathetic.
- Extrovert, outgoing, dynamic, expressive.
- Anxious and sensitive, company >.
- Fears disease & death.
- Startles easily.

Miasmatic analysis of Phosphorus is Psora +++, Sycosis ++, Syphilis +++, Tubercular +++.

Phosphorus covers the case miasmatically as well.

Final Prescription

Phosphorus 30 C. A 30 C potency was used initially based on the patient's low vitality. Unfortunately a detailed prescription chart is not available for this case.

Remedy Reaction

Within 8 months of treatment (I started the case in May, 1992, which can be confirmed in the web picture under after treatment written by the patient) the patient was very much improved. The patient no longer showed signs of an ulcer although duodenitis was noted after a barium meal investigation. The patient was noticing acidity occasionally, but was no longer experiencing the acid vomiting. There was still gas formation but to a lesser extent than before. The patient no longer experienced symptoms of dysentery and sleep was much better.

Authenticity of Cure

CD Reference: GA009-DUODENAL ULCER-RD

10. A CASE OF DUODENAL ULCER: MR T.D.

Case No. GA010

30 year-old, Hindu male, brought to me first on 25th of November 1986 with the following complaints:

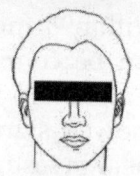

Photo of the patient, Mr. T.D

Present Complaints

- Pain abdomen: severe, excruciating: soon after taking milk products, followed by vomiting (++), which is more in the afternoon and evening. Patient is better after eating.
- Sensation of heaviness in abdomen especially in the morning with water brush.
- Total loss of appetite, fears after intake of milk (which the patient likes), pain will ensue again, which will end in vomiting.
- Whatever he eats, eructation of the same, even hours after eating, a little better by strolling in open air.
- < Morning and Evening. < From warm applications on abdomen. Wants cold showers. Pain abdomen > by pressure (though stomach is very sensitive to pressure). < From fatty foods (red meat, butter etc.), milk. Better after vomiting and stool. Likes consolation even during colic.
- Head – Frontal with sore eyes and blood vision. Congestive headache < in sun > by pressure, cold application.
- Eye - Occasional lachrymation with burning in the eyes > in open air.
- Ear - During childhood, had history of discharge per ear, cured by Homoeopathy.
- Nose - Cold settles in nose --> coryza with thick yellowish expectoration.
- Mouth - Bitter taste. Dryness of mouth.
- Tongue - Thick coating over the tongue.
- Lungs - Dry cough as a result from cold : < towards evening, lying > by sitting up.
- Chest - occasional chest pain > by lying over the affected area.
- Abdomen - (a) Distension of abdomen with heaviness. (b) Pressure in the abdomen with ineffectual desire for stool.
- Stomach - Extremely poor.

Gastro-Intestinal (G.I.) Diseases – Cured Cases

- Sweat - Average.
- Urine - (a) Stress incontinence : expulsion of urine while coughing or laughing. (b) Dark, turbid urine.
- Stool - (a) Ineffectual urging. (b) Stool 3-4 times a day, little relief of his distension and heaviness of abdomen, after stool. (c) Stools of various colours.
- Upper Extremities - Occasional joint pains > by hard pressure.
- Palm - Burning in the palms and soles > by cold application.
- Joints - Occasional erratic joint pains > by hard pressure.
- Lower Extremities - Burning of the soles.
- Male Genital Organs - (a) Extremely strong desire. (b) Frequent wet dreams. (c) Thinks of sexual pleasure frequently.
- Skin Disease - Skin heals okay. Nothing Abnormal Detected.
- Mild, Quarrelsome, Fault-finding. Irritability after eating. Jealous. Silent, Peevish. Morose in the afternoon. Neat and clean. Fear of death, disgusted with life. Memory: weak. Weeping mood, involuntary sighing. Sympathetic. Active. Fear of ghosts, darkness, and incurable disease and of failures. H/O Jaundice : twice in 1980 and 1983. H/O Measles and mumps: during childhood. Has not had chicken pox. Vaccinated. Prolonged History of intake of rich, spicy and fatty foods → indigestion → distension and acidity → dyspepsia --> Pain started in abdomen.
- Hot person. Desires open air. Catches cold easily.
- Food Preference:- (i) Sweet + (ii) Sour ++ (iii) Pungent and hot : average (iv) Salt : No (v) Salty + (vi) Bitter : No (vii) Bread : No (viii) Milk : Loves but aggravates his symptom. (ix) Potato + (x) Vegetables and Spinach + (xi) Onion + (xii) Fruits : Average (xiii) Fish + (xiv) Meat/Chicken + (xv) Egg (Boiled/Fried) : Average (xii) Rich, spicy and fat food : Loves fat but cannot tolerate these days (xvii) Warm food : No (xviii) Cold food + (xix) Warm drinks : No (xx) Cold drinks : ++ and lemonade (xxi) Ice cream +.
- Thirst - Average.
- Sleep - (a) Wide awake at night. (b) He lies in bed for prolonged period, in the morning. Dreams of daily business. Married with one child.
- Family History - H/O Rheumatism in the family.
- Had allopathic and homoeopathic medicines: without any appreciable change. (Prescription not available).

Investigations Carried Out Before/After Dr. Banerjea's Treatment

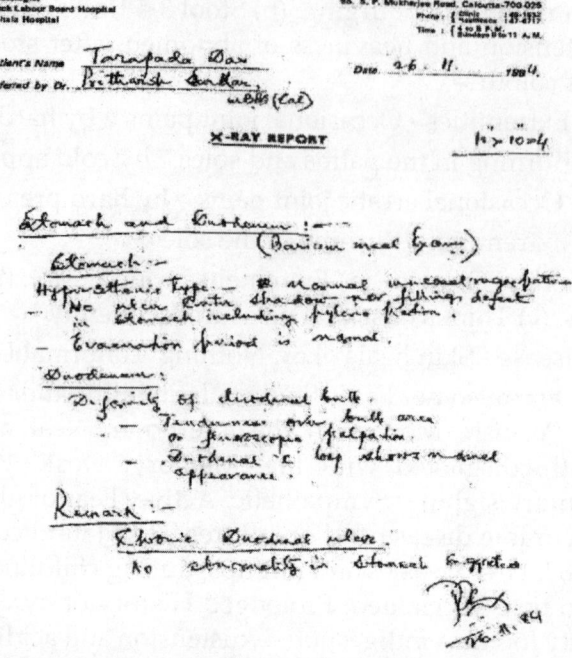

Barium meal report of stomach and Duodenum of Mr. T.D., before treatment.

Barium meal report of stomach and Duodenum, 7 months after treatment.

Barium meal report of Stomach and Duodenum after treatment.

26th Nov'84: Barium Meal Stomach and Duodenum: Remark:- Chronic duodenal ulcer. No abnormality in stomach suggested.

20th Apr'88: Barium Meal Stomach and Duodenum: Remark:- Radiologically no organic lesion seen either in the stomach or in duodenum.

CASE ANALYSIS, MIASMATIC DIAGNOSIS AND FINAL PRESCRIPTION

Miasmatic Analysis

- Pain and vomiting (++) < after taking milk better after eating: Psora.
- Sensation of heaviness with distension: Psora.
- Acidity: Psora.
- Loss of appetite: Psora.
- Stomach, joints and head pain > pressure: Sycotic.
- Cold shower, < warm applications: Syphilis.
- Aggravation from fatty foods: Sycosis.
- Headache with sore eyes, generally frontal, aggravation from sun: Psora-Syphilis.
- Eyes: occasional (lachrymation) with burning Psora-syphilitic.
- Nose: thick yellowish expectoration: Syco-tubercular.
- Mouth: Bitter taste, dryness: Psora.
- Dry cough as a result of cold: Psora.
- Cough aggravation in the evening, by lying down: Tubercular.
- Chest pain > lying on affected area: Sycosis.
- Pressure in abdomen with ineffectual desire for stool: Psora.
- Urine: stress incontinence, dark urine: Psora.
- Joints: erratic joint pains, > hard pressure: Sycosis.
- Extremely strong sexual desire: Sycosis.
- Nocturnal emissions (frequent wet dreams): Tubercular.
- Mental: Quarrelsome (Sycosis); Irritability (Syco-psoric);
- Jealous (Sycosis); Silent (Psora);
- Morose in the afternoon: Psora-sycotic.
- Neat and clean: Sycotic.
- Fear of death: Psora.
- Disgusted with life – (love for one's own life destroyed): Syphilitic.

- Weakness of memory: Psora.
- Fear of ghosts, darkness, incurable disease and of failures: Psora.
- Catches cold easily: Psora- Tubercular.
- Desires: Sour (Psora-Syphilitic); cold food and drinks: Syphilitic.
- Sleep: awakening with weariness: Tubercular.

It is a mixed miasmatic case with Psora-Syco-Tubercular preponderance.

Reasons for Prescription

Aggravation from milk is a strong indication for Homarus.
Other indications are:
- Deranged digestion;
- Sexual excitement;
- Disturbed sleep;
- Lack of appetite;
- < after sleep in the morning;
- Lachrymation and smarting in eyes;
- Burning soles of feet.
- Miasmatic analysis of Homarus is Psora ++, Sycosis ++, Syphilis ++, Tubercular ++.
- Homarus and Pulsatilla covers the case miasmatically as well.

Remedy Reaction

I started this case with Homarus 30 C, a good potency for a physical complaint of duodenal ulcer. Homatus is an interesting medicine prepared from the digestive fluid of Lobster. The triad symptomatology for prescribing this medicine is (a) dyspepsia with belching, aggravation from milk and milk product better after eating; (b) frontal headache with sore eyes; (c) sore throat with rawness and scraping sensation. In my opinion, it is a deep acting medicine as well. The remedy was changed to Pulsatilla, as a new remedy picture emerged (details of the symptoms are given under the prescription done on the basis of column, when I changed to Pulsatilla), beginning with 200C potency and finishing the case with 50M. The patient was cured of his ulcer in just less than 2 years of treatment.

Gastro–Intestinal (G.I.) Diseases – Cured Cases

Prescription Chart

Dates	Prescription Done on the Basis of	Treatment
25th Nov'86	As the patient's presenting symptom is (1) Vomiting, (2) Dyspepsia, (3) Indigestion, (4) Milk aggravation, (5) better after eating (6) Frontal headache with sore eyes (7) With two consecutive attacks of jaundice.	Homarus 30: 2 doses: alternate mornings.
3rd Jan'87	Vomiting to some extent relieved and the milk intolerance; but indigestion, dyspepsia and heaviness of the stomach persists.	Sac lac.
6th Feb'87	No further change. Went higher in potency.	Homarus 200: 2 doses: alternate mornings.
5th Mar'87	Can have milk now which is tolerable but (1) Pain in abdomen, (2) Dyspepsia, (3) Indigestion, (4) Heaviness etc. persists.	Homarus 200: 2 doses: alternate mornings.
16th Apr'87	No further change. So change in the plan of treatment: Considering (a) pain sometimes after eating, (b) Pain followed by vomiting, (c) Heaviness of abdomen especially in the morning, (d) Eructation of the food eaten > by strolling, (e) Loves fat but cannot tolerate, (f) Pain < from fatty foods, warm application > by pressure and somewhat relieved after vomiting, (g) Congestive sun-headache better by cold application, (h) Bitter taste, (i) Stress incontinence, (j) Ineffectual urging for stool, (k) Burning palms and soles, (l) Strong sexual desire, (m) wide awake at night in mild, amiable silently peevish person, who likes consolation and has had prolonged H/O taking fatty, spicy food; (n) Desires open air.	Pulsatilla 200: 2 doses: alternate morning.
24th May'87	Dramatically better in terms of appetite but (1) Pain, (2) Distension, (3) Heaviness still persists: wait and watch with wisdom.	Sac lac.
16th Jun'87	(1) Appetite, (2) Vomiting, (3) Eructation less but (a) Pain, (b) Heaviness persists.	Pulsatilla 200: 2 doses: alternate mornings.
29th Jul'87	No further change.	Prescription done on the basis of
6th Sep'87	Pain is a little better, but still heaviness of abdomen and ineffectual desire for stool.	Pulsatilla 10M: 2 doses: alternate mornings.
18th Oct'87	Pain much better. No vomiting in the last month. Patient is much happier.	Sac lac.

Dates	Prescription Done on the Basis of	Treatment
14th Nov'87	Patient doing much better in every regard. (i) Pain in abdomen, (ii) Vomiting, (iii) Heaviness of abdomen, (iv) Gas and distension, (v) Eructations, (vi) Burning palms and soles better, but (a) Ineffectual urging for stool, (b) Stress-incontinence, (c) Strong sexual desire: hyper sexuality and (d) Strong love for fatty – greasy foods are still unaffected. Wait and watch with wisdom for further movement of symptoms.	Sac lac.
Jan'88	Pains etc. doing better, but above noted things are unchanged. Repeat.	Pulsatilla 10M: 2 doses: alternate mornings.
3rd Feb'88	Standstill in aforestated status, though pain, distension and heaviness better.	Pulsatilla 50M: 2 doses: alternate mornings.
4th Mar'88	Better in every regard (1) Not a single episode of pain and vomiting, (2) Ineffectual desire for stool less, (3) Sexual desire is also to some extent modified, (4) Stress incontinence 50% better.	Sac lac.
2nd Apr'88	Doing much better (a) Ineffectual desire for stool, (b) Stress incontinence gone, only love for fatty food is still persistent. Asked to do follow-up Barium-meal X-ray of the Stomach and duodenum for re-assessment.	Sac lac.
28th Apr'88	X-ray shows healed up ulcer. CURED of the problem : though I have asked him to continue the treatment for some time more : to evaluate if the medicine can change the innate love for fatty food, but the patient refused to continue the treatment any more, as he thinks himself completely cured and that also radiologically assessed as we established : and more-over he likes to enjoy his fatty-meal.	

Authenticity of Cure

CD Reference: GA010-DUODENAL ULCER-TD

11. A CASE OF GIARDIASIS : MASTER A.D.

Case No. GA011

Age : 5 years as on 27th June, 1995.
Sex : Male
Height : 3'7"
Weight : 14 kgs.

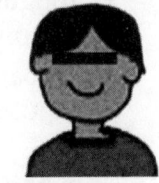

Photo of the patient, Master. A.D

Presenting Complaint

1. (a) History and Development

- The boy had a normal digestive system until 11 months old when he had his first attack of gastroenteritis and vomiting.
- Since then he has had loose motions off and on and at the age of 1 year 9 months, he had to be hospitalised with severe diarrhoea, vomiting and dehydration.
- Since then he cannot have milk, any milk products or wheat products (even biscuits].
- He had now become a patient of chronic indigestion.
- Being strictly on rice, rice products and regular allopathic medicines he still suffers from indigestion, almost the whole year.
- The boy consumes only boiled vegetables, stews and very bland foods [of which he is utterly disgusted] even though he gets frequent attacks of loose stools with distension of abdomen.
- His stool has been tested and since 1993 he is suffering from Giardiasis and has had lots of allopathic medications, without appreciable results. Thus became a chronic sufferer of Giardia problem, over three years, and as a result of this, being a kid, his digestive system has been totally altered.
- At present he is under allopathic treatment, but came to me because they are totally frustrated and would like to try Homoeopathy !

(b) Modalities: Aggravation and Amelioration of the Presenting Complaints

- Urging for stool aggravated by milk and milk products.
- Wheat product intolerance.
- Indigestion and heaviness of abdomen : better by vomiting.

2. Physical Generals [Head to Foot Scanning of Symptoms]

- Teeth: Sometimes the boy grinds his teeth at night during sleep.
- Tongue: During loose motions the boy has a thick white coating on his tongue.
- Throat: Occasionally the child gets swollen tonsils from cold exposure.
- Cough: Cough : non-productive, causing constant tickling sensation in the throat. History of breathing trouble, allopathic treatment carried out at the age of 3 months, lots of antibiotics taken.
- Abdomen: There is a distension of the whole abdomen and there is continuous passing of flatus (offensive +++).
- Appetite: During loose motion the child has decreased appetite.
- Sweat: All over the body. No bad odour.
- Urine: Clear urine, quantity fair, no bad odour.
  - Stool:
  - Colour: Dirty – yellow
  - Odour: Offensive [+++]
  - Urging: Ineffectual [+++]
  - Development: History of asthma when the boy was 3 months old allopathically treated - asthma got better [suppressed] but he has never been well since. - amelioration but severe diarrhoea since -amelioration associated with abdominal pain.
  - Type of stool: Mucussy [++]. Occasionally bloody.
  - Associated symptoms: Crampy pains in the abdomen during and after. A little better after passing stool, but do not abate totally.
- Extremities: Sometimes the child complains of pain in the legs.
- Skin: Nothing abnormal detected.

3. Mind

- Mild, but at times obstinate. Anxious and apprehensive, thinks about his disease, seems to be incurable to him.
- Talkative at home, passive amongst strangers.
- Desires company, but takes time to be friendly, wants to be alone at times.
- Weeping mood, craves consolation.
- He cannot tolerate blood letting.
- Does things in a hurry.
- Fear of : darkness, thunderstorm, failure.

4. Signs of Grief or Past History of Emotional Suppression

Working mother - unable to provide proper attention and sufficient time to the child. Child feels lonely, may have some grief or depression for not getting parents' attention, but even when asked has not opened up. Mother has tendency to conceal inner grief [?]:

5. Treatment, He Had in Past

He was under allopathic medication since birth. [This is the first time, they are visiting a Homoeopath] !

Stool report of Mast A.D., before treatment.

Stool report of Mast A.D., 6 months after treatment.

6. Past Medical History

No severe illness, not even the common childhood diseases. Could be due to the prolonged and continuous course of antibiotic treatment throughout childhood, which has suppressed the expression of other manifestations.

7. Vaccination

Child has been thoroughly vaccinated [full course].

8. What Is the First Cause of Break-Down of Health

Attack of gastroenteritis with vomiting at 1 year 9 months of age.

9. Homoeopathic Generalities

- Heat and cold relation: Chilly person, does not catch cold easily.
- Desire and aversion for food-stuffs:
- Desire: Sweet [++], Salt [+++], Salty [+], Bread [+], Milk [++], Potato [++], Fish [+], Chicken [+], Egg [++], Warm food [+], Cold drinks [++], Ice-cream [++].
- Aversion: Sour. Vegetables and Spinach. Rich & spicy food. Cold food.
- Thirst: Thirsty [++] in all weathers.
- Sleep:
  - Sleeps well during the first hours of night
  - Dreams of daily work, dead people.
- Sweat: Sweats profusely [+++], all over the body mainly on face.

10. Family History

- Father and mother alive : no serious illness.
- Paternal side: Hypertension.
- Maternal side: Rheumatism.

Investigations Carried Out Before/After Dr. Banerjea's Treatment

17th Mar'93: Faeces: Mucus present. Occult Blood Test = weakly +ve (positive). Cyst: Giardia Lambia, undigested starch +, vegetable cell ++.

6th Nov'95: Faeces: Mucus: slight, Occult Blood Test = +ve (positive), Occasional Giardia Cyst., undigested starch +, vegetable cell +.

7th Nov'95: Faeces: Mucus – nil, Vegetable cell +, Cyst not found.

8th Dec'95: Faeces: Brownish, soft, formed. Alkaline.

11th Dec'95: Faeces. Report clear, cyst : nil.

CASE ANALYSIS, MIASMATIC DIAGNOSIS AND FINAL PRESCRIPTION

Provisional Diagnosis: Giardiasis.
Miasmatic Diagnosis: Syco-Psoric.

Miasmatic Analysis

- Giardiasis: Syco-tubercular.
- Vomiting: Psora.
- Loose stool, diarrhoea: Sycosis.
- Aggravation from milk and milk products: Tubercular.
- Wheat intolerance: Tubercular.
- Indigestion and heaviness of abdomen : better by vomiting: Sycotic (abnormal discharge ameliorates).
- Grinding of teeth during sleep: Psora.
- White coating on tongue: Tubercular.
- Swollen tonsils from cold exposure: Tubercular.
- Non-productive cough, tickling sensation: Tubercular.
- Distension of the whole abdomen (Psora) and there is continuous passing of flatus (offensive +++]: Tubercular.
- Decreased appetite during loose motion: Psora-sycotic.
- Stool: Yellow: Sycotic; Offensive: Syphilitic; Ineffectual urging: Psora.
- Mucus in stool: Sycotic; occasionally bloody: Tubercular.
- Crampy pains: Sycotic.
- Mental: Mild, anxious and apprehensive: Psora. Obstinate: Tuberculo-syphilitic.

- Talkative: Sycotic; passive amongst strangers: Psora.
- Wants to be alone at times: Psora-syphilitic; weeping mood: Psora-sycotic.
- Cannot tolerate blood letting: Psora.
- Do things in a hurry: Sycotic.
- Fear of: darkness, thunderstorm, failure: Psora.
- Desires: Sweet: Psoric; Salty: Syco-tubercular; Cold drinks: Syphilitic.
- Aversion: Green leafy vegetables: Sycosis; Cold food: Psora.
- Sleep: Dreams of dead people: Syphilis.
- Sweat: Profuse sweat: Sycosis.

It is a mixed miasmatic case with Syco-Psoric preponderance. As diarrheoa is one of the presenting problem which is Sycotic (constipation is psoric, dysentery is syphilitic, bloody stool is tubercular) therefore, sycotic miasm is in the surface.

Reasons for Prescription and Remedy Reaction

The reasons to support the prescriptions are given in the prescription chart below. 200 C followed by 1M potency of Nux Vomica was used to remove the effects of suppression from the allopathic medication given in the past. Miasmatic breakdown of Nux Vomica is Psora +++, Sycosis ++, Syphilis +, Tubercular ++.

Prescription Chart

Date	Prescription Done on the Basis of	Treatment
27th Jun'95	• Considering prolonged history of allopathic Medication and strong drugging. • Ineffectual desire for stool. • Pain is a little better after defecation. • Indigestion – amelioration by continuous passing of flatus. Indigestion and heaviness of abdomen, relieved by vomiting. • Fear of thunder. • Chilly person. • Miasmatic opening of Psora.	Nux Vomica 200: 2 doses followed by 1M: 1 dose
19th Aug'95	Noappreciable change. Wait & watch for movement of symptoms.	Sac lac.
9th Sep'95	No appreciable change. Complementary of Nux Vomica given.	Sulphur 30: 2 doses

Date	Prescription Done on the Basis of	Treatment
26th Sep'95	Aggravation [++]. Severe bouts of loose stool. Mucus [++], blood [+], indigestion increased. Seems to refuse almost all foods, scared of getting loose stool from the simplest food. Frustrated. Anxious [++]. Change in the plan of treatment. Prescribed Morgan on the basis of: • Nux Vomica - Sulphur cycle was well indicated, but it was not holding the case. Bowel nosode thought of as the nearest analogue of Sulphur prescription. • Prolonged Irritable Bowel Syndrome [I.B.S.] - congestion [++] of gastro-intestinal mucosa. • Chronic indigestion - affections of liver - liver function altered. • Indigestion: better by vomiting. • Anxious and apprehensive of his state of health.	Morgan Pure 200: 2 doses in distilled water [1] globule divided into 2 doses]
21st Oct'95	No appreciable change, but gained weight. Now 16 kg. Wait and watch. Asked to repeat stool tests.	Sac lac.
14th Nov'95	Doing a little better. Stool is semi-formed but occasional bouts of loose stool, still poor appetite. Stool report: better; Giardia cysts: occasional in one report and in the other: absent.	Sac lac.
12th Dec'95	Child is dramatically better. • Energy is remarkably better. • Stool formed, mucus almost non-existent. • No distension of abdomen and not feeling any heaviness. • Anxiety, fears of incurability totally disappeared. • Parents got excited and repeated the stool test. No Giardia in three consecutive days.	Sac lac.

Authenticity of Cure

CD Reference: GA011-GIARDIASIS-AD

12. A CASE OF SPLENOMEGALY: MASTER M.S.

Case No. GA012

Age : 12 years-old.

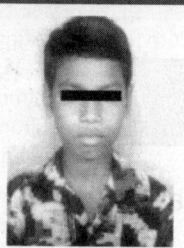

Photo of the patient, Mast. M.S.

Presenting Complaints

- Pain in abdomen, left sided (in the spleen area).
- Pain better by pressure and gentle rubbing.
- Recurrent sinus trouble, more during the rainy season. Sinus pain aggravated by change of weather.
- During the abdominal pain sometimes the patient have an urge for frequent micturition.
- Sweat more during sleeping; rarely sweats when he is awake.
- Makes up stories about friends, tendency to concealment. Lives in a lie.
- Withdrawn. Occasionally melancholic and indifferent.
- Tendency to conceal; possessive, suppressive.
- Past History: Neglect in upbringing, mistreatment in child-hood with socio-cultural stress.
- Food Desires: Desires salty, sour, cold food (++)
- Aversion: Green leafy vegetables.
- Thirst: Average.
- Sleep: Average.
- Thermal: Chilly Patient.

Date treatment started 21st September, 1993. Investigations are inconsistent. Cured in just over 3 years.

Investigations Carried Out Before/After Dr. Banerjea's Treatment

6th Mar'96: Ultra Sonography upper abdomen: Remark:- Suggestive of hyperechoic splenomegaly.

3rd Aug'99: Ultra Sonography abdomen: Remark:- Echogenic patterns are normal.

CASE ANALYSIS, MIASMATIC DIAGNOSIS AND FINAL PRESCRIPTION

Miasmatic Analysis

- Pain better by pressure and gentle rubbing: Sycotic.
- Sinus problems: Sycotic.
- Sinus problems aggravated during rainy season: Sycotic.
- Frequent micturition: Sycotic.
- Withdrawn: Syphilitic.
- Secretive: Sycotic.
- Possessive: Sycotic.
- Tendency for concealment: Sycotic.
- Lives in a lie (negative falsification): Sycosis

This is a Syco-Syphilitic case.

Reasons for Prescription

- Left sided pain.
- Pain better by pressure.
- Sinus trouble = Sycosis.
- Aggravate during rainy season and aversion to green leafy vegetables = Hydrogenoid constitution.
- Sinus pain aggravated by change of weather = Sycosis.
- Frequent micturition accompanies pain.
- Sweat when he sleeps, stops when he wakes: PQRS for Thuja.
- Live in lie (tendency to be deceitful is an interesting character of Thuja).
- Tendency to conceal; suppressive = Sycosis.
- Possessive.
- Chilly patient but desires cold food. Desires salt/salty.
- Past History: Neglect in upbringing, mistreatment in child-hood with socio-cultural stress. (this is also an important background in Thuja development).

Miasmatic breakdown of Thuja is Psora ++, Sycosis +++, Syphilis ++, Tubercular ++.

Final Prescription

Unfortunately a detailed prescription chart is not available for this case. The patient was given the remedy Thuja 200 C, a good potency for complaints such as splenomegaly, with the patient having good vitality. The patient was cured of his complaint in just over 3 years.

Authenticity of Cure

CD Reference: GA012-SPLEENOMEGALI-MS

Gastro-Intestinal (G.I.) Diseases – Cured Cases

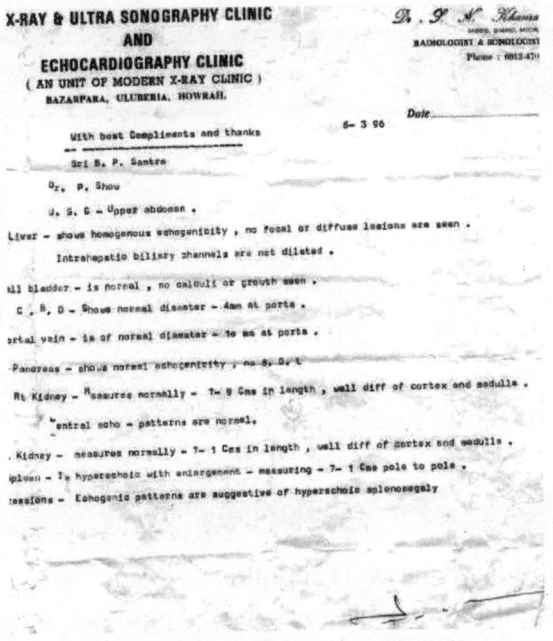

Sonography report, before treatment.

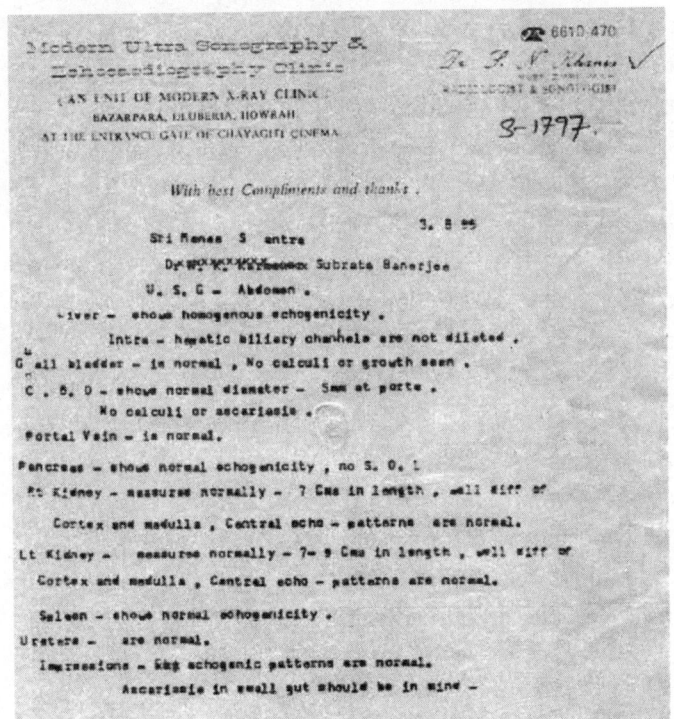

Sonography report, after treatment.

13. A CASE OF CHOLECYSTITIS (THICKENED NON FUNCTIONING GALL BLADDER) : MR. J.S.

Case No. GA013

50 year-old male (as on 24th May, 1995)

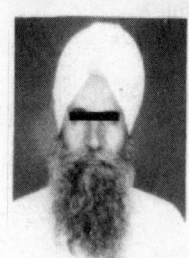

Photo of the patient of Mr. J. S.

Presenting Complaints

- Pain in abdomen, since 11 months.
- Pain at right hypogastrium region. Aggravate on empty stomach. Ameliorated by eating banana.
- Distension of abdomen due to gas. Aggravates in empty stomach.
- Had history of irregular diet habit.
- Stool – Regular, not clear, constipation.
- Homoeopathic Generalities – Hot patient.
- Desires – Vegetable and spinach, pungent, sweet, banana, cucumber, warm food, salty food.
- Aversion – Sour,
- Thirst – Excessive.
- Appetite – Decreased. Sleep: Normal.
- Urine – clear.
- Sweat – Average.
- Pain in the calf muscles worse motion; better rest & pressure.
- Mind – (a) Angry and irritable. (b) Mental tension. (c) Gradual loss of memory. (d) works hurriedly.
- Pain: Darting, stitching type of pain, better by pressure.
- ECC: Easily catches cold.
- Pain in calf muscles < motion > pressure
- Gas & Acidity.

Gastro-Intestinal (G.I.) Diseases – Cured Cases

Investigations Carried Out Before/After Dr. Banerjea's Treatment

8th Apr'95: X-ray OCG(Oral Cholecystography): Remark:- Mild chronic cholecystitis.

21st Aug'97: OCG (Oral Cholecystography):- Remark:- Normal functioning gall bladder.

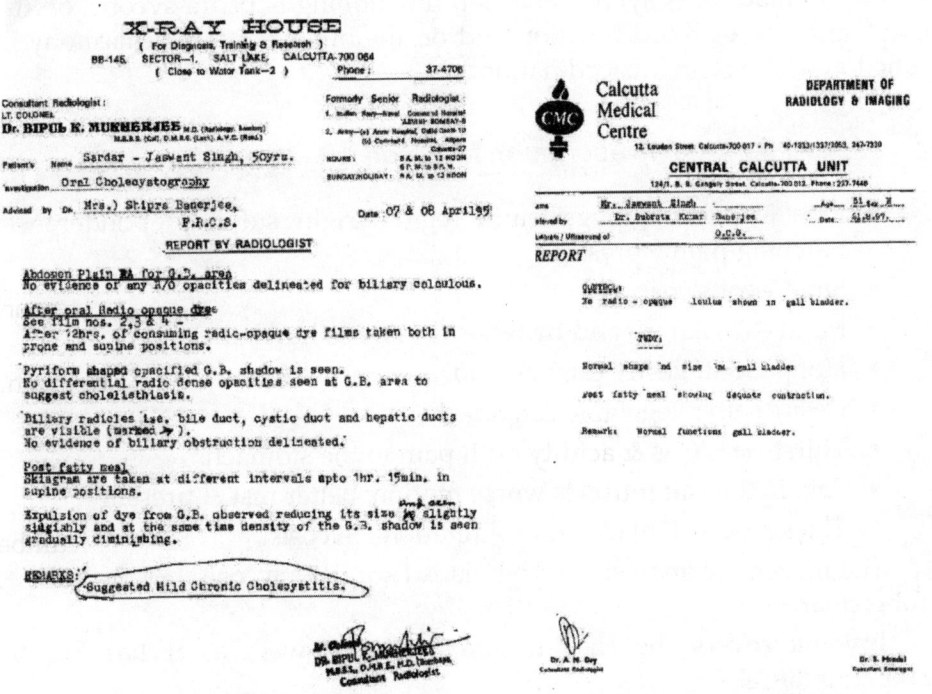

O.C.G. report of Mr. J. S. before treatment.

O.C.G. report of Mr. J. S., aftertreatment.

CASE ANALYSIS, MIASMATIC DIAGNOSIS AND FINAL PRESCRIPTION

This case is another good example of how Classical Homoeopathy can take care of pathological changes and here the thickened (non functioning) gall bladder has been reversed to normal.

Miasmatic Analysis

- Pain in abdomen aggravated on an empty stomach: Psora.
- Distension of abdomen due to gas: Psora.
- Stool – constipation: Psora.
- Mind – (a) Angry and irritable: Sycosis. (b) Gradual loss of memory: Sycosis. (d) Works hurriedly: Sycosis.

This is a case with Sycotic preponderance. As thickening of the wall of the gall bladder is sycotic and non functioning is psora-sycotic, on the one hand lack or hypo function and on the other hand mal-harmony in function which is an incoordination.

Final Prescription Made on the Basis of

- Pain at right hypogastrium region; right sided preponderance. Stitching pain > pressure.
- Stool – constipation.
- Mind – (a) Angry and irritable. (b) Works hurriedly.
- Hot patient; Easily catches cold.
- Desire salty; vegetable & spinach.
- Thirst- +++. Gas & acidity with pain in the stomach.
- Pain in the calf muscles worse motion; better rest & pressure.
- Thickened gall bladder: Proliferation : Sycosis.

The miasmatic analysis of Bryonia is Psora ++, Sycosis +++, Syphilis +, Tubercular ++.

Bryonia covers the case miasmatically as well, as it has Sycotic preponderance.

Final Prescription

BRYONIA, 30C/2: 1 globule in sugar of milk sachet dissolved in pure water and sipped slowly over 10 days. Then 10 days of no medicine, followed by another dose to be shaken and sipped for 10 days. The remedy was given in 30C potency on the basis of the patient's vitality and also that Bryonia in this potency is suitable for gall bladder complaints.

Remedy Reaction

Unfortunately a detailed prescription chart is not available for this case, however the patient improved over roughly three years and the follow-up

Sonography report was normal. So, in this case of pathological gall bladder characterised by thickening, Homoeopathy was capable of taking care of the thickening and reducing the inflammation of the gall bladder and the cholecystitis was simultaneously improved.

Authenticity of Cure

CD Reference: GA013-CHOLECYSTITIS-JS

14. A CASE OF CHRONIC DUODENAL ULCER: MR. J.A.

Case No. GA014

Age : 62 years-old as on 28th December, 1989
Sex : Male

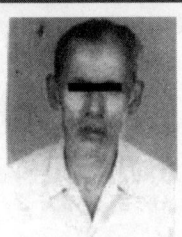

Photo of the patient
Mr. J. A.

Presenting Complaints

- Pain in upper abdomen, for 20 years agg. after eating; spasmodic pain > bending forward; > pillow pressure; previous – Allopathic. Homo. treat. Habit of taking rich and spicy food. Patient has been diagnosed as a case of Chronic Duodenal Ulcer. Suffering from pain and discomfort in upper part of abdomen, on and off for last 20 years or so. Patient has a good appetite → hungry → eats → pain → cannot eat anymore. Lot of gas (+++) goes downwards. After eating → patient feels weak (++).
- Stool: Constipation. Difficult evacuation. Feels like more will come and has to sit for long time. Not finished feeling (++).
- Occasionally headache, < sun heat; > Rest.
- Occasionally pain in neck, back; legs; right knee (more) → all the time, > heat application. > massage.
- Pain in epigastric region while pressing with hands. > after eating.
- Urine:- Ok.
- Pain in knee joint → tearing (more in right knee). Sensation of tearing < by bending the knee. < pressure. > rest.
- Appetite – Normal.
- Thirst – Scanty.
- Chilly patient.
- Catches cold easily.
- Sweat – scanty.
- Heals – Ok.
- Sleep:- Good. Dreams of various things.
- Desire:- Sweet++; Sour; Bitter; Vegetables & Spinach+; Milk; Fish, warm food (+++). Aversion to bread. Patient really prefers warm food though he feels it might not be good for his abdominal complaints.

- Mind:- Mild; Silent – habit; Desire for company; Weepy mood; Sympathetic. Sensitive (++).
- Past Medical History:- Typhoid in childhood. Treat – Allopathy. Skin disease – 20 years back. Treat – Allopathy. Chicken pox.
- Family Medical History:- Father – Leucoderma. Asthma. Mother died of paralysis. Mother Asthma. Brother – Cancer.
- Pain right knee joint. Cramping pain in calf muscle. < folding of leg. > Extension of knee joint.
- Occasional toothache. Pain in upper and lower mother tooth. < touch of any food.
- Sweat:- Profuse perspiration throughout the body.

Investigations Carried Out Before/After Dr. Banerjea's Treatment

30th Jul'90: Barium X-Ray: Chronic Duodenal Ulcer. Stool – Pus cell 3-4 hpf (high power field).

20th May'92: Barium X-Ray of Stomach & Duodenum: No filling defect. Duodenal bulb is slightly deformed.

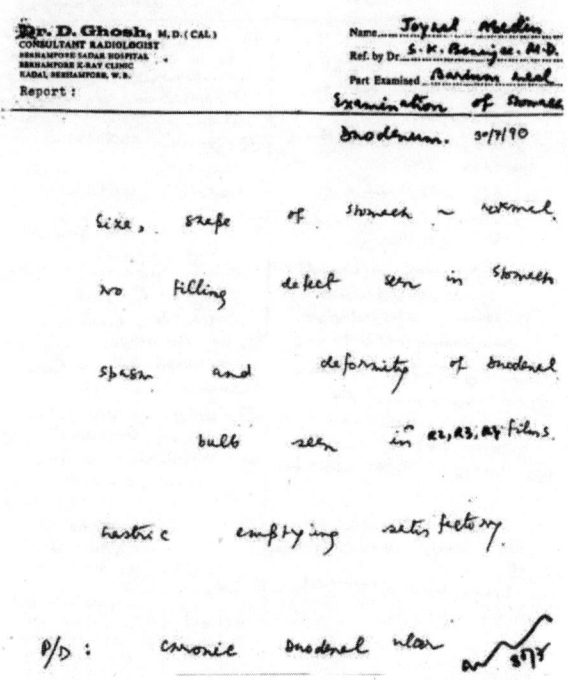

Ba-meal report of Mr. J. A. during homoeopathic treatment.

Dr. Kanai Lal Chatterjee
M.B.B.S., D.M.R.O., M.D. (CAL)
CONSULTANT RADIOLOGIST
SADAR HOSPITAL, BERHAMPORE

Name: Toynal Abedin
Ref. by Dr.: S. K. Banerjee
Part Examined: Ba-meal x-ray of stomach and duodenum

X-RAY REPORT

Mucosal pattern of the stomach appears slightly coarse. No obvious filling defect is seen in the stomach. Spasm is noted in the region of gastric antrum. Duodenal bulb is slightly deformed. C-loop and remaining parts of the small gut appear normal.

20/5/92

Ba-meal report of Mr. J. A. during treatment.

Before treatment of Dr. S.K. Banerjea	After treatment of Dr. S.K. Banerjea
① Gastralgia, M.T. Stomach Pain. After eating relief.	① 1989 1st Treatment of Dr. S. K. Banerjea at Computer treatment. Suggested by Chronic ulcer.
② ½/1 hour rest for again pain. Fish, Meat & Reich food after pain.	② Your advise Xray. Report. ulcer.
③ One hour going to latrine in the middle of dysentery.	③ 2nd years treatment. Again you are advise Xray. Report - No ulcer (normal).
④ My day to local Doctor treatment. You are the advise the Xray - the Xray. Xray Report ulcer.	④ Dr. Banerjea suggested no ulcer. You report I cured & fit.
⑤ 9 treatment of Local Doctor temporary relif after pain.	⑤ But I was wind & gas trouble.
⑥ Weight Less day to day.	⑥ I present eating to meat, fish & Sour But Reich food mostly.
⑦ Next Advise Ba-Xray of the Stomach & Duo. Report - Normal.	⑦ A intervals stick to Coryza. But I have to before Coryza.
	⑧ Left knee & Right elbow pain. But as Something Relif.

Patient's comments after treatment.

Gastro-Intestinal (G.I.) Diseases – Cured Cases

CASE ANALYSIS, MIASMATIC DIAGNOSIS AND FINAL PRESCRIPTION

Miasmatic Analysis

- Pain in upper abdomen, > bending forward: Sycotic; > pillow pressure: Sycotic;
- Lot of gas (+++) goes downwards: Psora. After eating → patient feels weak (++): Psora.
- Stool: constipation. Difficult evacuation: Psora.
- Not finished feeling (++): Syco-Psoric.
- Occasionally pain in neck, back; legs, > heat application: Psora.
- Chilly patient. Catches cold easily: Tubercular.
- Mild: Psora; Desires for company: Syco-Tubercular; Weepy mood: Sycotic.
- Prescription Made On The Basis Of:
- Pain in upper abdomen, for 20 years agg. after eating; spasmodic pain > bending forward; > pillow pressure; previous – Allopathic. Homo. treatment. Habit of taking rich. Spicy; food. Patient has been diagnosed as a case of Chronic Duodenal Ulcer. Suffering from pain and discomfort in upper part of abdomen, on and off for last 20 years or so. Patients have good appetite → hungry → eats → pain → cannot eat anymore. Lot of gas (+++) goes downwards. After eating → patient feels weak (++).
- Stool: constipation. Difficult evacuation. Feels like more will come and has to sit for long time. Not finished feeling (++).
- Occasionally pain in neck, back; legs; right knee (more) → in all time, > heat application. > massage.
- Chilly patient.
- Catches cold easily.
- Desire:- Sweet++; Sour; Bitter; Vegetables & Spinach+; Milk; Fish, warm food (+++). Aversion to bread. Patient really prefers warm food though he feels it might not be good for his abdominal complaints.
- Mind:- Mild; Silent – habit; Desires for company; Weepy mood; Sympathetic. Sensitive (++).

The miasmatic breakdown of Lycopodium is: Psora+++L, Sycotic+++, Syphilitic++, Tubercular+++.

Final Prescription and Remedy Reaction

LYCOPODIUM 200C.

Prescription Chart

I started the case with Lycopodium 200C and patient improved dramatically. I waited for 11 months after the 1st prescription and patient was steadily improving with this single dose of Lycopodium 200C; I did not have to repeat. Another wonderful example of classical homoeopathy, right prescription: Wait and Watch with wisdom (WWW)!

Authenticity of Cure

CD Reference: GA014-CHRONIC DUODENAL ULCER-JA

15. A CASE OF SALIVARY DUCT CALCULI: MR. A.N.

Case No. GA015

Age : 38 years as on 21st Jun, 1995
Height : 5 ft. 6 inches.

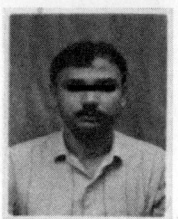

Photo of the patient Mr. A. N.

Presenting Complaints

- A stone in the right submandibular duct → since 1½ months back.
- Occasional swelling with pain in right mandibular region, better by warmth (++).
- Throat pain (right sided) and cannot eat food properly; cannot chew foods, better after taking allopathic medicine.
- Problem starts suddenly.
- Occasional burning tongue → since 8 years back.
- Pain in right testis → since ameliorated by hot applications.
- Knee pain (right) better by hot applications.
- Pain in hip (right).
- Occasional pain shifting in nature.
- Problems started after appendectomy (1994 February).
- Thermal: Chilly Patient.
- Sleep: Average.
- Appetite: Average.

Investigation Carried Out Before/After Dr. Banerjea's Treatment

5th Jun'95: X-ray mandible: Remark:- One small radio opaque stone is in submandibular duct in its lower end.

27th May'96: X-ray mandible: No evidence of calculus is demonstrated.

X-Ray report before treatment.

X-Ray report 11 months after treatment.

Patient's comments after treatment.

Gastro–Intestinal (G.I.) Diseases – Cured Cases

CASE ANALYSIS, MIASMATIC DIAGNOSIS AND FINAL PRESCRIPTION

Miasmatic Analysis

- Calculi: Sycosis.
- Swelling: Sycosis.
- Problem starts suddenly: Psora.
- Occasional burning tongue: Psora.
- Painful testis, amelioration by hot applications: Psora.
- Knee pain (right) (joint pains are Sycotic), better by hot applications: Psora.
- Shifting pains: Sycotic.

This is a mixed miasmatic case with syco-psoric preponderance.

Reasoning for Prescription

- Syco-Psoric nature of case.
- Right sided symptoms.
- Amelioration of pains of testis and sub-mandibular area by heat.
- Shifting pains.
- Pains come and go rapidly.

Miasmatic breakdown of Mag. phos. is Psora ++, Sycosis +++, Syphilis +, Tubercular ++.

Mag Phos covers the case miasmatically as well.

Remedy Reaction

This case was started with Mag. phos. 10M, the high potency being given on the basis of the patient's vitality and the strong similarity of the symptom picture. The case was finished in just over a year by Mag. phos. 50M.

Prescription Chart

Date	Prescription Done on the Basis of	Treatment
21st Jun'95	Sycotic remedy with pain better by warmth and right sided symptoms.	Mag. phos., 10 M, 2 doses.
9th Aug'95	Doing better. Testicular pain aggravates at new moon, at full moon had malaria and took allopathic medicine.	Sac lac.
11th Sep'95	Testicular pain (right)	Mag. phos., 10 M, 2 doses.
18th Oct'95	Stand still – still ameliorated hot application.	Mag. phos., 50 M, 2 doses.
20th Dec'95	Wait and watch.	Sac lac.
5th Apr'96	Better.	Sac lac.
31st May'96	Wait and watch.	Sac lac.
15th Jul'96	Cured. Patient states he can now eat any food and suffers no pain.	Sac lac.

Authenticity of Cure

CD Reference: GA015-SUB-MANDIBULAR DUCT CALCULI-AN

16. A CASE OF CHOLESTEOMA OF GALL BLADDER: MRS. M.D.

Case No. GA016

Age : 45 years-old as on 11th February, 2009
Sex : Female

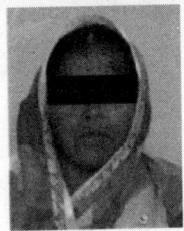

Photo of the patient, M.D.

Presenting Complaints

- Cholesteoma of Gall Bladder. Had history of trauma in right side of abdomen – 4 months back. Then again another trauma. Cow hit her abdomen with her horn. Soreness in the abdomen. Pain aggravated from touch and exertion.
- Sleeplessness.
- Burning head and abdomen.
- Palpitation aggravation exertion.
- Pain < weight carrying. < exertion.
- Gas(+++) and Acidity(++) - > taking water.
- H/O irregular diet.
- Burning vertex and occasional burning in the abdomen.
- Abdominal pain, > cold application.
- Occasional vertigo.
- Stool – Regular.
- Pain right side of abdomen < touch. Sensitive (++).
- Trauma in right side of abdomen 2 times.
- Head:- Burning. > cold. Occasionally giddiness.
- Occasionally dry cough. < cold.
- Stomach:- Sour mouth, < at 4 p.m. Nausea.
- Abdomen:- Distension (+++).
- Bowels:- Regular.
- Perspiration:- All over the body.
- Joints/Extremities:- Pain both knee. Occasional pain in knee. Pain sore to touch → later on little swelling (++).
- Thick and dry nails. Some warts in the covered area, gradually increasing in size.

Prescription of allopathic physician.

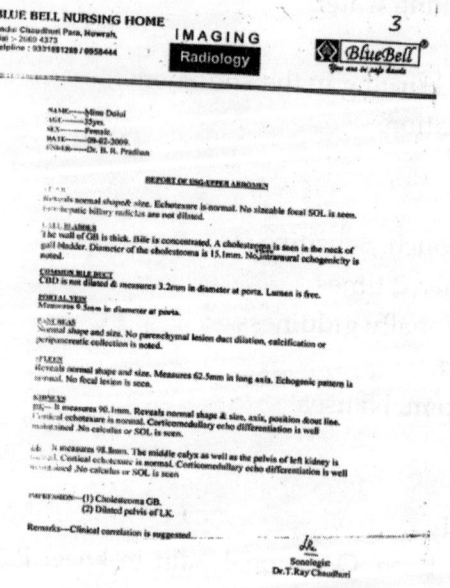

Sonography before homoeopathic treatment.

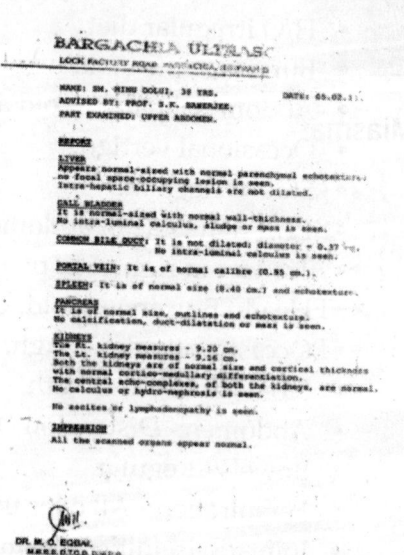

Sonography after homoeopathic treatment.

Gastro-Intestinal (G.I.) Diseases – Cured Cases

- Menstruation starts on 14 years of age. Number of children – 4. Nature of delivery – Normal.
- Temperament:- Absent minded; Amiable; Likes Company; Mild(++); Neat/clean; Sentimental; Sympathetic; Weepy.
- Fears from:- Accident, Animals, Darkness(+++), Death, Dogs, Diseases, Thunderstorm.
- Hot patient.
- Food Preferences:- Sweet(++), Savoury(++), Chicken(++), Green leafy(++), Cold food(++).
- Past Medical History:- Chicken pox, Measles, Tonsillitis.
- Family Medical History:- Mother – Gastric; Father – Gastric; Grandmother – Asthma; Brothers - Tb

Investigations Carried Out Before/After Dr. Banerjea's Treatment

9th Feb'09: Ultra Sonography (USG) upper abdomen:- Cholesteoma Gall Bladder. Dilated Pelvis of Left Kidney.

5th Feb'11: Ultra Sonography (USG) upper abdomen – NAD (Nothing Abnormal Detected).

CASE ANALYSIS, MIASMATIC DIAGNOSIS AND FINAL PRESCRIPTION

Miasmatic Analysis

- Soreness in the abdomen: Psora. Pain aggravated from touch: Sycotic.
- Abdominal pain, > cold application: Syphilitic.
- Pain both knee: Sycotic.
- Pain sore to touch → later on little swelling (++): Sycotic.

Final Prescription Made on the Basis of

- Cholesteoma of Gall Bladder. Had history of trauma in right side of abdomen – 4 months back. Then again another trauma. Cow hit her abdomen with her horn. Soreness in the abdomen. Pain aggravated from touch and exertion.
- Pain < weight carrying. < exertions.
- Abdominal pain, > cold application.

- Pain right side of abdomen < touch. Sensitive (++).
- Joints/Extremities:- Pain both knee. Occasional pain in knee. Pain sore to touch → later on little swelling (++).

The miasmatic breakdown of Arnica is: Psora++, Sycotic++, Syphilitic++, Tubercular+++

Final Prescription and Remedy Reaction

ARNICA 200C followed by 1M.

The prescription was made on the basis of Aetiology - H/O Injury, so two potencies were given.

Prescription Chart

Dates	Points in Favour of the Prescription	Prescribed Medicine
11th Feb'09	H/O Injury to Right hypochondrium → Injury to GB tissue → Cholesteoma.	Arnica 200C, 2 doses → 1M 1dose.
18th Feb'09	Passes mucussy stool. Gas acidity – Pain abdomen: stand still.	Sac Lac
4th May'09	Pain abdomen: little better.	PL (Sac Lac)
14th Jul'09	Pain abdomen – Less but present. < empty stomach > after eating. Gas++ and acidity++. < evening. Burning oesophagitis – palpitation with headache. > passing flatus & stool. After vomiting – feels better (Sour vomiting). Stool – Regular. Occasional Eructation. Appetite – Ok. Thirst – Less. Sleep – average. Wait and Watch.	PL (Sac Lac)
9th Oct'09	Doing better. Wait and Watch.	PL
2nd Aug'10	Pain was better, now stand still. So went for higher potency. Patient did not come for consultation for 9 months, was feeling Ok and financial problems.	Arnica 1M,1 dose → 10M, 1 Dose.
5th May'10	Stand still status.	Wait & Watch. PL
20th Aug'10	Was improved. But again < 20 days back. Occasional pain abdomen. < over exertion. < gas. Gas and acidity → pain epigastric. > taking water. H/O irregular food. > passing flatus. Occasional palpitations. Stool – not clear, mucussy stool. Sleep –poor. Thirst – Ok. Appetite – Ok. H/O Allergy – itching with swelling. < sweating. Warts – 50% >>.	Arnica 10M, 1dose → 50M, 1dose.

Dates	Points in Favour of the Prescription	Prescribed Medicine
28th Oct'10	Doing better.	PL
9th Feb'11	G.B. Stone:- USG report. All the scanned organs. Appear normal. At present, no problems. Stool – Regular. Appetite – Normal. Occasionally Gas forms. Thirst – Normal. Sleep – Ok.	PL

Authenticity of Cure

CD Reference: GA016-CHOLESTEOMA OF GALL BLADDER-MD

6 Gynaecological Diseases - Cured Cases
CHAPTER

1. A CASE OF BILATERAL POLYCYSTIC OVARIES: MRS K.B.

Case No. GY001

Age : 31 year-old as on 28.11.1988.
Age : 26 year-old young lady as on 24th March, 1992
Height: 5 ft.

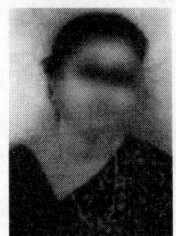

Photo of the patient,
Mrs. K.B.

Presenting Complaints

- Irregular menstrual cycle; at an interval of 3 – 4 months. Menstruation is profuse and long continued, when it happens. Menstrual pain aggravated from exertion, during full moon (if it occurs); better by lying on painful side. Menstrual flow more during day. Menstrual pain aggravated by jar. Sometimes she becomes very anxious and scared about the menstrual cycle and the pain.
- Black clotted blood.
- Excruciating pain (ovarian origin) during period. Pain in the lower abdomen, radiating towards thighs, followed by weakness (++) during and after menstruation.
- Leucorrhoea: watery, debilitating.
- Appetite poor.
- She was married in May 1989 and had been trying for a child since, but could not conceive.
- Head: Occasional headache; aggravates in the sun.
- Tongue: Moist.
- Stomach: Appetite average.

CASE ANALYSIS, MIASMATIC DIAGNOSIS AND FINAL PRESCRIPTION

This case is another good example of how Classical Homoeopathy can take care of pathological changes and the ovarian cyst has been taken care of.

Miasmatic Analysis

- Irregular menstrual cycle: Sycosis.
- Menstruation is profuse and long lasting, clotted: Tubercular.
- Leucorrhoea: watery, debilitating: Syco-Tubercular.
- Pain followed by weakness: Tubercular.
- Appetite poor: Psora.
- Stool : Constipation: Psora.
- Does everything in a hurry: Sycosis.
- Fear of dogs: Tubercular.
- Desires sweet: Psora.
- Chilly patient: Psora.
- Ovarian cyst, polycystic ovaries: Sycotic.
- Neat and clean: Sycotic.
- Mild: Psora; weepy: Psora - Sycotic.
- It is a mixed miasmatic case with Syco-Tubercular preponderance.

Final Prescription Made on the Basis of

- Irregular menstrual cycle; at an interval of 3 – 4 months.
- Menstruation is profuse and long lasting, when it happens.
- Menstrual pain aggravated from exertion, during full moon.
- Sometimes she becomes very anxious and scared about the menstrual cycle and the pain.
- Excruciating pain (ovarian origin) during period. Followed by weakness (++) during and after menstruation.
- Leucorrhoea : watery, debilitating.
- Mental Symptoms : Mild. Weepy, likes consolation.
- Chilly patient.
- Desires: Sweet+++,

Miasmatic breakdown of Thyroidinum is: Psora ++, Sycosis +++, Syphilis ++, Tubercular +++.

Thyroidinum covers the case miasmatically as well.

Final Prescription

THYROIDINUM, 1 M : 1 globule (No. 10: poppy seed size) in sugar of milk sachet, asked the patient to dissolve the powder in half or one litre of pure water and sip it slowly throughout the day, save a little at the bottom, top it up next morning, keep sipping throughout the next day. Generally I give instruction to my patient to dilute the medicated water (top it up with water) as many times as s/he likes. Continue like this for 10 days. Then 10 days of no medicine. Followed by another dose to be shaken and sipped for 10 days.

Remedy Reaction

Patient improved and all menstrual symptoms alleviated. Unfortunately a detailed prescription chart is not available for this case. However, in just over a year the follow-up sonography report was normal. So, in this case of cysts in the ovaries, Homoeopathy was capable of handling such a pathological condition and made the cysts disappear, this was proved and confirmed by the follow-up ultra-sonography.

Authenticity of Cure

CD Reference: GY001-BILATERAL POLYCYSTIC OVARY-KB

2. A CASE OF INFERTILITY ASSOCIATED WITH PELVIC INFLAMMATORY DISEASE & BILATERAL LARGE OVARIAN CYSTS COMPLETELY CURED BY HOMOEOPATHY

Case No. GY002

Mrs. S. D. K., aged about 32 years first came to me on 9th October, 1995 with the following complaints -

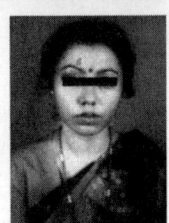

Photo of the patient, Mrs. S.D.K.

Presenting Complaints

- Irregular menstruation, delayed, profuse and clots.
- Trying to conceive for last three years, but not happening.
- Clinically diagnosed by Gynaecologist as a case of large right ovarian cyst and also left ovarian enlargement with cyst, associated with P.I.D. (Pelvic Inflammatory disease) Confirmed by Ultrasonography.

Head to Foot Scanning of Symptoms

- Head- No headaches. Sweat on back and front of head; sour smelling.
- Eyes- Nothing particular.
- Nose- Stoppage of nose < night. Catches cold easily and has a tendency of profuse and yellow discharge.
- Mouth- Foetor oris.
- Tongue- Blackish, prominent papillae.
- Throat- Prone to swelling of tonsils < cold (this symptom since childhood).
- Lungs- Nothing particular.
- Heart- Palpitation from least exertion.
- Chest- Whenever catches cold → cold extends downwards → tickling cough << warm room, << indoors.
- Abdomen- Can not bears tight clothing around abdomen.
- Appetite- Average.
- Sweat- Profuse perspiration, especially on head and back. Sour smelling.

- Urine- 8 - 10 times per 24 hours. Occasionally offensive or sourish smell.
- Stool- Constipated. Dry and occasionally with mucus. Sour smelling.
- Upper Extremities- Nothing particular.
- Lower Extremities- Backache < on sitting, < stooping.
- Female Genital Organs-
  - Sexual desire- Poor.
  - Menstruation - Puberty - 12 years of age. Onset - delayed.
    Duration - 4 - 5 days. Character - fishy, darkish. Quantity - profuse. Clots.
    Frequency - 40 days apart generally.
    Associated symptom during menses – (i) Profound weakness, (ii) Sharp cutting pain in the right ovarian region.
  - Leucorrhoea- Occasional yellowish discharge < before period.
- Rectum- Nothing particular.
- Skin Diseases- Occasional allergy from jewellery, contact allergy, small rash with itching.
- Mental Symptoms- (a) Mild, (b) Fault finding, (c) Absent minded, (d) Shy, (e) Wants to be alone, (f) Memory weak, absent minded, (g) Sympathetic, (h) Fears thunderstorms, accidents, failure.
- Exciting Causes/Causative Factors- No history of- (i) Injury, (ii) Mental grief or disappointments, (iii) Handling chemicals, (iv) Sexual excesses, (v) Excessive mental labours, (vi) History of S.T.D. etc.
- Past Medical History- Nothing particular.
- First Cause of Breakdown of Health- Cannot correlate.
- Homoeopathic Generalities-
  - Heat and Cold Relationship- Hot patient; but catches cold easily.
  - Desires and Aversions to Food Stuffs
    Desires: (i) Sweet++, (ii) Sour +, (iii) Salt +, (iv) Salty +, (v) Fruits +,(vi) Egg +++, (vii) Cold food +, (viii) Cold drinks +, (ix) Ice-creams +,
  - Aversions- (i) Bitter, (ii) Meat.
  - Thirst- Average.
  - Sleep- Okay. No particular dreams.
  - Discharges- Sweat, stool and urine all have a sourish smell.
- Marital Status-

- Married for four years and trying to conceive for last three years, but cannot conceive.
- Family History-
  - Paternal side- Cancer
  - Maternal side- Heart and rheumatic problems.
- Previous Medical Treatment-
  - Allopathic (conventional medicine) mainly hormonal drugs but reacted with feeling of discomfort and hot flushes → so stopped.
  - Homoeopathic Pulsatilla, Graphites, Sepia etc. in various potencies from other homoeopaths.

Investigations Carried Out Before/After Dr. Banerjea's Treatment

17th Apr'95: Ultra Sonography (USG) - Pelvis Good sized right ovarian cyst. 8.3 x 6.0 cm. Uterus normal. Left ovary enlarged and cystic.

Sonography report, before treatment.

27th Sep'95: H.S.G. (Hystero-Salpingography). Patent both fallopian tubes. Ultra Sonography (USG) Bilateral ovarian cyst.

9th Oct'96: Ultra Sonography (USG) pelvis. Remark:- Right ovarian Cyst. 5 cm x 2 cm & P.I.D. (Pelvic Inflammatory Disease).

23rd Jan'98: Ultra Sonography (USG) Pelvis. Remark:- Right ovary 4.5 x 3.9 cm (Just bulky, no cysts). Left ovary 2.5 x 2.5 cm (Normal).

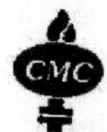

Sonography report, after 12 months of treatment.

Miasmatic Diagnosis: Syco-Tubercular

Psora	Sycosis	Syphilis	Tubercular
• Sour smelling sweat • Catches cold easily • Stool dry and constipated • Mild • Shy • Wants to be alone • Fear of thunderstorms, accidents, failure • Desires sweet • Sweat, stool, urine – sourish smell	• Sweat on back and front of head • Profuse and yellow discharge from nose • Blackish papillae on tongue, (hyper pigmentation) • Cannot bear tight clothing around abdomen (hypersensitivity) • Urine increased • Menstruation has fishy odour • Cutting pain in the right ovarian region during menstruation • Irregular menstruation (hormonal imbalance, in-coordination, sycosis) • Cystic mass and ovarian enlargement • Yellowish leucorrhoea • Absent minded • Married four years, trying to conceive for last three but cannot conceive (in-coordination also, fallopian tubes are patent, so no blockage; yet inability to conceive, therefore hormonal imbalance, sycotic) • From ultrasound (USG) report – ovarian cyst • Pelvic inflammatory disease (diagnosed by Gynaecologist)	• Stoppage of nose, < night • Foetor oris	• Recurrent swelling of tonsils < cold • Palpitation from least exertion • Menstrual blood – profuse and clots • Profound weakness during menstruation • Allergy from jewellery (nickel) • Fault finding • Desires cold food • Tendency to catch cold easily

Psora 9   Sycosis 14   Syphilis 2   Tubercular 8

This patient couldn't conceive even after three years of trying. This could be due to hormonal imbalance or in-coordination which is Sycotic. From the Gynaecologist's point of view the patient has patent fallopian tubes (H.S.G. report) and has bi-lateral ovarian cysts, this is Sycotic. So from the clinical and pathological point of view Sycotic miasm is coming as the surface miasm, and from the miasmatic totality we can see it is a mixed miasmatic case with Sycotic preponderance. Accordingly we need a mixed miasmatic medicine with Sycotic preponderance and here Calcarea Iodata entirely fits such miasmatic dyscrasica as well as covering the totality.

After the action of Calcarea Iodata, in the follow up sonography report one can see that not only the cysts have improved but the patient has conceived which reflects the wonderful capability of homoeopathy in changing lives.

Remedy Diagnosis: Calcarea Iodata.

(A) Remedy Discussion

- Features of Calcarea Carbonica -
  - Sweat on back of head, sour smelling.
  - Yellowish nasal discharge.
  - Tendency to catch cold easily.
  - Cannot bear tight clothing around abdomen.
  - Profuse perspiration, head and back, sour smelling.
  - Constipated, sour smelling stool.
  - Profuse menses with clots.
  - Fearful temperament.
  - Desires sweet, sour, egg, cold food, ice-creams.
  - Aversion to meat.

(B) Features of Iodum

- Offensive odour from month.
- Catches cold easily → cold extends downwards → tickling cough → << warm room and indoor (Ref. Dr. Boericke).
- Palpitation from least exertion.
- Profound weakness during menses.
- Irregular period.
- Sharp pain in right ovarian region.
- Hot patient.

(C) Features of Calcarea Iodata

- Nasal discharge has a tendency to be profuse and yellow.
- Takes cold easily.
- Prone to swelling of tonsils predisposition to glandular enlargements.
- Yellowish leucorrhoeal discharge.
- Allergic skin rash with itching.
- Ovarian enlargement = interpreted as glandular swelling.

Calcarea Iod. has the miasmatic breakdown: Psora ++, Sycosis +++, Syphilis +, Tubercular +++.

Gynaecological Diseases – Cured Cases

Calcarea Iod is one of the medicines I have developed by using it frequenty in clinic. I want my fellow homoeopaths to use this medicine when you will find some symptoms of Calcarea Carb and some symptoms of Iodum in either Calcarea (4F: Fair, Fat, Flabby, Freezing) or Iodum (Scrawny, Cachectic, Emaciated) constitution. Calcarea Iod has special affinity in all glands of the body, including tonsils, adenoids, thyroid, breast, lymph glands, prostrate, testis, ovaries, etc. So any tumour or swelling of these glands comes under the domain of Calcarea Iod. It is a hot patient with strong desire for fresh open air. I have given a detailed description of this medicine in my book "CLASSICAL HOMOEOPATHY FOR AN IMPATIENT WORLD".

Prescription Chart

Date	Prescription Done on the Basis of	Treatment
9th Oct'95	Features of Calcarea in hot constitution (other points in favour of prescription discussed earlier).	Calc. Iod., 200 C 2 doses. To sip (with water) the 1st dose for 7 days; 7 days off; then the 2nd dose to sip for 7 days.
17th Nov'95	Menses – 4 days, normal, regular, L.M.P. 28th Oct '95.	Wait and watch
20th Dec'95	L.M.P(Last Menstrual Period) - 18th Nov'95 L.M.P. - 17th Dec'95	Wait and watch
2nd Feb'96	L.M.P. 19th Jan'95 menses regular.	Wait and watch
1st Mar'96	Occasional pain in left side of abdomen. L.M.P. 17th Feb'96	Calc. Iod., 200 C 2 doses
12th Apr'96	As a whole doing better.	Wait and watch
3rd May'96	As a whole doing better.	Wait and watch
17th Jun'96	L.M.P. - 16th Mar'96 L.M.P. - 16th Apr'96	Wait and watch
15th Jul'96	Delayed menses L.M.P. - 20th May'96 L.M.P. 27th Jun'96	Wait and watch
14th Aug'96	L.M.P. - 4th Aug'96	Calc. Iod, 200 C 2 doses
20th Sep'96	No problem externally. Regular menses L.M.P. – 4th Sep'96	Wait and watch.
9th Oct'96	Menstruation regular. L.M.P. – 4th Oct'96	Wait and watch.
29th Nov'96	L.M.P. - 27th Oct'96 L.M.P. - 20th Nov'96	Calc. Iod., 1 M 2 doses
13th Jan'97	L.M.P. - 20th Dec'96	Wait and watch.

Cured Cases

Date	Prescription Done on the Basis of	Treatment
7th Feb'97		Calc. Iod., 1 M 2 doses, 10 M 1 dose
28th Mar'97	Threaten abortion happened 19th Mar'97. L.M.P. 20th Dec'96. Now physically fit.	Wait and watch.
12th May'97		Wait and watch.
23rd Jun'97	Menstrual cycle regular	Wait and watch.
18th Aug'97	M.C. regular L.M.P. 27th Jul'97. Trying to conceive, but not happening, dropped.	Calc. Iod., 200 C/2 doses
3rd Oct'97	Wait and watch.	Wait & watch.
21st Nov'97	Wait & watch.	Wait and watch.
22nd Dec'97	M.C. → regular. L.M.P. - 26th Nov'97	Wait and watch.
16th Feb'98	M.C. → 28th Jan'98 OVARIAN CYST CURED	Wait and watch.
6th Apr'98	Menstrual cycle → 28th Jan'98, 3rd Mar'98, 2nd Apr'98	Wait and watch.
1st Jun'98	L.M.P. – 9th May'98	Calc. Iod., 50 M 2 doses
13th Jul'98	L.M.P. – 7th Jun'98 & 7th Jul'98	Wait and watch.
19th Aug'98	L.M.P. – 5th Aug'98	Wait and watch.
23rd Sep'98	No change of anything → standstill L.M.P. – 9th Sep'98	Calc. Iod., CM 2 doses
30th Oct'98	L.M.P. – 8th Oct'98	Wait and watch.
14th Dec'98	L.M.P. - 10th Nov'98, 10th Dec'98 Normal cycle. Stool - one daily – clear. Sleep – sound. Appetite - normal.	Wait and watch.
3rd Feb'99	L.M.P. - 8th Jan'99 Stool - clear. Appetite - normal. M.C. On regular time.	Wait and watch.

Patient got pregnant in March'99 and delivered a normal healthy baby.

*Readers may view the pictures of the case (before and after treatment) in our website under Gynaecological Diseases (**Case No. GY 002**- A case of Ovarian Cyst in a 32 years old married woman, completely cured by Calcarea Iodata.).*

Authenticity of Cure

CD Reference: GY002-OVARIAN CYST-SDK

3. A CASE OF FIBROID & RENAL STONE MRS K.S.

Case No. GY003

Age – 32 years as on 14th October, 1988.

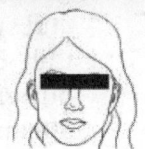

Photo of the patient, Mrs. K.S.

Presenting Complaints

- Pain in the right side of abdomen with burning sensation and associated with some shivering; pain aggravates after eating, especially after rich & fatty food→ pain as from pressure with occasional throbbing→ ameliorated by rest, cold application on abdomen.
- Backache aggravated by first motion, ameliorated by continued slow motion.
- Pain in right side of the body (hand, chest, leg) → began 15 days back; dull aching.
- Urine: Frequent urination worse when lying down; offensive odour; burning in the urethra during micturition – yellow in colour.
- Stool: Stool not clear; constipated stool.
- Menses: Time – Regular. No pain in abdomen. Scanty bleeding. Stays – 4 days. Dark, clotted blood.
- Anorexia (++) for last 6 months. Taste of food remains long after.
- Vertigo → aggravated by motion, ameliorated by rest and in fresh open air.
- Redness of eyes.
- Itching hip → vesicular ulcer → after itching, bleeding – itching aggravated due to perspiration.
- Thirstless.
- Hot patient.
- Perspiration all over the body.
- Burning sensation in palms.
- Disturbed sleep; wide awake at night.
- Desires: Pungent & hot ++, sour ++, vegetables & spinach, chicken, cold food +.

- Mind: Calm & amiable, can be silently angry and irritable but does not explode. Can be stubborn & obstinate, talkative, likes company and sympathy. Memory – Weak. Fear of dark & impending disease. Can be romantic ← or in phases → withdrawn. Sympathetic, but gives to receive back; can be demanding, needs support and attention.

Investigations Carried Out Before/After Dr. Banerjea's Treatment

10th Dec'87: Ultra Sonography: Gall bladder, liver, pancreas & kidney. Remark:- Small calcified nodule in the upper pole of right kidney.

15th Dec'90: Urine : Sediment – Trace. Ultra Sonography: lower abdomen:- Remark:- Cervical fibroid – measures 3.7 cm in diameter.

30th Apr'91: Ultra Sonography Abdomen: Remark:- Nothing Abnormal Detected.

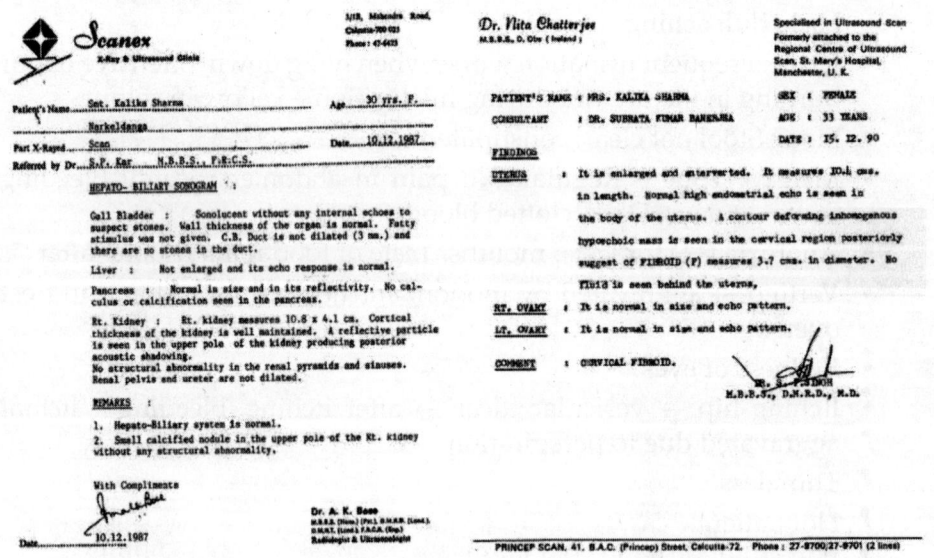

USG report of Mrs. K. S. before treatment.   USG report during treatment.

Gynaecological Diseases – Cured Cases

Dr. Nita Chatterjee
M.B.B.S., D. Obs (Ireland)

Specialised in Ultrasound Scan
Formerly attached to the
Regional Centre of Ultrasound
Scan, St. Mary's Hospital,
Manchester, U. K.

PATIENT'S NAME : MRS. KALIKA SAIMA
CONSULTANT : DR. S. K. BANERJEE

SEX : FEMALE
AGE : 33 YEARS
DATE : 30. 4. 91

FINDINGS

KIDNEYS : Right kidney length is 10.6 cms. and left kidney length is 11.1 cms. Renal parenchyma is normal. Echogenic renal sinuses are seen in the mid part. No stone, hydronephrosis or mass lesion is seen.

URETERS : No dialation or calculi is seen.

URINARY BLADDER : Normal capacity of the bladder is seen. Wall is smooth. No calculi or mass is seen.

UTERUS : It is anteverted and abnormal in size. It measures 8.6 cms. in length, 5 cms. in Tr. dimension and 4.2 cms. in A.P. dimension. High endometrial echo is seen in mid part. Echo pattern is homogenous. No fluid is seen behind the uterus. No focal abnormality is noted.

RT. OVARY : It is normal in size, position and echo pattern. A 2 cms. follicle is seen.

LT. OVARY : It is normal in size and echo pattern and lies postero lateral to the uterus.

COMMENT : NORMAL KIDNEYS, URETERS, BLADDERS, UTERUS AND OVARIES.

DR. S. P. SINHA
M.B.B.S., D.M.R.D., M.D.

PRINCEP SCAN, 41, B.A.C. (Princep) Street, Calcutta-72. Phone : 27-9700/27-9701 (2 lines)

USG report 4 months after treatment.

CASE ANALYSIS, MIASMATIC DIAGNOSIS AND FINAL PRESCRIPTION

- Miasmatic Analysis:
- Fibroids and renal stone: Sycotic.
- Burning sensation in abdomen: Syphilitic.
- Aggravation of pain after eating: Psora.
- Aggravation from fat food: Sycotic.
- Amelioration from cold applications on abdomen: Syphilitic.
- Backache ameliorated by continued slow motion: Sycotic.
- Urine: offensive odour: Tubercular.
- Urine: burning in urethra during urination: Psora.
- Urine: yellow colour: Psora-sycotic.
- Constipation: Psora.
- Menses: scanty bleeding: Psora. Clotted blood: Tubercular.

- Anorexia: Psora.
- Vertigo: aggravated by motion: Psora; ameliorated by rest: Psora-tubercular; amelioration in open air: Tubercular.
- Redness of eyes: Psora-tubercular.
- Vesicular ulcer: Syphilitic; aggravation from perspiration: Syphilitic;
- Itching followed by bleeding: Psora-tubercular.
- Thirstless: Psora.
- Burning sensation in palms: Psora.
- Disturbed sleep at night: Syphilitic.
- Desires: Pungent & hot: Sycotic; Sour: Psora-syphilitic; Cold food: Syco-tubercular.
- Mental: Calm and amiable: Psora. Stubborn and obstinate: Tuberculo-syphilitic.
- Talkative: Sycotic; Likes company and sympathy: Sycotic.
- Memory weak: Psora.
- Fear of dark and impending disease: Psora.

It is a mixed miasmatic case with Syco-Tubercular preponderance.

Reasoning for Final Prescription

- Sympathetic, but gives to receive back; can be demanding, needs support and attention.
- Calm & amiable, can be silently angry and irritable but does not explode.
- Stubborn & obstinate, talkative, likes company and sympathy.
- Vertigo ameliorated in the open air.
- Pain aggravates after eating, especially after rich & fatty food.
- Pains accompanied by chilliness (shivering).
- Pains better for cold applications.
- Thirstless.
- Taste of food remains a long time in mouth.
- Desires cold food.
- Increased desire to urinate when lying down.
- Burning in orifice of urethra during micturition.
- Scanty and clotted menses.

The miasmatic breakdown of Pulsatilla is Psora: ++, Sycosis +++, Syphilis +, Tubercular ++. This covers the Syco-tubercular preponderance of this case well.

Gynaecological Diseases – Cured Cases

Remedy Reaction

This case was started with Pulsatilla 200 C, the potency chosen on the basis of the patient's duration of suffering and the nature of the case. The case was finished with Pulsatilla 10M after just under 4 years of treatment.

Prescription Chart

Date	Prescription Done on the Basis of	Treatment
14th Oct'88	Right sided; pain associated with shivering (chilliness); pain aggravates after eating, especially after rich & fatty food; pain ameliorated by cold applications on abdomen. Backache aggravated by first motion, ameliorated by continued slow motion. Frequent urination worse when lying down. Menses: dark, clotted blood. Taste of food remains long after. Vertigo > in fresh open air. Thirstless. Burning sensation in palms. Disturbed sleep; wide awake at night. Likes cold food +. Mind: Calm & amiable, can be silently angry; does not explode. Likes company and sympathy. Fear of dark & impending disease. Can be romantic ← or in phases → withdrawn. Sympathetic, but gives to receive back; can be demanding, needs support and attention.	Pulsatilla, 200C, 2 doses. S.O.S: Hydrangia Q (if needed) for pain of stuck renal stone.
3rd Dec'88	No appreciable change; wait & watch.	Sac lac.
3rd Mar'89	Right hypochondrial burning — a little better. Occasional swelling sensation of the body. Lumbago -a little better. Wait & watch.	Sac lac.
3rd May'89	Improved.	Sac lac.
15th Jul'89	Pain in back aggravates when lying down at night.	Pulsatilla 200 C: Repeat
21st Jul'89	No appreciable change; wait & watch.	Sac lac.
29th Nov'89	Feels on the whole a little better, wait & watch for further movement of symptoms.	Sac lac.
6th Feb'90		Sac lac.
4th Apr'90		Sac lac.
21st May'90	Feels on the whole a little better, wait & watch for further movement of symptoms.	Sac lac.
3rd Jul'90	Acute pain of passing stone in the right side. [Ocimum Can. – pronounced symptoms of renal calculus in right side].	Ocimum Canum., 30 C/2
22nd Aug'90		Sac lac.
31st Oct'90	Feels on the whole a little better, wait & watch for further movement of symptoms.	Sac lac.

Date	Prescription Done on the Basis of	Treatment
14th Dec'90	Vertigo-came back. Itching in hip. Anorexia was a little better, but now again bad. Pain in extremities. Lumbago aggravated by motion ameliorated by rest. Perspiration in palms & soles (+++).	Pulsatilla, 1M...2 doses.
17th Dec'90		Sac lac.
19th Apr'91		Sac lac.
29th Apr'91	Feels on the whole a little better, wait & watch for further movement of symptoms.	Sac lac.
30th Apr'91		Sac lac.
18th Jul'91	Feels like a stand still status; so repeat.	Pulsatilla 1M.....2 doses.
20th Aug'91		Sac lac.
28th Aug'91	Feels on the whole a little better, wait & watch for further movement of symptoms.	Sac lac.
2nd Sep'91		Sac lac.
1st Nov'91		Sac lac.
4th Jan'92	Pain in right kidney, burning sensation, ameliorated by rest. Thirstless. Dry mouth. Pain aggravated by stretching the arms up, ameliorated by warmth.	Pulsatilla 10M....2 doses.
4th Feb'92		Sac lac.
6th May'92	Feels as a whole little better, wait & watch for further movement of symptoms.	Sac lac.
3rd Jun'92		Sac lac.
15th Jun'92	Cured of renal stone and fibroid (Vide USG – 12/6/92). Appetite when increased → Nausea. Thirst ++. Perspiration +++. Stool hard ++.	Sac lac.

Authenticity of Cure

CD Reference: GY003-UTERINE FIBROID
WITH RENAL STONE-KS

4. A CASE OF OVARIAN TUMOUR: MRS. M.G.

Case No. GY004

Age   : 24 years old as on 5th September, 2006
Sex   : Female
Height: 5 ft. 4 inches.
Weight: 64 kgs.

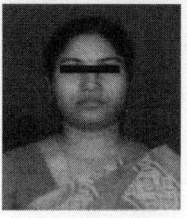
Photo of the patient
Mrs.M.G.

Presenting Complaints

- Menses prolonged, now continued for 1 month. Swelling and pain in both breasts, just before menses. Patient thinks hormonal balance is disturbed. She gets extremely anxious, worried (++) and irritable, before.
- Dysmenorrhoea for 1 month. More the flow, more the pain, Menarche at – 12 years of age.
- Pain on right side of lower abdomen during menses.
- Diagnosis P. C. O. D. (Right sided). [Polycystic Ovarian Disease]
- Irregular menses since July 2001 → PCOD. Now profuse menses bleeding and pain.
- Throat:- Hoarseness of voice due to excess cold. Cold affects voice.
- Stomach:- Appetite – Normal. Occasional Acidity. Acidity (++) with sour eructation.
- Stool – Constipated. 3 times a week.
- Perspiration – On hands, back of head, neck & feet, especially in summer. Sour smell of the sweat.
- Skin:- Rash on right hand after bee sting.
- Temperament:- Irritable; Weepy (+++); Anxious (++); Worried.
- Fear from darkness (++).
- Memory – Good.
- Hot patient. Dislike rainy.
- Food preferences:- Salty (+++); Bitter (++); Egg(++); Cold food. Aversion – Sweet; Spice.
- Thirsty (+++).
- Sleep:- Disturbed.
- Past Medical History:- Chicken pox.
- Family Medical History:- Mother – Cardiac problem.

Investigations Carried Out Before/After Dr. Banerjea's Treatment

2nd Aug'06 Ultra Sonography (USG) whole abdomen:- Ovarian Dermoid.

16th Oct'06 Ultra Sonography (USG) whole abdomen:- Bulky right ovary. Possibilities:- (1) Right ovary solid SOL. Right ovary – 40.0 x 42.0 mm; (2) Organised haemorrhage within right ovary. Left ovary 30 x 14 mm.

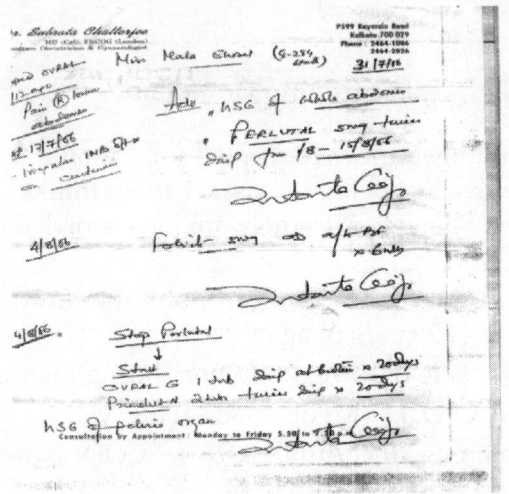

Allopathic Prescription of Mrs. M.G.

U.S.G. report of Mrs. M.G.
before treatment.

16th Jan'08 Ultra Sonography (USG) Pelvis:- Bulky right ovary – multiple small follicles.

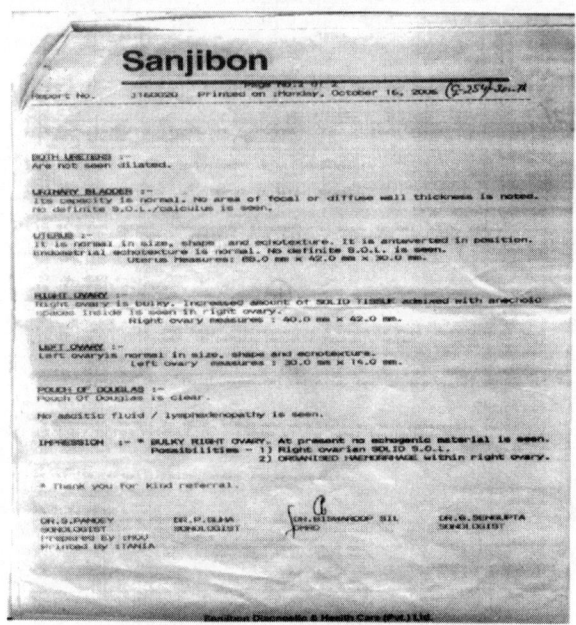

Continuation of U.S.G. report

U.S.G. (Pelvis) report of Mrs. M.G.
24 months after treatment.

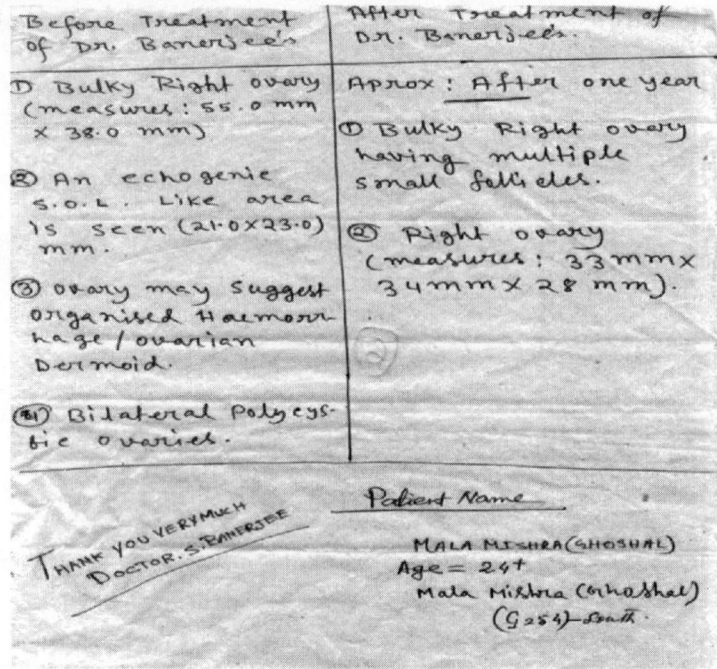

Remarks by the patient about treatment.

CASE ANALYSIS, MIASMATIC DIAGNOSIS AND FINAL PRESCRIPTION

Miasmatic Analysis

- Menses prolonged, now continued for 1 month: Tubercular.
- Swelling and pain in both breasts, just before menses: Tuberculo-Sycotic.
- Patients think hormonal balance is disturbed: Sycotic.
- She gets extremely anxious, worried: Psora.
- Irritable, before menses: Sycotic.
- Diagnosis P. C. O. D. (Right sided). [Polycystic Ovarian Disease]: Sycotic.
- Irregular menses: Syphilitic.
- Throat:- Hoarseness of voice due to excess cold. Cold affects voice: Psora-Tubercular.
- Stomach:- Acidity (++) with sour eructation: Psora.

- Stool – Constipated. 3 times a week: Psora.
- Temperament:- Irritable; Weepy+++: Sycotic.
- Fear from darkness (++): Psora.

Final Prescription Made on the Basis of

- Menses prolonged, now continued for 1 month. Swelling and pain in both breasts, just before menses. Patient thinks hormonal balance is disturbed. She gets extremely anxious, worried (++) and irritable, before.
- Diagnosis P. C. O. D. (Right sided). [Polycystic Ovarian Disease]
- Irregular menses since July 2001 → PCOD. Now profuse menses bleeding and pain.
- Throat:- Hoarseness of voice due to excess cold. Cold affects voice.
- Stomach:- Appetite – Normal. Occasional Acidity. Acidity (++) with sour eructation.
- Stool – Constipated. 3 times a week.
- Perspiration – On hands back of head, neck & feet especially in summer. Sour smell of the sweat.
- Temperament:- Irritable; Weepy+++; Anxious (++); Worried.
- Fear from darkness (++).
- Food preferences:- Salty+++; Bitter++; Egg++; Cold food. Aversion – Sweet; Spice.
- Hot Patient.

The miasmatic breakdown of Calcarea Iod is Psora++, Sycosis+++, Syphilitic+, and Tubercular+++.

Final Prescription and Remedy Reaction
CALCAREA IOD 200C

Prescription Chart

Dates	Points in Favour of the Prescription	Prescribed Medicine
5th Sep'06	PCOD Cyst. Desire – Salty. Anxious and worried. Fear of ghost. HOT.	Calcarea Iod 200C, 2 doses.
17th Oct'06	Weakness >. Dysmenorrhoea >. Bleeding >. As a whole 70% - 80%. Better.	PL (Sac Lac)
19th Dec'06	Doing better.	PL

Dates	Points in Favour of the Prescription	Prescribed Medicine
20th Jan'07	As a whole doing >. 90% >.	PL
7th Apr'07	As a whole doing much >.	PL
26th Jun'07	Patient feels stand still. So repeated.	Calcarea Iod 200C, 2 doses.
30th Oct'07	>	PL
22nd Jan'08	Dysmenorrheoa. Patient feels much better. Sonography done. Bulky right ovary: better. Right ovary SOL: better. Only few small follicles (which can be functional) are only present.	PL (Sac Lac)
6th May'08	As a whole >.	PL

Authenticity of Cure

CD Reference: GY004-OVARIAN TUMOUR-MG

7

CHAPTER

Uro-Genital (Male) Diseases - Cured Cases

1. A CASE OF ABDOMINAL TUMOUR: MR. A.R.

Case No. M001

A case of retroperitoneal pelvic mass (abdominal tumour) in a 39 year-old male.

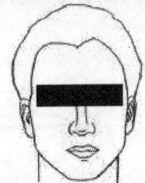

Photo of the patient, Mr. A.R.

Presenting Complaints

- Pain the left side of lower abdomen, better by pressure.
- Constipation. Occasional rounded ball like stool.
- Gas in abdomen.
- Pain from umbilicus towards lower abdomen, after urination.
- Pain feels at left side of lower abdomen during walking.
- In the month of March, 1995 at about 11.00 p.m., abdominal pain and vomiting started two hours after eating.
- Indigestion, stool not clear.
- Weakness++.
- Profuse wind forms in abdomen; aggravates in the afternoon; ameliorates by passing of flatus.
- Thirsty.
- Hot patient.
- Profuse sweating++ → bad odour to sweat.
- Desire for sour +++; salty++, pungent; bitter; vegetable and spinach; fish, luke warm food; cold drinks. Aversion to sweet.
- Mind: Irritable temperament (+++); talkative; desire for company; patient cries when reprimanded. Insecurity.

- Very business minded and materialistic. Mentioned a few times during the consultation and the follow-ups about insecurity and instability of the world economics. I felt like economy is the centre of all his conversations.

Investigations Carried Out Before/After Dr. Banerjea's Treatment

18th Apr'96 (before coming to me): Ultra Sonography of whole abdomen: Large retroperitoneal pelvic mass. Patient came to me for treatment at end of April 1996.

29th Mar'98 (after my treatment): Ultra Sonography of whole abdomen:- Nothing abnormal detected.

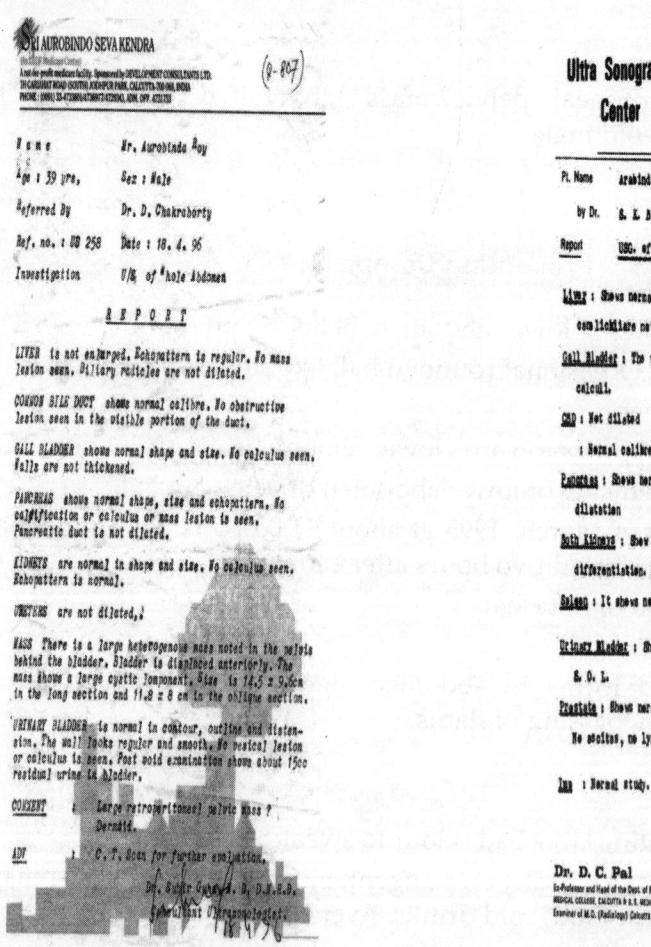

Sonographic Report of Mr. A.R., Abdominal tumour, before treatment

Normal Sonographic report, after 23 months of treatment

CASE ANALYSIS, MIASMATIC DIAGNOSIS AND FINAL PRESCRIPTION

This is an interesting case of a large abdominal tumour (according to ultra sonogram, can be cystic) and patient felt it was growing. Also pain and other discomforts were present.

Miasmatic Analysis

- Pain the left side of lower abdomen, better by pressure: Sycotic.
- Constipation. Rounded ball like stool occasionally: Psoric.
- Weakness: Mostly psoric, can be Psora-tubercular.
- Profuse wind forms in abdomen: Psora.
- Aggravation from movement: Syphilitic.
- Profuse sweating: Sycotic.
- Desire for sour: Psora; Salty: Sycotic; Pungent: Psora.
- Mind: Irritable temperament: Syco-tubercular;
- Talkative: Sycotic; Insecurity: Sycotic.
- Very business minded and materialistic: Sycotic.
- It's a mixed miasmatic case with Psora- sycotic preponderance.

Final Prescription Made on the Basis of

- Pain the left side of lower abdomen, better by pressure- Bryonia has amelioration from lying on the painful side.
- Constipation. Rounded, ball-like stool.
- Pain felt at left side of lower abdomen during walking – aggravation from motion.
- Thirsty.
- Hot patient.
- Profuse sweating++, bad odour to sweat.
- Desire for sour +++.
- Mind: Irritable temperament (+++). Insecurity.
- Very business minded and materialistic. Concerned about insecurity and instability of the world economics. I felt like economy is the centre of all his conversations.
- I have given emphasis on his mental essence which reflected materialism and was very much concerned about economy which in

turn reflected his insecurity and anxiety about the future. With such a mental essence in the background, he had this large abdominal tumour with pain better by pressure, etc. and accordingly Bryonia (the stock broker's remedy: no feelings or sentiments) was selected.

The miasmatics of Bryonia are: Psora ++, Sycosis +++, Syphilis +, Tubercular ++. This is a predominantly sycotic case with psoric and tubercular elements and therefore the miasmatic nature of the case is covered well by Bryonia.

Final Prescription

BRYONIA, 200 C: 1 globule (No. 10, poppy seed size) in sugar of milk sachet, asked the patient to dissolve the powder in half or one litre of pure water and sip it slowly throughout the day, save a little at the bottom, top it up next morning, keep sipping throughout the next day. Generally I give instruction to my patients to dilute the medicated water (top it up with water) as many times as s/he likes. Continue like this for 7 days. Then 7 days of no medicine. Followed by another dose to be shaken and sipped for 7 days.

The 200 C potency was used to begin with on the basis of the patient's vital energy and the totality of the case.

Remedy Reaction

Patient's response to Bryonia was very satisfactory. After 200 C, I waited for 2 months and constipation was better, pain was lessened and emotionally he was more relaxed. I repeated 200 C twice, and after 6 months from the initial treatment, I went to 1M and the changes were dramatic. Physical symptoms abated significantly. Pain and vomiting were 90% better including indigestion, gas and sweating. I waited for 4 months and then repeated 1M another time, but felt a stand still status and went to 10M. With the 10M dose the mental symptoms significantly improved, including the feelings of insecurity. The pain was totally absent, so I asked the patient to repeat the ultra sonography and the result was very satisfactory: large retroperitoneal tumour had disappeared with the action of homoeopathy! Patient was cured within 16 months.

Authenticity of Cure

CD Reference: M001-RETROPERITONEAL PELVIC MASS-AR

2. A CASE OF OLIGOSPERMIA : MR. S.B.

Case No. M002

A 31 year-old married male.

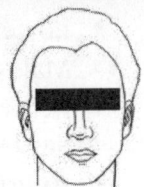

Photo of the patient, Mr. S.B.

Presenting Complaints

- Married for two years and nine months. Trying for a baby (18 – 20 months), but nothing is happening. Worried and concerned that problem belongs to him or his wife.
- Seminal fluid: scanty.
- Weakness++ and sticking pains.
- Pungent odour+++ of urine.
- Burning in rectum with occasional bleeding.
- Heart burn and eructations.
- Head: Hot vertex, burning.
- Eyes: Watery discharge from eyes.
- Ear: Otalgia – both ears sticky with occasional discharge.
- Nose: N.A.D (Nothing Abnormal Detected).
- Mouth: N.A.D.
- Teeth: Pain in teeth.
- Tongue: N.A.D.
- Throat: Occasional pain in throat on taking cold.
- Lungs: Occasional oppression in chest due to acidity and flatulence.
- Heart: N.P (Nothing Particular).
- Chest: N.A.D.
- Abdomen: Acidity aggravated on an empty stomach – sour eructation. Heartburn; on passing flatus both upwards and downwards.
- Stomach: Anorexia.
- Sweat: Profuse sweat all over the body. Offensive odour.
- Urine: Offensive and pungent odour in urine; burning sensation after micturition. No sediment after urination.
- Stool: Irregular and oily stool; bad odour; burning of rectum after passing of stool. Upper Extremities: Pain in extremities ameliorated by pressure and massage.

- Palms: N.A.D.
- Joints: Pain in joints aggravated in new moon and full moon.
- Lower Extremities: N.A.D.
- Male Genital Organs: Sexual desire – absent; testes: small; penis: lax.
- Anus: Burning in rectum after stool, occasional bleeding when a hard stool.
- Angry, stubborn +++.
- Talkative.
- Absent minded.
- Hopeless. Despair of recovery.
- Weak; gradual loss of memory.
- Gets angry when reprimanded.
- Sympathetic.
- Fear of thunderstorm.
- Grief especially for not having child.
- Chilly patient. Catches cold easily.
- Desires: Sweet++, sour+, salt+++, salty+, bitter: no, bread+, milk+, potato+, vegetables and spinach+, onion: no, fruits+, fish+, meat/chicken+, egg (boiled/fried)++, rich, spicy and fat food+, warm food: no, cold food++, warm drinks: no, cold drinks+, ice cream+.
- Thirsty.
- Disturbed sleep.
- Dreams of sex, daily work.
- History of masturbation.
- Typhoid in childhood, treatment – allopathy. Malaria in childhood, treatment – allopathy. Measles. Vaccination in childhood. Cannot correlate.
- Paternal – Tb, Diabetes, Gastritis.
- Treatment started in end-September 1990.

Investigations Carried Out Before and After Dr. Banerjea's Treatment

20th Jul'89: Semen: Motility: 20%; Count: 40 million; Pus cells: 1 – 2 HPF.
10th Sep'90: Semen: Motility: 10% Count: 25 million; Pus cells: 3 – 4 HPF.
21st Feb'92: Semen: Count: 170 million, Actively motile : 40 – 45%; Viability after 4 hrs.: 30 -35%.

Uro-Genital (Male) Diseases - Cured Cases

Semen report of Mr. S. B., before treatment

"X-RAY RELIEF" LABORATORY
2/1/B, BEPIN BEHARI GANGULY STREET, (1st Floor) CAL-12
(COLLEGE STREET & BOWBAZAR STREET, JUNCTION)
NEAR RUPAM CINEMA
Branch: 25/B/1/A, M. G. ROAD, CALCUTTA-9

REPORT ON EXAMINATION OF SPERMATIC FLUID

Pt's Name: Sri Swapan Bhowmick.
Date: 10. 9. 90.
Referred by Physician/Surgeon: Dr. N. Karmakar, D.M.S. (Cal.)

Physical Examination: White, opalescent, semi fluid.
 (a) Consistency: gelatinous
 (b) Viscosity: normal.
 (c) Liquefaction: normal.
Quantity: 2 ml.
Reaction: alkaline.

Microscopical Examination:
Motility:
 immediately after receiving — 10%
 after 2 Hours — 5%
 after 4 Hours — nil
 after 6 Hours — nil
 after 8 Hours — nil
 after 10 Hours — nil
 after 12 Hours — nil
 after 24 Hours — nil

Total Count: 25.0 millions per c.c.

Differential Count:
 Mature Form: 60%
 Immature Form: 25%
 Teratological Form: 5%
 Degenerated Form: 10%

Pus-cells: present (3+) per field
Epithelial-cells: present (+)

for "X-ray Relief" -Laboratory

Semen report of Mr. S. B., 17 months after treatment

Dr. Subir Kumar Dutta
MBBS, DCP, MD (Path & Bact)
Dr. Subhas Chandra Maitra
MBBS, DCP, MD, PhD (Canada)
Dr. Sunil Kumar Gupta
MBBS, DCP, MD, FRCPath (Eng.)

Scientific Clinical Research Laboratory Pvt. Ltd.
2, RAM CHANDRA DAS ROW
(OFF. 77, DHARMATALA STREET)
CALCUTTA-700012.
Phone: 24-1060

Date: 21. 2. 1992.

REPORT ON THE EXAMINATION OF

SEMEN

Patient's Name: Mr. S. Bhowmick.
Referred by Dr.: S. K. Banerjee.

Physical Examination:
 Colour — greyish white
 Quantity — 1 c.c.
 Viscosity — viscous just after discharge later thin mucoid opaque
 Blood — not visible

Chemical Examination:
 Reaction — alkaline (pH = 7.5)
 Occult blood test — negative

Microscopical Examination:
 Morphology — Mature forms — 65–70%
 Motility — Motile forms — 55–60%
  Actively motile — 40–45%
 Sperm count — 170 millions per c.c.
 Other features — Epith. cells — few R.B.C. — nil
  Leucocytes — 2–4 h.p.f.
 Viability — After 4 hrs. 30–35%

Normal specimen

CASE ANALYSIS, MIASMATIC DIAGNOSIS AND FINAL PRESCRIPTION

This is an interesting case of oligospermia where Homoeopathy has In azoospermia, I always try to open the case from a miasmatic point of view to clear up the deep-seated Syphilitic stigma, the destructive miasm destroying the spermatozoa.

Miasmatic Analysis

- Complete azoospermia is syphilitic and in oligospermia, as well, we have syphilitic preponderance, but psora (lack, scanty, denote psora) is also present in the background. Therefore my intention was to find an anti-syphilitic, which would cover the totality of symptoms as well.
- Lack of sperm in semen: Psora.
- Seminal fluid scanty: Psora.
- Weakness: Mostly psoric, can be psora-tubercular.
- Sensation of burning in rectum: Syphilitic.
- Bleeding from rectum: Tubercular.
- Oily stool: Sycotic.
- Heartburn: Psora.
- Sour eructations: Psora.
- Profuse sweat: Sycotic.
- Offensive perspiration, stool and urine: Syphilitic.
- Pains in extremities ameliorated by pressure and rubbing: Sycotic.
- Joint pains: Sycotic.
- Lack of sexual desire: Psora.
- Testes dwindling: Psora.
- Absent minded: Sycotic.
- Memory impaired: Syphilitic.
- Stubborn: Syco – Tubercular.
- Fear of thunderstorms: Psora.
- Catches cold easily: Tubercular.
- Talkative: Sycotic.
- Desires salt: Syco – Tubercular.
- Sexual dreams: Sycotic.

It's a mixed miasmatic case with Psora- syco-syphilitic preponderance.

Final Prescription Made on the Basis of

- Seminal fluid: scanty. Oligospermia.
- Sticking pains.
- Weakness++.
- Burning in rectum with occasional bleeding (haemorrhagic diathesis).
- Heartburn and eructations.
- Head: Hot vertex, burning.
- Sweat: Profuse sweat all over the body. Offensive odour.
- Urine: Offensive and pungent odour in urine; burning sensation after micturition. Boericke says of Nitric acid: "Scanty, dark, offensive. Burning and stinging."
- Male Genital Organs: Sexual desire – absent; testes: small; penis: lax.
- Anus: Burning in rectum after stool, occasional bleeding when hard stool.
- Angry, stubborn +++.
- Talkative.
- Absent minded.
- Hopeless. Despair of recovery – Nitric acid is anxious about health and a worrier. Boericke says "Hopeless despair".
- Weak; gradual loss of memory.
- Gets angry when reprimanded.
- Fear of thunderstorm.
- Grief, especially for not having a child.
- History of masturbation.
- Typhoid in childhood, Treatment – allopathy. Malaria in childhood, Treatment – allopathy. Measles vaccination in childhood.
- Chilly patient. Catches cold easily.
- Desires: Salt+++, egg (boiled/fried)++, rich, spicy and fat food+, [Nitric acid loves fat and salt – Boericke].
- Thirsty.
- Disturbed sleep.
- Dreams of sex, daily works.
- Paternal – TB, Diabetes, Gastritis.

The miasmatic breakdown of Nitric acid is Psora ++, Sycotic +++L, Syphilitic +++L, Tubercular +++, which covers the miasmatic nature of this case.

Personality and Appearance

Nitric acid is especially suited to thin, weak and debilitated persons with rigid musculature, dark complexion, black hair and eyes; ugly looking appearance; with broken down scrawny, cachectic constitution; anaemic and emaciated.

Temperament is usually nervous and irritable: excessive physical irritability. A very nervous, excitable, peevish individual who is easily angered by small things. Hateful and vindictive adamant and remains unmoved by any amount of apology because he is so rude and unsympathetic. He has great anxiety about his disease and is constantly thinking about his past troubles.

The 200C potency was chosen due to the nature of the case, a genito-urinary complaint, for which this potency of Nitric acid is particularly suited.

Nitric Acid covers the case miasmatically as well.

Final Prescription

ACID NITRIC, 200 C: 1 globule in sugar of milk sachet dissolved in pure water and sipped over 7 days. Then 7 days of no medicine, followed by another dose to be shaken and sipped for 7 days.

Remedy Reaction

I started the case with ACID NITRIC, 200 C. I waited for 4 months and in this period weakness and pungent odour of urine got slightly better. I repeated 200 C another time, but with the second dose of 200C there was no appreciable change. I was slightly confused at this stage, and felt like there was a pathological malfunction of the semen, so why not try a lower potency of Nitric acid. I decided to go down to 30C, 3 months later (placebos given in between). I waited for 2 months, but there was absolutely a standstill status, no movement of symptoms. I decided to do a semen analysis and the report was bad. I re-assessed the case, as I was questioning the choice of medicine. As 200C gave some improvement, I decided that the similimum must be in the higher potency in this particular case, so I decided to go for 1M of Acid Nitric. With 1M, the hot feeling in the vertex and burning, watery discharge from eyes and sticky discharge from the ears got better. Pain in teeth and throat improved, as also did the acidity, heartburn and flatulence. Appetite much improved (which I took as a remarkably positive sign). The odour of the sweat and bowels got better.

I waited for 2 months and then, when it got to a standstill status, I repeated 1M another time. I asked the patient to do a seminal analysis, and the result was much improved (54 million), but still not satisfactory. I felt there was no further movement in the case. I then went to 10M and with this dose the sexual and mental symptoms significantly improved, including the sexual desire (libido returned) and the laxation of the penis improved. Angry, stubborn, absent minded, hopelessness and despair of recovery all much improved almost to the extent of 80-85%. When it reached a status quo position after 6 weeks, I repeated another dose of 10M; the remaining 10–15% got better and the patient felt more positive and smiled. I asked him to repeat the test for semen count and this came out with a normal (spermatozoa count became normal) report.

After 6 months, he came back to inform me that his wife was pregnant!! Glory goes to Hahnemann and his beautiful Homoeopathy.

Authenticity of Cure

CD Reference: M002-OLIGOSPERMIA-SB

3. A CASE OF URETHRAL STRICTURE: MR. A.M

Case No. M003

Age : 36 Years

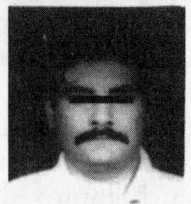

Photo of the patient
Mr. A.M.

Presenting Complaints

- Stricture urethra – operation done in February, 1995. Polyurea scanty, burning before and after micturition. Flow is slow; occ. retention. Pungent odour – urging to urinate.
- Pain in inguinal region, hypogastric region and waist, aggravate on stooping forward and backward. > Better by lying, massage.
- Head:- Sweat on forehead.
- Mouth:- Odour.
- Teeth:- Gum swollen, occasional blood comes out when pressed.
- White coated tongue.
- Palpitation < slight exertion, > by rest.
- Abdomen:- History of habit of taking rich and spicy food. Wind forms in abdomen; < after eating, better by passing flatus. Occasionally wind ascends upwards. Occ. acidity and sour mouth; and heaviness of abdomen. Chest pain – both sides better by eructation.
- Appetite – poor.
- Offensive odour in sweat.
- Urine – light yellow colour. Scanty but frequent. Odour in urine; burning.
- Stool – Regular, but not clear. Blackish yellow, sour smell. Ineffectual urging for stool. Whitish mucous in stool.
- Joints:- Occ. pain in waist < stooping, sitting for long period, > by lying, massaging.
- Skin – Heals fast. Itches both side of groin, no oozing.
- Mental – Calm and quiet. Talkative, desire company. Gloomy, fear of death.
- Memory – Active, Sympathetic.
- He does everything slowly. Fear of Dogs, accidents and incurable diseases.

Uro-Genital (Male) Diseases - Cured Cases

- Bad effects of masturbation – Break down of health.
- Habit of smoking.
- Past History:- Skin diseases – applied ointment. Tuberculosis in kidneys. Chicken pox – once. Chilly patient. Hates rainy weather. Likes open air, doors and windows open.
- Catches cold easily.
- Food Desire:- Sour+, Pungent and hot, Salty++, Onion, Chicken++, Egg+, Rich, Spicy and fatty food. Aversion to Sweet, Bitter, Vegetables and Warm food. Patient is thirsty.
- Sleep:- Disturbed. Sleepy in the late part of night. Dreams of various things.

Investigations Carried Out Before /After Dr. Banerjea's Treatment

28th Feb'90: Cystogram – Urethral Stricture. Micturating cystogram- (noted) narrowed segment is noted in the posteria urethra. Stricture urethra (posteria urethra).

10th Apr'04: Cystogram – Nothing abnormal Detected. Micturating Cystogram Investigation-is within normal limit, (normal cystogram report after 52 months of Dr.Banerjea's treatment.

Cystogram report of Mr. A.M. before treatment

MEDICARE IMAGES

Name: MR. A. MUKHERJEE **Sex:** M **Age:** 34 Years
Ref.by: DR. SUBRATA BANERJEE **Date:** 10.04.04

Thanks for referral

History of the patient: Check up.

M.C.U.

- Cystogram shows normal outline of bladder.
- No negative shadow or filling defect noted.
- Prostatic and penile part of urethra well visualised.
- Mild dilatation of penile part of urethra shown.
- No gross irregularity in neck of bladder.
- No mucosal irregularity noted.

The investigation is within normal limit.

DR. DIPANKAR DASGUPTA
D.M.R.D

DR. RAJEEV BISWAS
M.B.B.S., D.M.R.D.

Cystogram report after treatment

In the year 1994 I felt obstruction during urination. There was a burning sensation during urination. I went to a doctor for treatment. He examined me and said it's a case of stricture and suggested a operation. After operation he advised me for dilatation every six weeks. From 1995 I am under treatment of Dr. Ganguly. Dr. Banerjee.

My condition before meeting Dr. Banerjee	My condition after meeting Dr. Banerjee
1. Thin flow of urine	1. Thicker flow of urine
2. Burning sensation during urination.	2. Burning sensation has reduced markedly.
3. Amount urine is little and frequent urination.	3. Amount of urine is a little more.
4. I have to pressurise for urination	4. This trouble has reduced.
5. A feeling that urine has not fully discharged.	5. Now I feel this trouble sometimes.
6. A feeling of obstruction during urination	6. I still feel so.
7. I cannot control myself during it I feel	7. I still feel so.

Patient's comments after treatment

CASE ANALYSIS, MIASMATIC DIAGNOSIS AND FINAL PRESCRIPTION

Miasmatic Analysis

- Urethral Stricture: Syphilitic. Urethral stricture is a syphilitic problem, but many times sycosis joins in because of discharge.
- Polyurea: Sycotic. Scanty: Psora. Burning and pungent odour: Syphilitic.
- Pain in inguinal region and waist aggravation:-stooping forward and backward: Sycotic > lying: Psora.
- Gums swollen – occasional bleeding: Tubercular.
- White coated tongue: Sycosis.
- Palpitation: Tubercular.
- Abdomen – Gas, acidity, sour mouth: Psora, heaviness: Sycotic.
- Poor appetite: Psora.
- Sweat offensive odour: Syphilitic.
- Stool: Sour smelling: Psora, ineffectual urging: Psora, whitish mucous: Sycotic, blackish/yellow: Syco-Syphilitic.
- Mental: Calm,quiet,sympathetic: Psora. Talkative: Sycotic. Does everything slowly: Psora. Fears dogs: Tubercular. Fear of death, incurable diseases, accidents; Psora. Gloomy: Syphilitic.
- Chilly patient: Tubercular. Hates rainy: Sycotic. Chilly patient but catches cold easily: Tubercular. ECC-likes open air: Tubercular.
- Desires: Sour: Psora. Pungent, hot: Psora-Tubercular. Salt/salty: Syco-Tubercular. Aversion vegetables: Sycotic.
- Thirsty: Sycotic.
- Tuberculosis in kidneys: Tubercular.

It's a mixed miasmatic case with Syco-syphilitic preponderance.

Final Prescription Made on the Basis of

- Urethral Stricture.
- Urine-Polyuria scanty, burning before and after urination.
- Urging to urinate-pungent odour.
- Stool-Blackish yellow, ineffectual urging-mucus+++, bad odour.
- Occ. Bleeding before stool, burning in rectum after.
- Sweat-offensive odour from axillae, profuse perspiration-espcially. forehead.

- Mind- Fear of death, Gloomy.
- Thirst-Poor –due to polyuria.
- Appetite-Poor, Desires Fatty food, Salty++.
- Sleep Disturbed, Late night sleep.
- Dreams, Terror,Police.

Mixed Miasmatic case chiefly Syphilitic. Acid Nitric is a leading Tri-Miasmatic remedy.

The miasmatic breakdown of Acid Nitric is Psora ++, Sycosis +++L, Syphilis +++L, Tubercular+++.

Nitric Acid covers the case miasmatically as well.

Final Prescription

ACID NITRIC: 200C, 2 doses.

Remedy Reaction

Acid nitric has been prescribed which is a deep acting anti-syphilitic and anti-sycotic (reference Boericke's Materia Medica) as well as leading tri-miasmatic. Urethral stricture is a syphilitic problem, but many times sycosis manifests it's presence because of the yellowish discharge.

Prescription Chart

Date	Prescription Done on the Basis of	Treatment
22nd Dec'98		Nitric-Acid 200C, 2 doses
18th Feb'99	Urinary problem – was > from previous medicine now S/S.	Acid- Nit, 200C, 2 doses.
28th Apr'99	Wind formation. Epigastric pain. Belching gives relief. < from gas. Burning micturation. Lumbago < motion > rest. Burning abdomen – pain < from loss of appetite. Thirsty. Urine – strong odour. Stool – not clear, dysentery. Wait and Watch	Sac lac
23rd Jun'99	Wait and Watch	Sac lac

Uro-Genital (Male) Diseases - Cured Cases

Date	Prescription Done on the Basis of	Treatment
1st Sep'99	Stool – mixed with blood. Took allopathic medicine. Internal Piles. Itching of anal orifice during and especially after passing stool. Burning. Yellow, blackish, offensive. Obstinate constipation. Great straining, white shreddy particles. Urine – flow frequent and scanty must hurry, > after eating. Testicular pain. Urinary stream split. Difficult starting must wait a long time. Must strain before flow comes; flow intermits. Chilly patient. Thirst+++. Sweat+++. Appetite – poor. Dreams of various kinds. Disturbed sleep. Desire – cold food, mutton, egg. Pungent sour. Excess worry. Aversion to sweets.	Acid Nit, 1M, 2 doses.
23rd Nov'99	Obstructed flow of urine but have not been dilated since. Piles with bleeding.	PL15, Cynodon Q (given to control the acute bleeding piles).
9th Feb'00		Acid Nit, 1M, 2 doses
6th Jun'00	Stricture urethra – obstruction. Burning during and after urine. Frequent. Piles – Blood mixed and stool. Burning during, after stool. Stool – regular not clear. Mucus, gas whole abdomen > after stool. Appetite – scanty. Sleep – last part of night, Sweat – offensive. Desire – Veg. **A?** – Fish, Meat, Egg.	Sac lac.
14th Sep'00	Stricture urethra, piles – same as before. No other problem.	Acid Nit, 10M, 2 doses.
5th Nov'00	Flow normal when urging more, otherwise flow thin. Piles+. Thirst+. Appetite – poor. Sleep – poor. Sweat++.	PL15
18th Jan'01	Urinary flow normal. Improvement continued frequency of micturition + < after eating. Bleeding piles+. Constipation+. Thirst++. Appetite – poor. Sleep+. In this way I carried on the prescription and finished the case with Acid Nitric CM.	Sac lac.
10th Apr'04	Cystogram – Nothing Abnormal Detected. M.C.U. Investigation-is within normal limit, (normal cystogram report after 52 months of Dr.Banerjea's treatment).	

Authenticity of Cure

CD Reference: M003-URETHRAL-STRICTURE-AM

4. A CASE OF RECURRENT HERPES GENITALIS: MR. K. C. M.

Case No. M004

Age : 36 Years
Age : 35 years as on 10th November, 1993
Height : 5 ft. 5 inches.
Weight : 63 kgs.

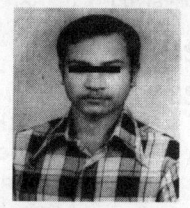

Photo of the patient
Mr. K. C. M.

Presenting Complaints

- Occasional penile eruptions appear at 10 – 11 days interval/bimonthly. Dry.
- Occasional pain.
- Initially rash also appeared, with pimples on penis, on body especially the back, then cleared.
- Now occasional pimple-like eruptions, which appear on the extremities.
- Itching → watery discharges.
- Patient is unmarried.
- History of promiscuity.
- Stool: Regular & okay.
- Urine: Okay.
- Appetite: Normal.
- Thirsty.
- Hot patient. Likes: winter, Hates: rainy weather.
- Profuse perspiration all over the body. No bad odour in sweat.
- Heals okay.
- Sound sleep.
- Dreams: Nothing.
- Desires: Sweet+, pungent, bitter, vegetables and spinach, fish, lukewarm food, cold drinks. Aversion to sour.
- Mind: Mild, talkative, desire for company, emotional, consolation ameliorates; sympathetic, weepy mood, cannot tolerate blood letting. Fear of being alone.
- Past History: Measles, chickenpox, cancer.
- History of diphtheria in childhood. Treated allopathically.

Investigations Carried Out Before/After Dr. Banerjea's Treatment

25th Aug'93: Blood: VDRL - + ve.
23rd Aug'95: Blood: VDRL – ve.

Allopathic prescription of Mr. K. C. M. before treatment

Blood report Mr. K. C. M. before treatment

Blood report 23 months after treatment

Patient's comments after treatment

CASE ANALYSIS, MIASMATIC DIAGNOSIS AND FINAL PRESCRIPTION

Miasmatic Analysis

- Herpes Genitalis: Sycotic; whereas Recurrent Herpes Genitalis is Syco-Tubercular.
- Occasional penile eruptions appear at 10 – 11 days interval: Tubercular.
- Dry eruptions: Psora.
- Itching: Psora.
- History of promiscuity; visiting prostitutes.
- Aggravation from rainy weather: Sycotic.
- Profuse perspiration all over the body: Sycotic.
- Cannot tolerate blood letting: Psora.
- Desires: Sweet+: Psora; Pungent: Sycotic; Luke warm food: Sycotic; Cold drinks: Syphilitic.
- Fear of being alone: Psora.

It's a mixed miasmatic case with Psora-sycotic preponderance.

Final Prescription Made on the Basis of

- Periodic attacks.
- Weepy mood.
- Profuse perspiration.
- Desire for warm food.
- Hydrogenoid – hates rainy weather.
- Thirsty for cold drinks.
- Eruptions that itch and discharge a watery fluid: Boericke says "watery blisters".

Miasmatic breakdown of Natrum Sulph. is: Psora ++, Sycotic +++L, Syphilitic +, Tubercular +.

Natrum Sulph covers the case miasmatically as well.

Constitution and Personality

Natrum Sulph. is particularly indicated where complaints are due to living in damp houses, basements, cellars etc. Changes from dry to damp seasons aggravate the symptoms.

There is much sadness and gloom in Natrum Sulph., music makes this patient melancholic and inclined to weep. Great loathing of life with suicidal tendencies.

Remedy Reaction

The treatment was begun with Natrum Sulph. 1m, moving to a prescription of Thuja as the symptom picture changed. The patient's symptoms were dramatically improved over 7 years of treatment.

Prescription Chart

Date	Prescription Done on the Basis of	Treatment
10th Nov'93	Aggravation from change of season, which is strongly sycotic. Recurrent Herpes Genitalis is Syco-Tubercular. Syco-Syphilitic with cancer in the background. Felt there is a good match so went for high potency!	Natrum sulph., 1M, 2 doses, sipped in water.
6th Dec'93		Sac lac.
7th Feb'94	Emotional feeling lifted but physically unchanged. Wait and watch with wisdom (WWW).	Sac lac.
5th Mar'94	Gap between attacks is increasing.	Sac lac.
30th Mar'94		Sac lac.
4th May'94	Much better, but mucus in stool.	Sac lac.
1st Jun'94		Sac lac.
6th Jul'94		Sac lac.
17th Aug'94	Standstill, not improving further.	Natrum sulph., 1M, 2 doses.
14th Sep'94	Much better. Occasional eruption.	Sac lac.
9th Nov'94	Had eruption once only. Still felt standstill, not improving properly.	Natrum sulph., 10M, 1 dose.
14th Dec'94		Sac lac.
25th Jan'95		Sac lac.

Uro-Genital (Male) Diseases - Cured Cases

Date	Prescription Done on the Basis of	Treatment
8th Mar'95	Was better, occasional R.H.G (Recurrent Herpes Genitalis). Rash: once in 10 days. Still felt standstill, not improving properly.	Natrum sulph., 10M, 2 doses.
26th Apr'95	Better than before 85%.	Sac lac.
7th Jun'95	Penile eruption. Almost ceases then freshens up again. A prescription was needed to clear up the case. Occasional pain in the penis.	Natrum sulph., 1M, 2 doses → 10M, 1 dose.
31st Jul'95		Sac lac.
9th Oct'95	Doing better. Now okay. Blood report: negative of herpes genitalis (23/8/95).	Sac lac.
25th Nov'95	Now okay.	Sac lac.
8th Jan'96	Standstill.	Natrum sulph., 50M, 1 dose
19th Feb'96		Sac lac.
10th Apr'96	As a whole better.	Sac lac.
5th Jun'96	Standstill.	Natrum sulph., 50M, 2 doses
25th Jul'96		Sac lac.
24th Aug'96	Pimple like eruption in penis ameliorated. Now pain occasional, no itching. No other problems. Thirst+, Appetite+, Sleep+, Sweat: profuse, offensive. Prescription made to move case forwards.	Natrum sulph., CM, 2 doses
3rd Oct'96	Now pimples appear at 3-month intervals. Now no problem. Change in prescription, following the sycotic chain of remedies.	Thuja, 1M, 2 doses
1st Nov'96	Patient feels better. No new problem. Thirst+, Appetite+, Sleep+.	Sac lac.
4th Dec'96	Doing better. Thirst+, Appetite+, Sleep+, Occasional pain in penis.	Sac lac.
4th Feb'97	Patient as a whole feels better.	Sac lac.
31st Mar'97		Thuja, 1M, 2 doses.
14th May'97	As a whole better occasional pimples appear.	Thuja, 10M, 2 doses.
2nd Jul'97	Doing better.	Sac lac.
13th Aug'97	Was aggravated now better. No other problem. New pimples have appeared again.	Thuja, 1M, 2 doses → 10M, 1 dose.

30th Sep'97	Now as a whole feels better.	Sac lac.
1st Dec'97	Doing better. Occasional pain in penis. No other problem.	Sac lac.
9th Feb'98	Doing better 90% better.	Sac lac.
8th Apr'98	Now always slight pain in penis.	Thuja, 1M, 2 doses → 10M, 1 dose.
6th Jun'98	Sores appeared after 3 months, but subsided after 10 days. Now better.	Thuja, 50 M, 2 doses.
25th Jul'98	Better; occurred once some days before, but at moment it is normal.	Sac lac.
12th Sep'98	Better but low pain occurring, sometimes.	Sac lac.
17th Oct'98	Better.	Sac lac.
4th Dec'98	Improved.	Sac lac.
9th Feb'99	Doing better.	Sac lac.
23rd Mar'99	Doing better. Occasional mild pain in penis.	Sac lac.
22nd May'99	Doing better. Problems appeared one time after taking medicine. Stayed 4 – 5 days.	Sac lac.
19th Jul'99	Doing much better.	Sac lac.
13th Sep'99	Doing better. Waited for 15 months.	Sac lac.
22nd Nov'99	Doing better.	Sac lac.
25th Jan'00	Doing much better.	Sac lac.
15th Mar'00	Doing better. Eruptions on penis slightly appear → one time.	Sac lac.
13th May'00	Doing better.	Sac lac.
26th Jun'00	Doing much better.	Sac lac.
28th Aug'00	Doing much better.	Sac lac.
17th Oct'00	Doing better.	Sac lac.
27th Nov'00	Doing better. Oozing one time after taking medicine, ameliorated automatically. Otherwise no problems.	Sac lac.
1st Feb'01	Doing better. Eruptions appeared one time, stayed 3 – 4 days, better automatically.	Sac lac.
28th Mar'01	Doing much better.	Sac lac.

Authenticity of Cure

CD Reference: M004-RECURRENT HERPES GENITALIS-KCM

5. A CASE OF HYPERTROPHY OF PROSTATE WITH RECURRENT- U.T.I.

Case No. M005

MR. T. C.

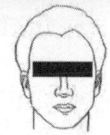

Photo of the patient, Mr. T.C.

Presenting Complaints

- Recurrent Urinary tract infection with urine retention. Diagnosed as enlargement of Prostate.
- Difficulty in urination, interrupted flow.
- Regular indigestion and flatulence.
- History of Jaundice 12 years back – Gas forms all the time.
- Repeated urge of stool – with mucus.
- Knee pain, shoulder pain, muscle pain especially lower extremities – right sided. Heaviness of the extremities, pain better by motion and pressure. Worse lying down.
- During U.T.I. severe pain in lower abdomen, better by pain killer/ antibiotic. Heaviness of lower abdomen.
- Head – Perspiration ++, more than normal, more during sleep rarely during daytime. Occasional vertigo.
- Abdomen: Appetite – Normal. But indigestion and flatulence is there. Distention both sides of abdomen. Get temporary relief by passing flatus.
- Bowels: Regular – 2-3 times/day. Semi-liquid. Pungent and bad odour. Not satisfactory evacuation. Stool after meal, nervous diarrhoea. Pain before bowel movement. Weakness after evacuation.
- Rectum: Excessive gas formation, sometimes cause pain in rectum.
- Urine: Normal; Recurrent attack of U.T.I. Frequent urination – sometimes. Interrupted flow of urine.
- Excessive sweating: Odour under arm. Sometimes stains.
- Joints: History of Tennis elbow – twice, frozen shoulder once.
- Skin: Dry, dandruff ++. Itching sometimes in groin sticky discharge. Very rare use of ointments, lotions.
- High sexual desire, inconsistency in erection, premature ejaculation.
- Temperament: Absent minded++, Introvert+++, Negative, Punctual++, Stubborn++, occasionally withdrawn ++.
- Depression: Failure in 1997/98 in his professional and personal life.

- Nature: Pessimism, lack of trust etc.
- Accompanying Symptoms: Become totally quiet, introverted, do not like to be disturbed.
- In 1997 – Left job and started business – Business failed – also marriage failed in 1997 – UTI – Pain lower abdomen.
- Chilly patient, dislike rainy season. Likes winter.
- Food desire: Sweet+++, Salt+++, Salty+, Savoury++. Meat++, Egg+++, Spice++. Likes warm food.
- Thirst – Likes drinks long interval. The patient is Thirstless.
- Sleep – Ok. Dreams of sex.
- Odour in stool and sweat.
- Past Medical History: Chicken pox, Tonsillitis, Glandular Tb, Typhoid, Skin diseases.
- Family History: Mother – Osteoarthritis, Hysterectomy. Father – Death by heart failure.

Investigations Carried Out Before/After Dr. Banerjea's Treatment

14th Sep'00: Ultrasonography of Urinary system and Prostate. Remark:- Prostate is enlarged in size, multiple scattered echogenic

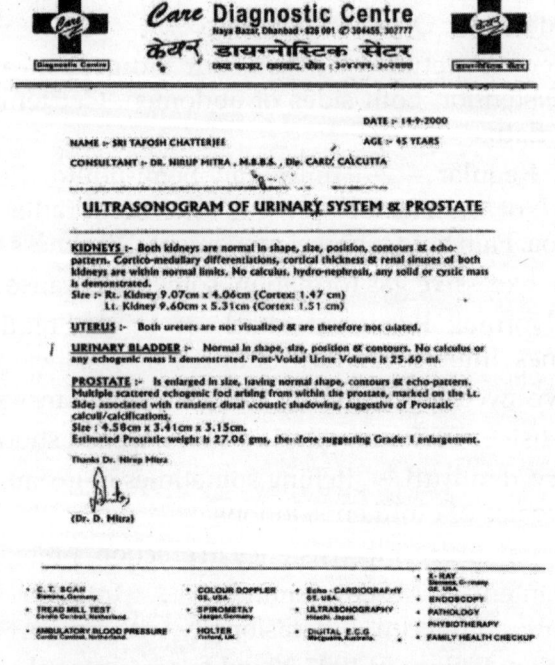

U.S.G report of Mr. T.C. before treatment

foci – suggesting, grade 1 enlargement. Estimated Prostatic weight is 27.06 gms.

14th Jan'05: Ultra Sonography (USG) lower abdomen:- Impression – Normal study.

CDP Medicare Private Limited

Shri. Tapash Chatterjee.   14.1.2005.
Dr. Subrata K. Banerjee.

ULTRASONOGRAPHY OF LOWER ABDOMEN INCLUDING KIDNEYS

KIDNEYS : Both the kidneys appeared normal in shape and size. The cortical echogenicity and the central echocomplex appeared normal. The pelvicalyceal systems were no. dilated.

BLADDER was normally distended and contained no sizeable lesion within. Almost no residual urine (about 5ml) left after voiding.

PROSTATE appeared normal in shape and size.

IMPRESSION : Normal study.

(DR SUBRATA DAS)
D.M.R.D, M.D.

U.S.G report, 9 months after treatment

Progress report regarding treatment of Tapash Chatterjee under Dr. Subrata Kumar Banerjea commencing March 2004

Before treatment started	Since treatment started
1. Virulent attack of urinary tract infection, the frequency which was once in 2 & 1/2-3 yrs round about 1997 when the problem first started, increased to about once a year by Feb/March 2004. USG done of lower abdomen in 2000 revealed Grade I prostrate enlargement resulting in retention of 25ml. of urine.	1.USG done in Dec2004, 9 months after commencement of treatment of Dr Subrata Banerjea, showed Prostrate to be of normal size and urine retention of 4ml which is standard. No pain attack has occurred for almost one yr; although the pathologist conducting USG opined that pain attack for U.T.I. can happen even other than Prostrate enlargement.
2. Weak sexual performance in terms of inconsistent and not full erection inspite of urge being more than normal. Hormone tests revealed no abnormalities.	2. Problem still persists
3. Occasional bout of acute amebiosis which is hereditary.	3. Problem increased of late, subsides only by regular use of S.O.S. medicine prescribed by Dr Banerjea.

Comments of patient, before and after treatment

CASE ANALYSIS, MIASMATIC DIAGNOSIS AND FINAL PRESCRIPTION

Miasmatic Analysis

- Enlargement of prostrate: Sycotic.
- Recurrent U.T.I.: Syco-Tubercular. Frequent urination: Sycotic. Intermittent flow of urine: Psora-Sycosis.
- Abdomen – Excessive gas, distention: Psora-Sycotic (excess), Heavy lower abdomen: Sycotic.
- Mucous in stool: Sycotic. Weakness after evacuation: Psora.
- Joint pains: Sycotic.
- Excessive sweating; odour: Sycotic.
- Nervous diarrhea: Sycotic.
- Skin – Dry, itching, dandruff: Psora.
- High sexual desire: Sycotic. Inconsistency – erection and premature ejaculation: Psora-Sycotic.
- Temperament – Absent minded, Punctual ++: Sycotic. Introvert+++: Syphilitic. Stubborn: Tubercular. Pessimistic: psora. Withdrawn: Syphilitic.
- Dislikes rainy: Sycotic. Likes winter: Syphilitic.
- Desires- Sweet: Psora, Salt/salty: Syco-Tubercular. Desire meat: Tubercular. Warm food: Sycotic.
- Thirstless: Psora.
- P/H Tonsillitis, glandular T.B: Syphilitic. Scrofulous: Tubercular.

It's a mixed miasmatic case with Psora-sycotic preponderance.

Final Prescription Made on the Basis of

- Prostrate enlarged.
- Difficulty in voiding urine; interrupted flow of urine.
- Indigestion.
- Introvert +++ Absent minded, withdrawn.
- Heavy lower abdomen.
- Joint pains with heaviness of muscles aggravation:-lying down better by motion, better by pressure.
- Salt/salty +++.
- Sweat ++ on sleeping not during waking hours. Weakness after evacuation.

Uro-Genital (Male) Diseases - Cured Cases

- High sexual desire, inconsistency in erection and premature ejaculation.
- Recurrent U.T.I.
- Sleep – Dreams of sex.
- Thirstless.

The miasmatic breakdown of Conium is Psora ++, Sycosis ++, Syphilis+, Tubercular + C++

Conium covers the case miasmatically as well.

Final Prescription

Preponderance of the Sycotic miasma and considering the overall totality, Conium Mac 200C was the first prescription of choice.

Prescription Chart

Date	Prescription Done on the Basis of	Treatment
13th Apr'04	Prostate enlarged. Indigestion. Introvert. Heavy lower abdomen. Desire: - Salt+++, Salty. Sweat++.	Conium 200C, 2 doses.
26th Jun'04	As a whole >>. But patient generally gets the UTI attack at an interval of 12 – 13 months. Wait and watch	Sac lac
7th Sep'04	NAC. Occ. pain abdomen with mucus stool. Sac lac. For emergency SOS (mucus stool)	Holarrhoeana antidysenterica (Kurchi) Q, 10 drops 8 hourly SOS
6th Nov'04	Appetite less. Occ. Dull pain in urinary organs. Others Standstill. Now Ankle pain esp. early morning. Occ. knee pain, pain disappear spontaneously. Wait and watch	Sac lac.
22nd Jan'05	Urinary problem >. USG – Prostate : Normal. ENLARGEMENT GOT CURED, ALSO NO RESIDUAL URINE.	

Authenticity of Cure

CD Reference: M005-HYPERTROPHY OF PROSTATE-TC

8 Neoplastic Diseases – Cured Cases
CHAPTER

1. A CASE OF BRAIN TUMOUR: MRS P.R.

Case No. NEO001

Mrs. P.R.J., 23 years, Hindu Female, brought to me first on 8th of August 1988 with the following complaints:

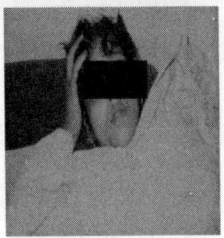

Mrs. P.R.J., Brain Tumour, before treatment.

Presenting Complaints (Started in February, 1988.)

- Recurrent vomiting followed by sweat. Sweat also on little exertion.
- Loss of sleep.
- Slurring of speech aggravated in the morning and night, ameliorated after warm drinks.
- Dimness of the vision, aggravated by excitement and better by rest.
- Vertigo with dizziness especially while walking.
- Loss of appetite.
- Dull, heavy headache.
- Aggravation in the morning and night (esp. vomiting and vertigo).
- Aggravation from motion, exertion, better by rest.
- Better in open air.
- Worse from warmth in general.
- Headache ameliorated by pressure.
- Better by sleep.

- Better by consolation.
- Dull and heavy ache, giddiness.
- Occasional apthous ulcers.
- Occasional dry cough with pain right side of the chest.
- Occasional palpitation especially after emotion.
- Gas and distension in the upper abdomen.
- Extremely poor appetite, though slight hunger felt between 9 a.m. to 10 a.m.
- Sweat ++, especially in the back parts. No odour. Sweat on exertion. Vomiting followed by sweat.
- Stool - White mucus. No ineffectual urging. Neither diarrhoeic nor constipated. Mucus present +.
- Coldness of the extremities especially after the vomiting.
- Sexual desire ++, history of masturbation during youth, before marriage.
- Menses - Started at 14 years of age, occasional pain, menstruation is scanty, occasional flow with scanty periods.
- White discharge after periods.
- Mind was at first clear – then there was gradual stupefaction.
- Gloomy ++; absent minded +; forgetful ++. Wants to be alone. Fear of death (occasional).
- Memory weak.
- Weepy +. Sympathetic +. Slow & dull.
- Fear of darkness, incurable disease.
- Past History- History of- Recurrent vomiting at 7 years. of age; also H/O school going diarrhoea treated allopathically; H/O measles in childhood.
- What is the first cause of breakdown of health? Cannot co-relate.
- Chilly patient. Sensitive to cold and damp. Likes to take baths regularly. Does not catch cold easily.
- (34)   Desire and aversion for foods - Sweet +, sour +, pungent and hot +, salt +, salty +, bitter No. Bread +, milk No, potato +, vegetables and spinach +, onion No, fruit +, fish ++, meat and chicken +, egg (boiled/fried) +. Rich, spicy and fat food +, warm food No, cold food ++. Warm drinks No, cold drinks +. Ice cream +.
- Thirstless.
- Loss of sleep may be from worry.

- Married for four years.
- Family History- (i) Mother – rheumatism, (ii) Father - asthma.
- Treated by one Calcutta's leading Homoeopath's with Causticum without effect.

Investigation Done Before Dr. Banerjea's Treatment

20th Jul'88: Electro Encephalogram (E.E.G.) - Mildly abnormal Electro Encephalogram (E.E.G.) indicating interseizure pattern of left temporal region.

20th Jul'88: C.T. Scan of Brain C.T.study reveals an irregularly enhanced cystic midline S.O.L. (space occupying lesion) in the posterior fossa. Findings are suggestive of Haemangioblastoma. Cystic astrocytoma cannot be ruled out on these findings.

6th Nov'89: C.T.Scan of Brain - Normal Scan. Provisional diagnosis - Brain Tumour ? (Haemangioblastoma or Cystic Astrocytoma). Miasmatic diagnosis - Psora-Sycotic. Constitutional remedy – Gelsemium.

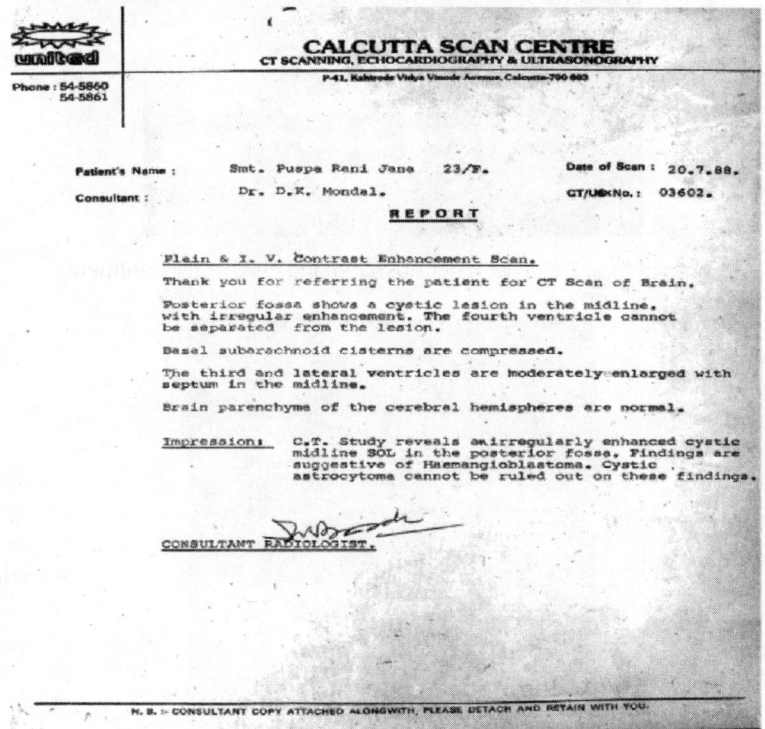

Scan report, before treatment.

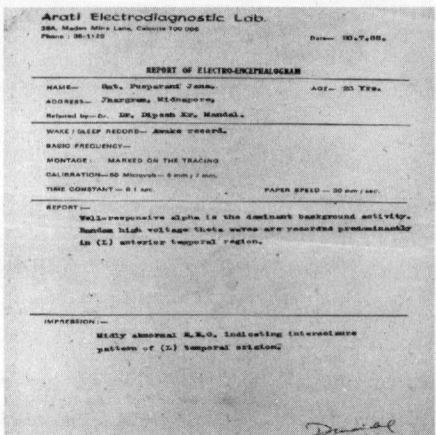

EEG report, before treatment.

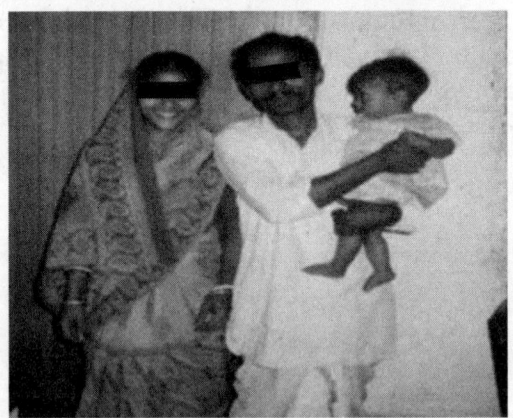

Photo of Mrs. P.R.J. with her husband and child, after treatment.

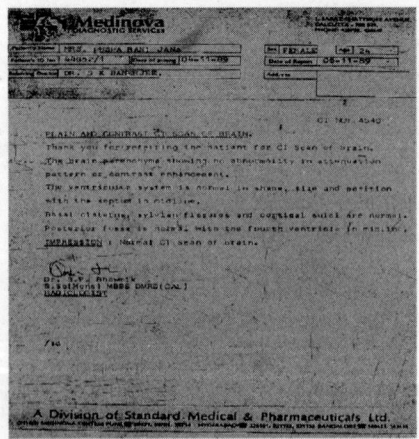

Scan report, after 15 months of treatment.

Miasmatic Interpretation & Discussion

General nature of the Sycotic miasm

Sycosis produces in-coordination everywhere; over-production, growth infiltration in forms of warts, condylomata, tumours & fibrous tissues etc.

Organs/tissues are affected by this stigma (Sycosis)

Entodermal tissues, soft tissues etc. (-- whereas Psora affects ectodermal tissues, Syphilis affects mesodermal tissues).
Psychic manifestations of Sycotic stigmata in relation to the case in concern Sycosis the in-coordinating miasm, manifests in-coordination in psychic sphere also. As if the association fibres of the cerebrum and the linking fibres of the autonomic nervous system with central nervous system have become out of gear. This in-coordination is manifested in the field of memory by forgetfulness of what she has just thought, said and done.

General manifestations of Sycotic Stigmata

All "hypers" are Sycotic or (-- whereas "hypos" are generally Psoric and "dyses" are generally Syphilitic). Hyperplasia of the tissues of the case in concern is Sycotic.

This is a case of brain tumour which was diagnosed by C.T. scan as a case of haemangioblastoma or astrocytoma. Haemangioblastoma is Syco-Tubercular and it is a tumour of vascular origin, whereas astrocytoma is Syphilo-Sycotic and it is a space occupying lesion in the brain with degenerative changes. The neurologist and neurosurgeon were of the opinion that as the patient had deteriorated so quickly and was almost bedridden within a few months, it was more likely to be an astrocytoma which is a malignant tumour of Syco-Syphilitic variety.

One can observe the Syco-Syphilitic preponderance of the case in a Psoric background, from the above miasmatic assessment therefore we have to think of a medicine which covers Syco-Syphilitic dyscrasia. Gelsemium covers the totality including the emotional state of the case as well as the miasmatic background. One can see the wonderful results of Gelsemium in this case and with the right selection of the medicine and the dose a patient of such advanced pathology has improved so dramatically which reflects the powerful penetrating dynamic capabilities of homoeopathy.

SYCOTIC TAINT OF GELSEMIUM Dr.Clarke refers a case of Hydrosalpingitis of gonorrhoeal origin cured by Gels 1M.

Miasmatic Interpretation

Psora	Sycosis	Syphilis	Tubercular
• Dimness of vision better by rest • Loss of appetite • Vertigo aggravated by movement and ameliorated by rest • Headache better by sleep • Dry cough • Gas and distension in upper abdomen • Coldness of extremities • Scanty menstruation • Gradual stupefaction • Fear of death • History of school going diarrhoea (during childhood) • Loss of sleep from worry • Wants to lie down day and night which ameliorates her trouble • Weepy and depressed • Various fears, of darkness, of incurable disease • Anamnesis from P/H • Craves sweet + • Craves pungent & hot food • Aversion to milk • Paresis and functional paralysis (Sycosis joins)	• Recurrent vomiting • Sweats on little exertion • Slurring of speech • Vertigo while walking • Headache ameliorated by pressure • Sweat ++ especially on the back • Sexual desire ++ • Leucorrhoea after menses • Absent-minded • Weepy + • Sensitive to damp • Rheumatism with mother (F/H) • Asthma with father (F/H) • Absentminded • Desires salt (can be tubercular as well) and salty food • Anamnesis from F/H (family history of Rheumatism with mother and Asthma with father).	• Vertigo worse at night • Apthous ulcers • White mucous • Gloomy ++ • Forgetful • Slow and dull	• Vertigo better in open air • Palpitation • Desires cold food

Psora 20   Sycosis 16   Syphilis 6   Tubercular 3

Points In Favour of Gelsemium

- Slurring of speech which was > by warm drinks (patient as a whole was not fond of warm drinks, but she found sipping warm water relieved (particular modality of the complaint Dr.Clarke refers stimulants ameliorate).
- Dim vision < from excitement (In Gelsemium we have general < from emotion & excitement).
- Vertigo > in open air (Boericke).
- Dull headache > by pressure and compression.
- Complete relaxation and prostration of the whole muscular system lack of muscular coordination (Clarke).
- Coldness of extremities (Kent).
- Insomnia from worry (Clarke).
- Dr. Harvey Farrington refers weakness and languors are the earliest symptom to appear. Patient feels tired and weary and wants to lie down. Dr. Farrington clearly emphasized that the excessive weakness is the prodromal state of practically all the complaints where Gelsemium is indicated. Dr.Clarke refers that the lassitude is expressed by the patient (--not expressed, Mur.Acid.).
- Desire to be let alone.
- Thirstless.
- Mind was first clear - gradual or insidious stupefaction.
- Listless attitude. Wants to lie down and rest (Clarke).
- Apathy regarding illness.
- Anamnesis of the P/H of school-going diarrhoea.
- Dr. Clarke refers functional paralysis (paresis) of all descriptions.
- Appearance: Heavy, dull appearance of the face (expression) of the countenance (Clarke). Apathy regarding her illness; "discernings are lethargic" (Ref.Boericke).

Notes on Gelsemium

- **When there is presence of many group of symptoms of various ailments and if according to the indications Gelsemium being prescribed at the outset, it can really abort the entire disease. (Ref. Ghatak).**

- Due to absence of deep-acting anti-Psoric base, Gelsemium cannot prevent the frequent relapse of the complaints due to Psoric stigmata. Dr. Nilmoni Ghatak refers that one might think that when Gelsemium has the capability to cure many deep-seated diseases, like paralysis, then how can it be possible that the medicine does not posses deep-seated anti-Psoric stigmata, but this may be noted that when the exciting cause excites the latent/dormant Psora to explode and thereby occurs manifestation of paralytic symptoms, Gelsemium having inability to prevent the said explosion of latent Psora and thereby annihilating the problem permanently like, Sulphur, Causticum, etc., does, which also corresponds miasmatically to the case. But Gelsemium has the capability of aborting the ailment when indicated by its totality, especially at the outset.

Gelsemium has the miasmatic breakdown: Psora +, Sycosis ++, Syphilis +, Tubercular +.

Prescription Chart

Date	Prescription Done on the Basis of	Treatment
8th Aug '88		Gelsemium 200C - 2 doses. To sip (with water) the 1st dose for 5 days; 2 days off; then the 2nd dose to sip for 5 days.
25th Aug '88	No change.	Wait and watch
24th Sept '88	No change, standstill but no further deterioration.	Gelsemium 200C – 2 doses
12th Oct '88	Standstill, no worsening.	Wait and watch.
16th Nov '88	Standstill, so go higher	Gelsemium 1000 (1M) – 2 doses
13th Dec '88	Improved. Vomiting is less. Vertigo and weakness are better.	Wait and watch
15th Feb '89	Better in every way. Patient has conceived. L.M.P. 18/12/88	Wait and watch
27th Mar '89	Better in every way. Pregnancy is progressing nicely and there are no complications.	Wait and watch
26th April '89	More or less cured, no major presenting complaints. Weakness occasionally, headaches etc. Patient is reluctant to continue any further treatment as she has to travel about 120 km to get to the city.	Wait and watch

*Readers may view the pictures of the case (before and after treatment) in our website under Neoplastic Diseases (**Case No. NEO 001**- A case of Brain Tumour in a 23 years young married woman, completely cured by Gelsemium).*

Authenticity of Cure

CD Reference: NEO001-BRAIN TUMOUR-PRJ

2. A CASE OF CYSTIC HYGROMA OF THE NECK: MASTER S.M.

Case No. NEO002

Name of the Patient Mast. S.M., 3 months old baby (as on 17th November, 1998)

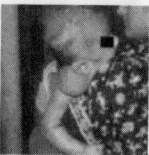

Photo of the patient, Master. S.M.

Presenting Complaints

- A large lump on the right side of neck. At birth there was a nodule of the size of a small lime which rapidly grew and by the age of 2 months it was almost the size of a large grapefruit. The mass was not painful but soft, cystic in texture.
- The paediatric surgeon gave the diagnosis and advised surgery but also mentioned there were chances of recurrence afterwards. The parents have decided not to opt for surgery but elected Homoeopathy.
- The baby had had an acute cough, for the last 15 days which might be due to exposure to cold, also occasional vomiting with expectoration of white mucous.
- Stool - Offensive, dry, hard, occasionally contained mucous.
- Temperament- Mild, generally quiet and appeared to be in his own world, not very much communication. The mother of the baby said he was decidedly hot, tended to kick off coverings; if covered, and became cranky.
- Cervical lymph gland on the other side (left) of the neck was swollen+++.
- Food desire - Sweet++, sour+, salt+, cold food+. (This was not revealed initially because he was a tiny baby and did not have any particular preference for flavours but this was established at the age of 16 months).
- Thirsty +.
- Sleep- Nothing to report.
- Sweat – Profuse on head. Occasionally smelled sour.

CASE ANALYSIS, MIASMATIC DIAGNOSIS AND FINAL PRESCRIPTION

This case is a wonderful example which illustrates the depth and beauty of Classical Homoeopathy which can handle such pathology. As the parents of the baby were not happy with the prognosis given by the surgeon, therefore Homoeopathy accepted the challenge.

Psora	Sycosis	Syphilis	Tubercular
Acute cough from exposure to cold Expectoration of white mucus Stool, dry, hard Mild, generally quiet and appears to be in his own world Desires sweet Sweat smells sour	Large lump Lump soft, cystic in texture Sweats profusely on head		Desires cold food Cervical lymph gland on the other side (left) of the neck was swollen

Psora 6   Sycosis 3   Syphilis 0   Tubercular 2

Mixed miasmatic case with Psora-Sycotic preponderance

This is a good example of a case of large tumour with Psora-Syco-Tubercular preponderance. As the surface miasm is predominately Sycotic (manifestation is tumour) and the second layer is Psoric therefore we have to think of a medicine which is either mixed miasmatic (covers all the miasms) or has similar Syco-Psoric-Tubercular preponderance. The Calcarea group is tri-miasmatic with Syco-Tubercular preponderance whereas the Iodum group is preponderantly tubercular. Therefore Calcarea Iod will exactly cover the miasmatic dyscrasia of the case. Calcarea Iod also has the capability of taking care of such cystic swellings and covers the totality, and is therefore an appropriate medicine covering the surface miasm as well as the surface symptoms.

Final Prescription Made on the Basis of

- Large lump of the neck.
- Started as a nodule, grew larger and became a soft cystic mass.
- Stool dry, hard.
- Mental Symptoms - Mild, generally quiet and appears to be in his own world, not very much communication (I understood this to be withdrawn).
- Hot patient.
- Cervical lymph gland on the other side (left) of the neck swollen+++. Glandular involvement.
- Desire - sweet++, sour+, salt+, cold food+

- Thirsty+.
- Sweats profusely on head. Occasionally smells sour.
- Miasmatic coverage.

Calcarea Iod. has the miasmatic breakdown: Psora ++, Sycosis +++, Syphilis +, Tubercular +++.

Final Prescription

CALCAREA IODATUM, 200C 1 globule (No. 10 poppy seed size) in sugar of milk sachet, the powder was dissolved in 8 ounces of pure water (preferably in his feeding bottle) The bottle was shaken and sipped throughout the day, some water was saved at the bottom, topped up the next morning, and sipped throughout the next day. Generally I give instruction to my patients to dilute the medicated water as many times as s/he likes. The patient will continue like this for 7 days. Then 7 days of no medicine. Followed by another dose to be shaken and sipped for 7 days in the same way.

Prescription Chart

Date	Prescription Done on the Basis of Watch this Chart Printer	Treatment
17th Nov'98	As discussed above.	Calc. Iod. 200C, 2 doses
25th Nov'98	Patient's parent thinks the baby is little better.	Wait and watch
15th Feb'99	Doing better. Mass is better; stool okay.	Wait and watch
12th Apr'99	Mass is reducing.	Wait and watch
15th Jun'99	Doing better. Mass is better. Some skin eruption appeared, could be surfacing of Psora. Wait and watch. Ask to apply some plain coconut oil and nothing else. Report to me if aggravation or if there is a spread.	Wait and watch
10th Aug'99	Mass decreased. Skin disease better. Emotionally more communicative and becoming restless. Sleep okay, stool okay. As a whole, swelling 60% better.	Wait and watch
12th Oct'99	Symptoms same as before. Wait and watch.	Wait and watch
4th Dec'99	Appears to be standstill status.	Calc. Iod, 200C 2 doses
4th Feb'00	No further appreciable change.	Calc. Iod, 1M, 1 dose
8th Apr'00	Little better. As a whole swelling, 70% better.	Wait and watch
3rd Jun'00	No further appreciable change.	Calc.Iod., 1M, 2 doses
15th Jul'00	Little better. As a whole swelling 80% better. Mentally more alert and reactive.	Wait and watch

Date	Prescription Done on the Basis of Watch this Chart Printer	Treatment
12th Sep'00	No further appreciable change. Mass – Standstill.	Calc.Iod. 10M, 1 dose
27th Oct'00	Mass is reducing in size. Wait and watch.	Wait and watch
22nd Dec'00	Mass is better almost 95% gone but appears to be standstill since mid November 2000.	Calc.Iod. 50M 1 dose
28th Jan'01	Mass completely disappeared.	

Remedy Reaction

I began with **CALCAREA IODATUM 200C** and gradually ascended up to **50M** in two years.. Within three months of starting homoeopathic treatment, the mass started reducing and within eight months, it came down to the size of a small lime. In two years, it had totally disappeared.

*Readers may view the pictures of the case (before and after treatment) in our website under Neoplastic Diseases (**Case No. NEO 002** - A case of Cystic Hygroma (massive swelling in the side of the neck) in a young 6 months old baby, completely cured by Calcarea Iodata).*

Authenticity of Cure

CD Reference: NEO002-CYSTIC HYGROMA-SM

Cured Cases

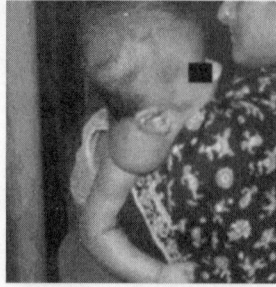

Baby S.M., massive swelling (diagnosed as Cystic Hygroma), before treatment.

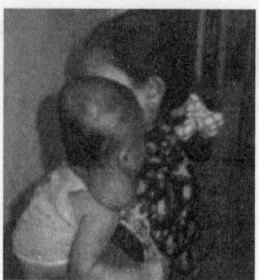

Before treatment.

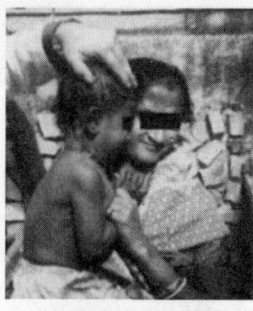

Decreased swelling, 3 months after treatment.

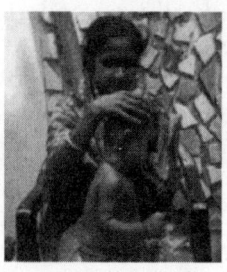

Swelling decreasing, 8 months after treatment.

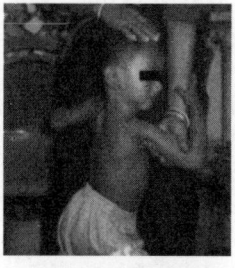

Swelling decreasing, 14 months after treatment.

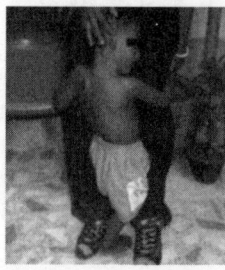

Swelling completely decreased 22 months

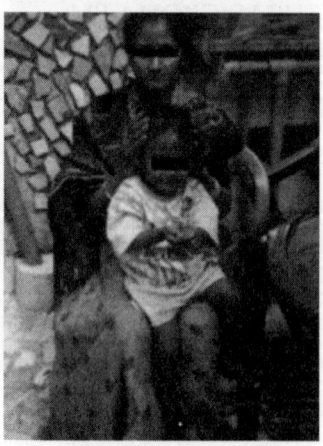

after treatment.

3. A CASE OF FIBROLIPOMA -INGUINAL REGION: MR. A. K. C.

Case No. NEO003

Age   : 39 years 8 months old as on 9th May, 1992
Sex   : Male
Height : 5 ft. 8 inches.
Weight : 89 kgs.

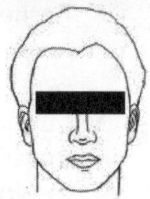

Photo of the patient,
Mr. A.K.C.

Presenting Complaints

- The lump appeared in the left abdomen on 1977. Initially Dr. Murari Mukherjee suggested Diverticulitis. But Barium Enema, found no colon blockage. Thereafter, patient became well after taking antibiotics and Banocide Forte. But problem recurred again. There was a lump like swelling in the left abdomen in 1977. After treatment of hetrazen and antibiotics, the swelling disappeared. Then from August, 1987, every six months, the swelling appeared and after treatment as above, the swelling disappeared. This frequency of appearance of the swelling has come down to every 3 to 4 months interval. From December 1989, he was under treatment of Dr. H. P. Chowdhury and up to August'90 he was okay. Thereafter, due to infrequent medication, the swelling appeared again in December'90, February'91 and Septemebr'91. Then after taking hetrazen and antibiotics, the swelling disappeared. The swelling again surfaced in March'92 and then he was under treatment of Dr. S. K. Banerjea.
- Then from Aug'87 onwards, the lump is appearing every 6 months. This cycle came down to 3 - 4 months in 1989. Reports indicate some infection but none of the doctors could pinpoint the infection. Also the lump disappeared after taking antibiotics and Banocide Forte but recurred again.
- From Dec'89 to Aug'90, patient was okay, when he was under treatment of Dr. H. P. Chowdhury. But from Aug'90 to Sept'91. He had irregular medication due to him being posted to Burnpur. Then the lump appeared n Feb'91 and Sept'91. From Oct'91. He was okay. In the 1st week of April'92, the lump appeared with active pain. Then after taking Terramycin, etc. for 10 days, the pain eased and this lump reduced. Then he took Dr. H. P. Chowdhury's medicine from 11.06.92. The pain started again from around 17.04.92. Then fresh medicine from Dr. Chowdhury has eased the pain only. Meanwhile

Dr. A. K. Roy Chowdhury suggested FNABC etc. But nothing could be found and he suggested surgical operation.

- Earlier, the lump used to appear with a throbbing pain and slight fever. But in April'92, the pain became very active and restricted every movement.
- Lump in left iliac fossa. Hard pain < press → < at night. > rest → throbbing pain. Previous treatment → Allopathy & Homoeopathy → No sustained improvement.
- Pain increased if any pressure was imported on the left abdomen, e.g., trying to get up from bed or sitting position, vice versa; running etc.
- Abdomen:- If pressure is given on the left abdomen then pain increases, e.g. trying to get up from a sitting position, etc. Hungry but can not eat much. Feels distended. Gas (++) especially lower abdomen, aggravated afternoon – evening time. Occasional acidity, mouth feels sour.
- Sweat:- Sweat on axilla and groin.
- Stool:- Constipated. Incomplete, not finished sensation.
- Mental symptoms:- Angry; Irritable temper; Talkative; Desires to be neat and clean; Disgusted with life; Active; Having involuntary sighing, gets more angry; Sympathetic, Cannot tolerate blood letting; Hurry; Fear of failures; Hallucinations; Mental worry. Sensitive (++).
- Habit:- Smoking and Pan chewing.
- Leucoderma in 1974-75 and Appendicitis was operated on, in December, 1967.
- Food preferences:- Sweet+++; Salty+++; Potato; Vegetables; Fruits; Chicken; Egg (Fried); Rich Spicy food; Cold drinks. Aversion to bitter. Patient prefers warm food (++).
- Thirsty.
- Chilly Patient.
- Sleep:- Sound. More deep in morning.
- Family Medical History:- Father has Blood Sugar from 1967 and Heart Problem (minor0 from 1971. Mother had history of Epiliptic till. Maternal Grandmother – Cancer.

Neoplastic Diseases – Cured Cases

Investigations Carried Out Before / After Dr. Banerjea's Treatment

24th Apr'92: Fine Needle Aspiration Cytology (FNAC) – from (Left) inguinal lymph gland. Fibrolipoma – A benign lesion. Blood Sugar Post Prandial (BSPP) → 114 mg/dl / 22.2.92 → 102.0 mg/100 ml. X-Ray Pelvis → NAD. (Nothing Abnormal Detected). Blood Sugar Fasting → glucose → 95.0 mg%. Cholesterol → 204 mg/. Triglycerides → 268 mg%.

10th Apr'93: Sonography – Lower abdomen. A hypo echoic SOL (Space Occupying Lesion) with irregular outline is noted in (Left) iliac fossa. Matted lymph nodes or thickened ? intestinal loops.

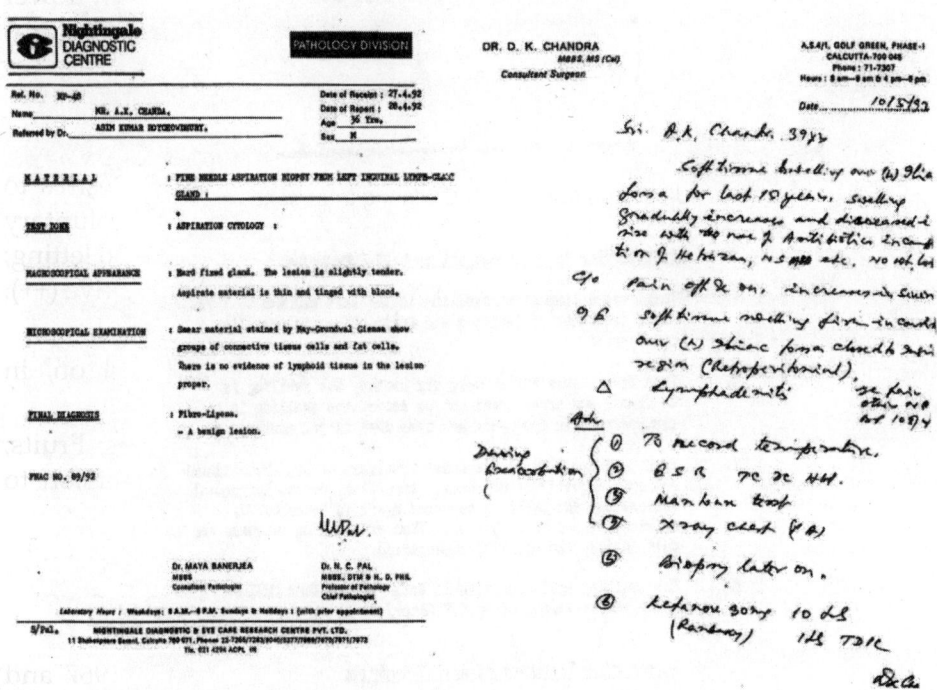

Biopsy report of Mr. A.K.C. before treatment.   Allopathic prescription of Mr. A.K.C.

Dr. S. K. Sharma
Sc. M.B.B.S. D.M.R.E. (BOM)
I.D. (RADIOLOGY), F.I.C.A. (U.S.A)
C.C.P. (U.S.A) MEMBER BMUS (U.K.) AIUM SI.S.AI
CONSULTANT RADIOLOGIST & ULTRASOUND SPECIALIST

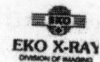
EKO X-RAY
DIVISION OF IMAGING

MR ARUP KR CHANDRA   39 yrs.   10.04.93
DR SUBRATA KR BANERJEA

SONOGRAPHY OF LOWER ABDOMEN:

URINARY BLADDER

Urinary bladder is normal in shape. Walls are smooth and regular. Lumen is clear. Post voiding sonogram shows considerable residual urine.

PROSTATE GLAND

Prostate gland shows heterogneous echotexture with regular margins. It measures:-

Antero-posterior - 2.6 cm.
Transverse   - 3.7 cm.
Cephalo caudal   - 2.7 cm.

Region of left iliac fossa shows a hypoechoic area with irregular margin - ? thickened intestinal loops ?? matted lymph nodes.

DR S K SHARMA MD

54, Jawaharlal Nehru Road, Calcutta - 700 071 Phone : 22 9246/8098/8105/8106

USG report of Mr. A.K.C. during treatment.

Status prior to the treatment by Dr.S.K.Banerjea.

1. There was a lump like swelling in the left abdomen in 1977. After treatment of hetrazan and antibiotics, the swelling disappeared.

2. Then from August 1987, every six months, the swelling is to appear and after treatment as above, the swelling is to disappear. This frequency had come down to 3/4 months.

3. From December 1989, I was under treatment of Dr.H.P.Chowdhury and upto August'90 I was okay. Thereafter, due to infrequent medication, the swelling appeared again in December'90, February'91 and September'91. Then after taking hetrazan and antibiotics, the swelling disappeared.

4. The swelling again surfaced in March'92 and then as I am under the treatment of Dr.S.K.Banerjee.

Status after treatment of Dr.S.K.Banerjea.

1   I am well and there has not any relapse

ARUP KUMAR CHANDA

Patient's comments 21 months after treatment.

CASE ANALYSIS, MIASMATIC DIAGNOSIS AND FINAL PRESCRIPTION

Miasmatic Analysis

- The lump appeared in the left abdomen: Sycosis.
- Abdomen:- If pressure is given on the left abdomen: Psora.
- Feels distended. Gas (++) especially lower abdomens: Psora (lack of digestion),
- Stool:- Constipated: Psora (slow peristalsis).
- Mental symptoms:- Angry; Irritable temper: Sycosis; Talkative: Sycosis; Desires to be neat and clean: Sycosis.
- Disgusted with life: Psora-Syphilis;
- Active, Hurry: Sycosis;
- Fears of failures: Psora.
- Hallucinations: Syphilis;

Final Prescription Made on the Basis of

- The lump appeared in the left abdomen on 1977. Initially Dr. Murari Mukherjee suggested Diverticulitis. But Barium Enema, no colon blockage was found. Thereafter, the patient became well after taking antibiotics and Banocide Forte. But problem recurred again. There was a lump like swelling in the left abdomen in 1977. After treatment of Hetrazen and antibiotics, the swelling disappeared. Then from August, 1987, every six months, the swelling appeared and after treatment with antibiotics, the swelling disappears. This frequency of appearance of the swelling has come down to every 3 to 4 months interval. From December 1989, he was under treatment of Dr. H. P. Chowdhury and up to August'90 he was okay. Thereafter, due to infrequent medication, the swelling appeared again in December'90, February'91 and September'91. Then after taking Hetrazen and antibiotics, the swelling disappeared. The swelling again surfaced in March'92 and then he decided to be treated by Dr. S. K. Banerjea.
- Lump in left iliac fossa. Hard pain < pressure → < at night. > rest → throbbing pain. Previous treatment → Allopathy & Homoeopathy → No sustained improvement.

- Abdomen:- If pressure is given on the left abdomen then pain increases, e.g. trying to get up from a sitting position, etc. Hungry but cannot eat much. Feels distended. Gas (++) especially lower abdomen, aggravated afternoon – evening time. Occasional acidity, mouth feels sour.
- Stool:- Constipated. Incomplete, not finished sensation.
- Mental symptoms:- Angry; Irritable temper; Talkative; Desires to be neat and clean; Disgusted with life; Active; Having involuntary sighing, gets more angry; Sympathetic, Cannot tolerate blood letting; Hurry; Fear of failures; Hallucinations; Mental worry. Sensitive (++).
- Food preferences:- Sweet+++; Salty+++; Potato; Vegetables; Fruits; Chicken; Egg (Fried); Rich Spicy food; Cold drinks. Aversion to bitter. Patient prefers warm food (++).
- Chilly Patient.

The miasmatic breakdown of Lycopodium is Psora+++L, Sycotic+++, Syphilitic++, Tubercular+++.

Final Prescription and Remedy Reaction

LYCOPODIUM 200C

Prescription Chart

I prescribed Lycopodium 200C in May, 1992. It took about 20 – 22 months and patient gradually improved. In my experience Lycopodium is one of the profoundly deep acting medicines and generally I wait for quite a long time, after a single dose. In this case after Lycopodium 200C was given in May'92, I waited 9 months as the recurrence of the swelling was lessening, therefore there was no need of repeating the medicine. Glory goes to Classical Homoeopathy of Hahnemann!

Authenticity of Cure

CD Reference: NEO003-FIBROLIPMA INGUINAL REGION-AKC

4. A CASE OF CHRONIC SUB-MENTAL LYMPH NODE ENLARGEMENT: MS. B.S.

Case No. NEO004

Age   : 19 years-old as on 11th January, 1995
Sex   : Female
Height : 4'-8"

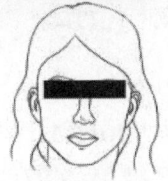

Photo of the patient, MS. B.S.

Presenting Complaints

- Sub mental lymph node enlargement, since about 1½ yrs back.
- No pain, no tenderness.
- Homoeopathic Generalities: Hot ++ patient; aggravation warmth and warm room. Likes fresh air.
- Desires: Salt ++, Sour ++, pungent ++, salty food, fish ++, egg, meat, cold food.
- Aversion: Bitter. Thirst: poor.
- Appetite: Average
- Sleep: Okay. Sweat: Average
- Stool: changeable colour; occasional pain.
- Urine: Clear
- Menstruation: Irregular, starts and stops again, can continue for 8 to 10 days;
- Menstrual discharge – average. Pain in lower abdomen – 1st day of discharge.
- Mind: Generally mild; timid; silent, can get irritable from trivial cause, but does not express irritability. Can be weepy, but more brooding (inward grief). Suspicious, desires company, works slowly, fear of darkness.
- Wants to please everybody.
- Past History: Chicken Pox (1 year ago)
- Family History: Elder sister – breast tumour. Parents: Okay.

Cured Cases

Investigations Carried Out Before / After Dr. Banerjea's Treatment

6th Jul'94: Haemoglobin - 9.7 gm%. Erythrocyte Sedimentation Rate - 22mm. White Blood Cell - 6,500. Neutrophil: 59; Lymphocyte:31; Eosinophil:9; Monocyte:1; Basophil: 0.

6th Jul'94: Mantoux Test: 20 x 20 mm. indurations, positive.

24th May'97: Mantoux Test: 20 x 20 mm. indurations positive.

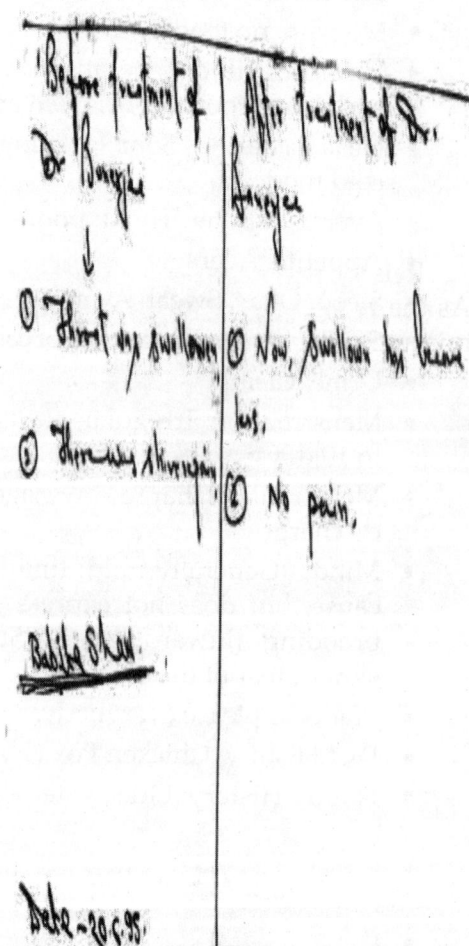

Allopathic prescription of Ms. B.S. before treatment.

Patient's comments 13 months after treatment.

CASE ANALYSIS, MIASMATIC DIAGNOSIS AND FINAL PRESCRIPTION

Miasmatic Analysis

- Sub mental lymph node enlargement: Syco-tubercular.
- Desires: Salt ++: Syco-tubercular. Pungent: Sycosis. Sour: Psora-syphilitic.
- Desires: Cold food: Syco-tubercular.
- Stool – Colour changeable: Tubercular.
- Menstruation: Irregular: Syphilis.
- Menses: Starts and stops again: Changeable: Tubercular.
- Mind: Generally mild, timid, silent: Psora.
- Can be weepy but more brooding (inward grief): Psora.
- Suspicious: Sycosis.
- Works slowly: Psora.
- Fear of darkness: Psora.
- Family History: Elder sister – breast tumour: Sycosis.

It is a mixed miasmatic case with Syco-Tubercular preponderance. As the presenting problem is lymph node enlargement, therefore Sycotic miasm is in the surface.

Prescription Made on the Basis of

- Sub mental lymph node enlargement.
- Hot (++) patient; aggravation warmth and warm room. Likes fresh air.
- Desires: Cold food.
- Stool colour: Changeable.
- Menstruation: Irregular. Starts and stops again, can continue for 8 to 10 days Intermittent.
- Mind: Generally mild; timid; silent, can get irritable from trivial cause, but does not express irritability: Passive irritability. Amiable; weak memory.
- Can be weepy, but more brooding (inward grief). Cries when reprimanded.
- Desires company.
- Fear of darkness.

- Wants to please everybody.
- Thirst-poor. Desire Salt & Salty (++).

The miasmatic breakdown of Pulsatilla is Psora ++, Sycosis +++, Syphilis +, Tubercular ++.

Pulsatilla covers the case miasmatically as well.

Remedy Reaction

The case was started with Pulsatilla 200 C and finished with Pulsatilla 50M. The 200 C potency was begun after taking into account the vitality of the patient and clarity of the symptom picture. The patient reported reduced swelling after 5 months of treatment. Unfortunately a detailed prescription chart is not available for this case.

Authenticity of Cure

CD Reference: NEO004-SUBMENTAL LYMPHNODE ENLARGEMENT-BS

5. A CASE OF SEBACEOUS CYST IN THE NECK: MR T.S.

Case No. NEO005

Age : 27 years as on 14th June, 1991
Height : 5 ft. 5 inches

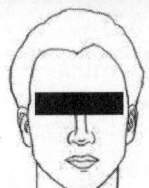

Photo of the patient, Mr. T.S

Presenting Complaints

- Lump (cyst) in throat (on side of the neck, clearly visible): since 2½ years back.
- Texture of lump: Soft: Occasional mild pain in the affected area.
- Weakness especially in the morning, after rising. Unrefreshed sleep. Cannot sleep until 1 am; tosses and turns in bed. Habit of going to the toilet (to pass stool) around 11pm; then finds it difficult to get up in the morning. Feels tired+++ in the morning.
- Dreams of various things.
- Stool: Regular, white mucus in stool. Habit of nocturnal evacuation (seminal emissions).
- Urine: Occasional yellow colour in urine. Frequent urination.
- Appetite: Normal.
- Thirstless. Has to force himself to drink.
- Chilly patient, but likes to be in fresh open air, even in the winter.
- Sweat: Scanty.
- Desires: Sweet ++; salty; potato; egg ++; onion; fried food +; cold food; cold drinks.
- Aversion to meat.
- Mind: Angry; irritable temperament, but gets frustrated inside; does not generally let it out; reserved displeasure from job (does not like the boss); suspicious and jealous mood.
- Silent habit; Gloomy; Absent minded; Wants to be alone; Fear of death; Weepy mood; patient gets angry when reprimanded; Fear of incurable diseases; snakes.
- Past History: Skin disease in childhood. Treated allopathically.
- Father died of gastric cancer.
- Uncle → T.B.
- Right sided preponderance.
- Pain: Shifting type. During pain patient feels chilly.

Investigations Carried Out Before/After Dr. Banerjea's Treatment

31st May '91: Mantoux test – Negative.

9th Jun '91: Blood: Haemoglobin 11.6, White Blood Cell 7,000, Neutrophil$_{90}$ Lymphocyte$_{25}$ Monocyte$_1$ Eosinophil$_4$ Basophil$_0$. Erythrocyte Sedimentation Rate-15.

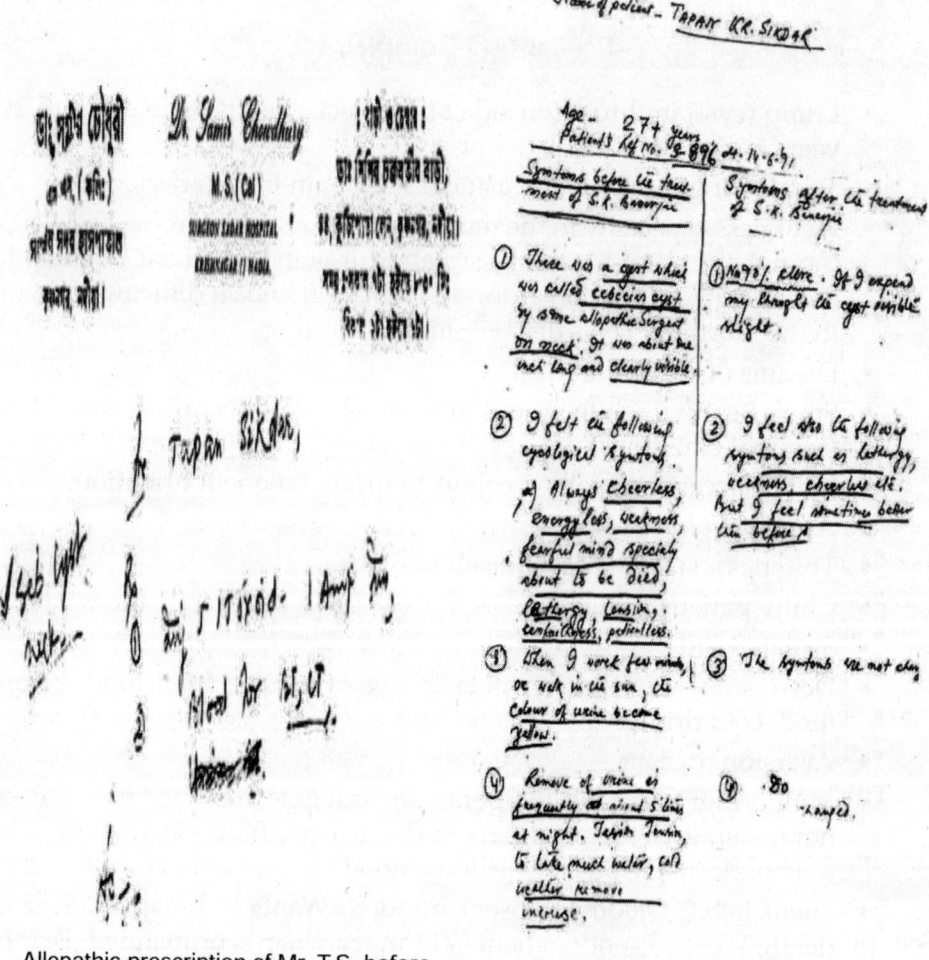

Allopathic prescription of Mr. T.S. before treatment.

Patient's comments 24 months after treatment.

Neoplastic Diseases – Cured Cases

CASE ANALYSIS, MIASMATIC DIAGNOSIS AND FINAL PRESCRIPTION

Miasmatic Analysis

- Cyst in the neck: Sycosis.
- Weakness especially in the morning: Psora.
- Unrefreshed sleep: Incoordination: Sycosis.
- Tosses and turns in bed: Sycosis.
- Habit of nocturnal evacuation: Syphilis.
- Frequent urination: Sycosis.
- Mucus in stool: Sycosis.
- Desires: Cold food: Syco-tubercular. Cold drinks: Syphilitic. Sweet: Psora.
- Aversion to meat: Syco-syphilitic.
- Chilly patient, but likes to be in fresh open air, even in the winter: Tubercular.
- Suspicious and jealous mood: Sycosis.
- Irritability: Syco-psoric.
- Silent habit: Psora.
- Absent minded: Sycosis.
- Wants to be alone: Psora.
- Fear of death: Psora.
- Weepy mood: Sycosis.
- Fear of incurable diseases and snakes: Psora.
- Past History: Father died of gastric cancer: Syphilis.
- Uncle → T.B: Tubercular.

This is a mixed miasmatic case with Syco-Tubercular preponderance.

Prescription Made on the Basis of

See prescription chart below. A remedy with sycotic and tubercular preponderance was chosen due to the miasmatic breakdown of the case.

Pulsatilla is a leading sycotic remedy, with miasmatic breakdown of Psora ++, Sycosis +++, Syphilis +, Tubercular ++.

Pulsatilla covers the case miasmatically as well.

Remedy Reaction

I started this case with Pulsatilla 200c, this potency was chosen on the basis of the vitality of the patient and clarity of the symptoms. I finished the case with Pulsatilla 50M in just under 2 years.

Prescription Chart

Date	Prescription Done on the Basis of	Treatment
14th Jun'91	Cyst (Sycotic); Weakness especially in the morning; Unrefreshed sleep. Can't sleep till 1 am; tosses and turns in bed. Feels tired+++ in the morning. During pain patient feels chilly (Dr. Nash says pain with chilliness is Pulsatilla). Habit of nocturnal evacuation. Frequent urination. Thirstless. Has to force himself to drink. Chilly patient, but likes to be in fresh open air, even in the winter. Desires: Cold food; cold drinks. Aversion to meat. Mind: Angry; irritable temperament, but gets frustrated inside, does not generally let it out; Reserved displeasure from job (does not like the boss); suspicious and jealous mood. Silent habit; gloomy; absent minded; wants to be alone; fear of death. weepy mood. Syco-tubercular preponderance.	Pulsatilla, 200C, 2 doses.
1st Jul'91	Standstill status	Sac lac.
2nd Aug'91	Wait and watch.	Sac lac.
4th Sep'91	No appreciable change. Repeat.	Pulsatilla, 200 C, 2 doses.
6th Dec'91	Patient had enteric fever (Typhoid) à had lots of allopathic medication. Standstill status now. So repeated again.	Pulsatilla, 200 C, 2 doses.
3rd Feb'92	No change in the cyst. Went to a higher potency.	Pulsatilla, 1 M, 2 doses.
20th Mar'92	Doing better; cyst has started decreasing in size.	Sac lac.
4th May'92	Much better.	Sac lac.
3rd Jun'92	Improved, but patient felt standstill status for 2 weeks.	Pulsatilla, 1M, 1 dose.
29th Jul'92	No further change, therefore went to a higher potency.	Pulsatilla, 10 M, 2 doses.
28th Oct'92	Further 15% improvement	Sac lac.

Date	Prescription Done on the Basis of	Treatment
6th Jan'93	No further change. Wait.	Sac lac.
17th Feb'93	No further change. Intuition and experience told me that a higher potency was needed.	Pulsatilla, 50 M, 2 doses.
3rd Mar'93	Almost 90% better. Patient reported that cyst still slightly visible if extends throat, urinary symptoms are unchanged and mood is still the same although sometimes he feels it is better than before.	Sac lac.
10th May'93	CURED	No prescription.

Authenticity of Cure

CD Reference: NEO005-SEBACEOUS CYST IN NECK-TS

6. A CASE BRONCHOGENIC CARCINOMA: MR. S.L.

Case No. NEO006
Age : 30 years old as on 17th October, 1992
Sex : Male

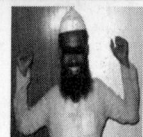

Photo of the patient, MR. S.L.

Presenting Complaints

- Dry cough aggravation early morning 2 – 3 a.m. and afternoon around 3 – 4 p.m. cough also aggravated during damp and rainy weather some discomfort in chest. Fever < evening. Body ache > massaging. Swelling in inguinal gland → < cold weather; < movement; > hot application.
- Stool: - 3/4 times. White mucus in stool.
- Joints: - Pain in joints. Pains < in damp weather. Creeping pain > lying on bed. < jerking.
- Had H/O immoral intercourse.
- Occasionally Bleeding per rectum → previously no treatment.
- Skin disease: - Delayed healing. Lots of brownish red spots all over the chest and back some itching dermatitis in the back, sensitive to touch.
- Mental Symptoms: - Gets more angry and irritable temper. Suspicious. Tendency to conceal his feelings. Jealous. Absent minded. Desires to be neat and clean. Memory – Weak. Weeping mood; occasionally have involuntary sighing. Mind: - Mild; Talkative; Desire for company; Fear of death; Fear of Ghost, Thunderstorm, Snake.
- Swelling of testis. Occasionally Lumbago, < sitting to standing. < jerking.
- Headache → Frontal headache → << Sun heat. Throbbing pain. > pressure.
- M.G.O. → premature ejaculation → quick discharge.
- Appetite – Normal.
- Thirst – Normal.
- Chilly patient.
- Catches cold easily.
- Delayed healing.
- Sleep – Good. Dreams of snake.
- Desire: - Salty food (++); Sweet (+); Cold food; Meat; Bitter; Milk.

- Past Medical History: - T.B.; Skin disease; Malaria; Measles; Chicken Pox.
- Family Medical History: - Skin disease; Rheumatism; High blood pressure; Piles; T.B.

Investigations Carried Out Before/After Dr. Banerjea's Treatment

22nd Jul'92: Thoraco Lumbar Spine: - Scoliosis dorsal spine. Erosion anterior surface Lumbar 4th vertebra. Koch's infection.

25th Jul'92: Chest X-Ray:- Left NAD (Nothing Abnormal Detected). Right – Dense opacity at para tracheal region? Enlarged gland, Encysted effusion.

22nd Sep'92: Chest X-Ray Dense homogeneous opacity of right para vertebral region. Growth? Encysted effusion.

7th Nov'92: Blood:- Haemoglobin – 11.8 gm%; White Blood Cell (W.B.C.) – 7200 cm Neutrophill 50 Lymphocyte 40 Eosinophill 6 Monocyte 4 Basophil 0 Erythrocyte Sedimentation Rate – 22 mm.

7th Nov'92: Chest X-Ray:- Growing mass in right. superior mediastinum. Bronchogenic CA. No destructive lesion in the ribs or in dorsal vertebral. Bony abnormality Lumbar 3rd vertebra. Bronchial CA.

20th Dec'93: Chest X-Ray:- Complete radiological regression of right Superior mediastinal mass since April, 1992.

CASE ANALYSIS, MIASMATIC DIAGNOSIS AND FINAL PRESCRIPTION

Miasmatic Analysis

- Dry cough aggravation early morning 2 – 3 a.m.: Psora.
- Afternoon aggravation around 3 – 4 p.m.: Sycosis.
- Cough also aggravated during damp and rainy weather: Sycosis.
- Swelling in inguinal gland: Syco-Tubercular.
- Joints: - Pain in joints: Sycosis. Pains < in damp weather: Sycosis.
- Skin disease: - Delayed healing: Syphilis.
- Lots of brownish red spots all over the chest and back: Sycosis (hyper-pigmentation).

Final Prescription Made on the Basis of

- Dry cough aggravation early morning 2 – 3 a.m. and afternoon around 3 – 4 p.m. cough also aggravated during damp and rainy weather some discomfort in chest. Fever < evening. Body ache > massaging. Swelling in inguinal gland → < cold weather; < movement; > hot application.
- Joints: - Pain in joints. Pains < in damp weather. Creeping pain. > lying on bed. < jerking.
- Skin disease: - Delayed healing. Lots of brownish red spots all over the chest and back some itching dermatitis in the back, sensitive to touch.
- Chilly patient.
- Desire: - Salty food (++); Sweet (+); Cold food; Meat; Bitter; Milk.
- Mental Symptoms: - Gets more angry and irritable temper. Suspicious. Tendency to conceal his feelings. Jealous. Absent minded. Desires to be neat and clean. Fear of death. Memory – Weak. Weeping mood.

The miasmatic breakdown of Thuja is Psora++, Sycotic+++, Syphilitic++, and Tubercular++.

Final Prescription and Remedy Reaction

THUJA 30C

Prescription Chart

I have prescribed Thuja 30C, 1 dose for this patient in October, 1992. Patient improved considerably after the medicine, fever, pain and discomfort in chest and cough gradually got better and I waited for 3 months after the first prescription. Thereafter I repeated Thuja 30C again after 3 months, when the patient reported a stand still status. My last prescription was Thuja 200C and in the ultra-sonography report of March 1993 the radiologist reported significant improvement!

Authenticity of Cure

CD Reference: NEO006-BRONCHOGENIC CARCINOMA-SL

Neoplastic Diseases – Cured Cases

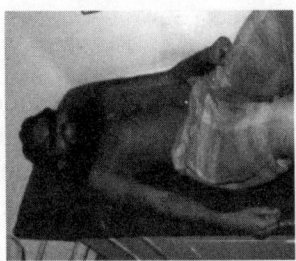

Photo Md. S. L with Brochogenic Carcinoma, before treatment.

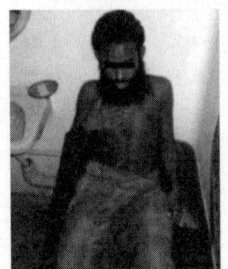

Md. S. L. before treatment.

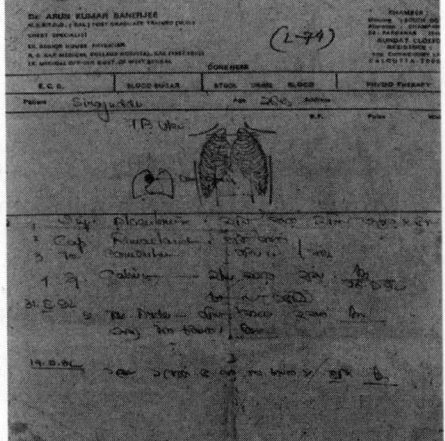

Allopathic prescription of Md. S.L. before treatment.

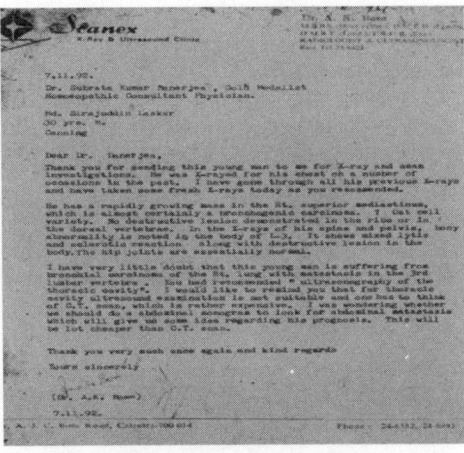

USG (sonography) report during treatment.

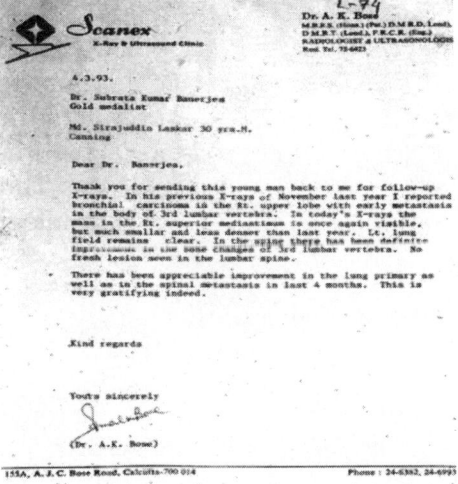

USG report 6 months after treatment.

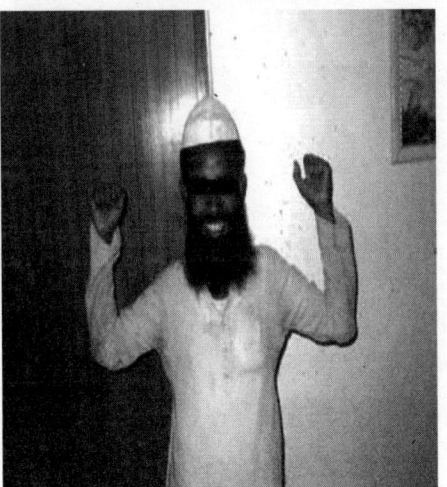

Md. S. L. after treatment.

9 CHAPTER
Neurological Diseases – Cured Cases

1. A CASE OF LONG STANDING CEREBRAL ATROPHY: MR. R.N.B.

Case No. NEU001

A 41 year-old married male at 28th September 1990.

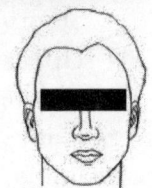

Photo of the patient, Mr. R.N.B

Presenting Complaints

- Vertigo: sensation as if everything around him is whirling around, with blurred vision; ameliorated in open air, ameliorated by fanning.
- Hemicrania: alternating sides. Sometimes the entire head feels heavy and aches violently. Mild pain in occipital region and forehead.
- Occasional oppression in breathing, with occasional creeping pain in right chest and feelings of uneasiness.
- Greasy, oily face.
- Talks loudly when asleep.
- Vertigo aggravated by motion, slightest exertion, and night; ameliorated by lying down. Aggravation from cold, noise (+++), jar (++), pressure, intercourse, anger, irritation, consolation, during full moon.
- Amelioration from bathing
- Head - Burning of vertex, which is sometimes hot.
- Eye - Blurred vision: cloudiness of sight with vertigo.
- Ear – N.P (Nothing Particular).
- Nose - Occasional blocked nose with thin watery coryza.
- Mouth - Occasional apthae.
- Teeth - Pain on left side of teeth, aggravated by cold drinks.

- Tongue - Coated tongue, looks like mapped.
- Throat - Sore throat from cold, most painful on the left side.
- Lungs - Very occasional dry cough from exposure to cold.
- Heart - Light feeling in chest especially during vertigo.
- Chest – Nothing particular.
- Abdomen - (a) Gas and distension with discomfort around umbilicus. (b) Eructation ameliorates. (3) The more the gas, the more the vertigo and giddiness.
- Stomach - Appetite: average.
- Sweat - Sweat: average.
- Urine - Stress incontinence - involuntary urination while laughing and sneezing
- Stool - (1) Hard stool. (2) Constipation with ineffectual desire.
- Upper Extremities - (1) Occasional joint pains, aggravated on waking.
- Palm – Nothing particular.
- Joints - Occasional pain in knee, more in the left. Pain in back: aggravation after long standing or sitting, relieved by hard pressure, pressing the back with a pillow.
- Lower Extremities – Nothing particular.
- Male Genital Organs - (1) Lax penis, (2) Sexual power: deficient.
- Anus - (1) Occasional rectal irritation and pain. (2) Irritation relieved by scratching.
- Skin Disease - Itchy groin, aggravated while undressing.
- Angry or irritable temper, fault-finding.
- Suspicious mood, jealous.
- Talkative.
- Neat and clean. Wants to be alone +++.
- Fear of death. Disgusted with life.
- Memory: Active.
- Weeping mood and does not entertain consolation, more angry.
- Hurried.
- Fear of ghosts, darkness, thunderstorm ++, incurable disease, failure ++.
- Mental worry, grief, death of dear ones.
- History of bronchitis during childhood.
- History of jaundice in 1984.

- Had chicken pox once.
- Hot person. Desires open air.
- Catches cold easily.
- (i) Sweet + (ii) Sour: No (iii) Pungent and hot: No (iv) Salt ++ (v) Salty +++ (vi) Bitter: No (vii) Bread: No (viii) Milk + (ix) Potato + (x) Vegetables and Spinach: Average (xi) Onion + (xii) Fruits + (xiii) Fish ++ (xiv) Meat/Chicken ++ (xv) Egg (boiled/fried) + (xii) Rich, spicy and fat food: Aversion (loathes) (xvii) Warm food +++ (xviii) Cold food: Aversion (xix) Warm drinks + (xx) Cold drinks + (xxi) Ice cream: Average.
- Thirst: Poor.
- Sleep - Disturbed sleep: head feels heavy: wakes up.
- Patient is occupied with dreams and thinks of them, even after waking in the morning; he behaves like the dream was reality.
- Married with two children (girls).
- Family History - History of Rheumatism in the family.
- Have had allopathic and homoeopathic medicines: without any appreciable change.

Investigations Carried Out Before/After Dr Banerjea's Treatment

2nd Feb 1990   Chest X-ray:- A small area of resolving congestion at the lower lobe of right hilum and right cardio-hepatic angle. No parenchymal infiltration seen. Cardiac silhouette normal.

11th May 1990   Skull X-ray:- Normal.

22nd May 1990   CT Scan Brain: - The CT scan of the brain reveals minimal diffuse cerebral atrophy.

29th May 1990   Chest X-ray:- Nothing abnormal detected.

3rd Nov 1992   CT Scan Brain: - Normal plain and contrast enhanced CT Scan of Brain.

Report of CT Scan Brain of Mr. R.N.B., a case of Cerebral Atrophy, before treatment.

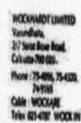

WOCKHARDT
Medical Centre

REPORT ON: ULTRASOUND/CT SCAN

Patient's Name: Mr. R. N. Bhattacharya
Patient No.: C 062157
Age: 41 yrs.   Sex: Male
Date: C 062157
Referred by: Dr. I. ROY
C.T. No. 2549

PLAIN & CONTRAST ENHANCED CT SCAN OF BRAIN

Thank you for referring the patient for CT scan of brain.

Brain parenchyma shows no focal abnormality in attenuation & contrast enhancement.

Lateral ventricles are mildly dilated with commensurate enlargement of bilateral cortical sulci.

Rest of the ventricular system & subarachnoid spaces appear normal.

No shift of midline structures noted.

Posterior fossa is normal.

IMPRESSION: The C.T. scan of brain reveals minimal diffuse cerebral atrophy.

DEPARTMENT OF ULTRASOUND/CT SCAN
DATE: 22.5.90
DR. S.P. BHOWMIK
RADIOLOGIST-IN-CHARGE

CT Scan Brain report, 21 months after treatment.

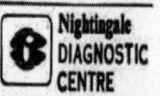
Nightingale DIAGNOSTIC CENTRE
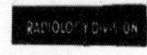

Ref. No. CT-IB11012669
Date: 3-11-92
Name: Mr. Rabindranath Bhattacharyya
Age: 42 Yrs.   Sex: M
Referred by: Dr. Subrata Kr. Banerjee
Examination: CT Scan of Brain

REPORT

Plain and I.V. Contrast Enhancement Scan

Thank you for referring the patient for CT Scan of Brain.

Posterior fossa, fourth ventricle normal.

Basal cisterns and subarachnoid spaces are normal.

Sylvian fissure, inter hemispheric fissures are normal.

Sulci are normal.

Ventricular system normal with septum in midline.

No parenchymal lesion shown.

IMPRESSION: Normal plain and contrast enhanced CT scan of Brain.

DR. P. K. CHAKRABORTY
MD DMRD
RADIOLOGIST

CASE ANALYSIS, MIASMATIC DIAGNOSIS AND FINAL PRESCRIPTION

There are two approaches in a case like this: e.g. Cerebral Atrophies, Senile Dementia, etc. where you can either open the case with a polychrest on the basis of the totality (if conspicuously available) or prescribe a lesser known medicine on the basis of the few symptoms available on the surface and the corresponding organopathic (the medicine having a predilection for action on the specific organ); by centrifugal action more symptoms will come to the surface. Here I found a good totality and accordingly prescribed a polychrest.

Miasmatic Analysis

- Vertigo: sensation as if everything around him is whirling around: Sycotic.
- Ameliorated in open air, ameliorated by fanning: Psora-tubercular.
- Hemicrania: alternating sides: Tubercular.
- Greasy oily face: Syco-syphilitic.
- (i) Vertigo aggravated by motion, slightest exertion: Psora; (ii) Night: Syphilitic; (iii) Ameliorated by lying down: Psora. Vertigo with loss of vision: Psora.
- Nose - Occasional blocked nose: Sycotic.
- Light feeling in chest (empty) with vertigo: Psora.
- Throat - Sore throat from cold: Syphilo-tubercular.
- Occasional ulcers in mouth: Syphilo-tubercular.
- Distention of abdomen from gas: Psora
- Urine - Stress incontinence - involuntary urination while laughing and sneezing: Syphilitic.
- Constipation, hard stool, with ineffectual desire: Psora.
- Joints - Occasional pain in knee, more in the left. Pain in back: aggravation after long standing or sitting, relieved by hard pressure: Sycotic. Pressing the back with a pillow: Sycotic.
- Male Genital Organs - (i) Lax penis: Psora, (ii) Sexual power: deficient: Psora.
- Skin disease aggravated by undressing: Tubercular.
- Angry or irritable temper, fault-finding: Sycotic.
- Suspicious mood, jealous: Sycotic.

- Talkative, neat and clean: Sycotic.
- Wants to be alone: Syphilitic.
- Fear of death: Psora; Disgusted with life: Syphilitic.
- Hurried: Sycotic.
- Talks during sleep: Psora.
- Fear of ghost, darkness, thunderstorm, incurable disease, failure: Psora.
- Mental worry, grief, death of dear ones: Psora.
- Weepy mood: Psora-sycotic.
- Desire: Salt, salty: Syco-tubercular. Warm food: Sycotic.
- Aversion to cold food: Psora.
- Catches cold easily: Psora-tubercular.
- Poor thirst: Psora.

It's a mixed miasmatic case with Psora-Sycotic preponderance. Atrophy (A=Absence/ Lack/ Deficient; Trophy= Growth) is Psoric; so need a medicine which obviously do cover Psora well.

Final Prescription Made on the Basis of

The reasoning for the choice of remedy is as stated below in the prescription chart. I began the case with the 200c potency as the patient's energy was good and, as Natrum Mur. is an inert substance in the crude form, a reasonably high potency is required.

The miasmatic breakdown of Natrum Mur. is Psora +++, Sycosis +++, Syphilis ++, Tubercular ++.

Natrum Mur covers the case miasmatically as well.

Remedy Reaction

NATRUM MURIATICUM, 200 C to begin with and finished with **10 M**. Patient was completely cured in just over 2 years as shown by the CT scan on 3rd November 1992.

Neurological Diseases – Cured Cases

Date	Prescription Done on the Basis of	Treatment
28th Sep'90	(1) Considering vertigo with blurred vision ameliorated by lying down, open air, aggravated by motion, exertion and noise (+++). (2) Appearance of the face: greasy and oily, (3) Dreams of robbers and fire and moreover occupied in the fantasy of the dream even after waking as if reality. (4) Appearance of the tongue. (5) Toothache aggravated by cold drinks. (6) Stress incontinence - in urine. (7) Temperament: irritable (++), fault-finding person. (8) Weepy, but does not entertain consolation. (9) Fears thunderstorm. (10) Desires - salt, salty, but loathes fatty. (11) Wants to be alone+++; (12) Hot patient; but takes cold easily.	Nat. Mur. 200: 2 doses: alternate mornings.
3rd Nov'90	No change in vertigo but temperamentally better; less irritation and tension: wait and watch.	Sac lac.
14th Feb'91	Temperamentally much better, but vertigo and reeling still persisting. Blurred vision little improved. Repeat.	Nat. Mur. 200: 2 doses: alternate mornings.
21th Feb'91	No further change. Stand still (wait for further movement of symptoms).	Sac lac.
13th Aug'91	Standstill status.	Natrum Mur. 1M: 2 doses: alternate mornings.
5th Dec'91	(1) Blurring of the vision: much better; but vertigo though 10% to 15% relieved still very much there.	Sac lac.
26th Mar'92	Standstill. Go higher in potency (as frontal and occipital pain was complained of also: advised to undergo an X-ray of para-nasal sinus).	
31st June'92	(1) X-Ray shows mild right maxillary sinusitis. (2) Vertigo dramatically (70%) better. (3) Dreams and stress incontinence much improved. (4) Hemicrania or oppressed breathing, loud talking during sleep, joint pains better. (5) Less fault finding, now easy-going, less fears and takes an interest in life (no feelings of disgust).	Sac lac.
8th Jul'92	Same as before (wait)	Sac lac.
5th Aug'92	No further change. Very slow movement of symptoms. Repeat.	Natrum Mur. 10 M: 2 doses: alternate mornings.
4th Sep'92	Patient feeling better.	Sac lac.
28th Oct'92	Much better. Vertigo and reeling almost gone. Doing much better. Wait. Asked the patient to repeat the CT scan.	Sac lac.

Date	Prescription Done on the Basis of	Treatment
5th Nov '92	Doing better in every regard: (1) Temperamentally a totally different person. (2) Happy, amiable, easy going, extrovert, likes to mix with people. (3) Headache and vertigo: all disappeared. (4) Food habit changed: he likes and enjoys his spicy Indian meal, these days! CT scan report normal.	Cured.

Authenticity of Cure

CD Reference: NEU001-CEREBRAL ATROPHY-RNB

10
CHAPTER

Psychiatric Disorders - Cured Cases

1. A CASE OF ANXIETY NEUROSIS: MS. F.K.

Case No. P001

Age – 24 years as on 2nd November, 1991.

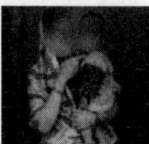

Photo of the patient, MS. F.K.

Presenting Complaints

- Feels depressed does not want to work, does not like to talk.
- Even, occasionally, stops taking food.
- At present: Suffers with this type of phase once or twice in a week; going on for the last 10 to 12 months.
- Sleep – very much disturbed.
- Cries silently.
- Black discolouration around the eyes.
- Palpitation: aggravated from motion.
- Leucorrhoea, watery, white, no bad odour.
- Dry (++) tongue.
- Acidity-- occasional.
- Allergy (skin rash) on bathing in pond.
- Itching in winter, ameliorates from sitting in sun.
- Temperament : Timid and gentle. Weepy, easily forgetful. Forgetfulness aggravated since age 17 (after the first attack of the disease).
- Shy, sympathetic. Likes to be with known people. Likes consolation.
- Can't bear to be alone, especially in evening and night.
- Dreams: Nothing particular.

- Sleep posture: Generally lies on back with hands over forehead.
- Desires: Salty ++, salt+, fish, cold food ++ & drinks, ice-cream.
- Before attack starts crying, blackish discolouration around the eyes and wants to lie down all the time.
- Always feels like crying. Fear of death during the attack.
- Heat - cold relationship: Hot patient.
- Susceptibility: To cold, but prefers windows open and to be in the fresh air.
- Thirst: Good, cold water.
- Stool: Nothing abnormal.
- Urine: OK.
- Sweat: +++, face & forehead. No odour, no staining.
- Menses: Regular. 5 days. No clots. No pains.
- Past History:- H/O: mental illness (diagnosed as anxiety neurosis) twice before: age 17 and age 19.
- First attack at the age of 17. Treated allopathically, recurred again at age 19 years. Again treated with conventional medicine but not fully recovered. She was on medication for 3 years, then stopped the medicines; 6 months later attacks started again. History of death of her best friend by a car accident → got extremely upset → cried for 3 months → attack started afterwards. H/O: Diphtheria at the age of 4½ years. H/O: Repeated attacks of high fever during childhood.
- Family History: Grandfather: Psychiatric problems.

CASE ANALYSIS, MIASMATIC DIAGNOSIS AND FINAL PRESCRIPTION

Miasmatic Analysis

- Depressed does not want to work, does not like to talk: Syphilis.
- Stops taking food: Syphilis (as this can be destructive).
- Cries silently: Psora-syphilis (silently is isolation, so syphilitic)
- Black discolouration: Hyper pigmentation: Sycosis.
- Palpitation: aggravated from motion: Tubercular.
- Leucorrhoea, watery: Tubercular.
- Dry (++) tongue: Psora.
- Acidity: Psora.

Psychiatric Disorders – Cured Cases

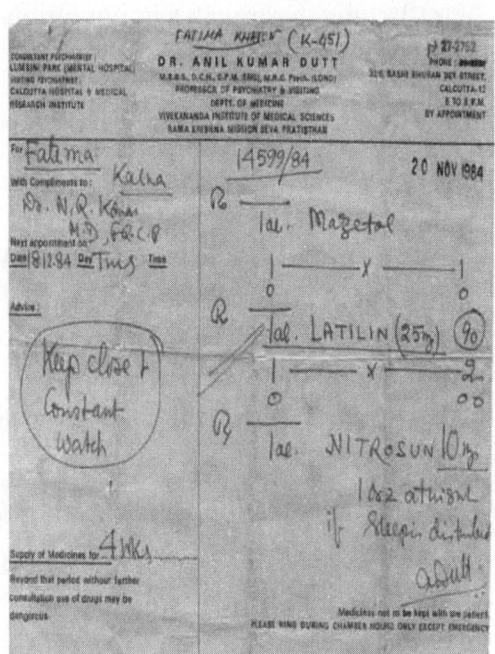

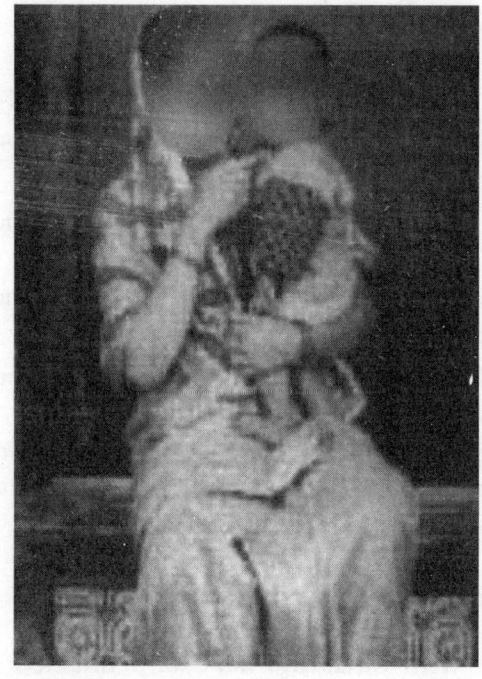

- Itching, aggravates in winter: Psora.
- Allergy: Tubercular.
- Timid and gentle: Psora.
- Forgetful: Psora-syphilis.
- Shy: Psora.
- Can't bear to be alone: Psora.
- Always feels like crying: Syco-syphilis.
- Fear of death: Psora.
- Susceptibility: to cold: Psora-tubercular.
- Sweat: +++: Sycosis.

It's a mixed miasmatic case with Psora-Sycotic preponderance.

Prescription Made on the Basis of

- Feels depressed, does not want to work and does not like to talk.
- Sleep – very much disturbed.
- Cries silently.
- Black discolouration around the eyes.
- Temperament: Timid and gentle. Weepy, easily forgetful. Forgetfulness aggravated since age 17 (after the first attack of the disease).
- Shy, sympathetic. Likes to be with known people. Likes consolation.
- Can't bear to be alone, especially in evening and night.
- Sleep posture: Generally lies on back with hands over forehead.
- Desires: Cold food ++ & drinks, ice cream.
- Before attack, starts crying, blackish discolouration around the eyes and wants to lie down all the time.
- Always feels like crying. Fear of death during the attack.
- Heat cold relation: Hot patient.
- Susceptibility: To cold, but prefers windows open and to be in the fresh air.
- Past History: Had history of death of her best friend by car accident → got extremely upset → cried for 3 months → attack started afterwards.

Final Prescription and Remedy Reaction

I started the case with **Pulsatilla 200C** and finished with 50M, a more detailed prescription chart, is unfortunately not available. 200 C potency was chosen on the basis of the patient's vitality and to minimise any aggravation of mental symptoms. The miasmatic breakdown of this remedy is Psora ++, Sycosis +++, Syphilis +, Tubercular ++. Pulsatilla covers the case miasmatically as well.

Patient improved steadily and was completely cured within 2 years. I asked the patient to visit me periodically once every 6 months, to make sure that, even after stopping the medicine, nothing recurred. She visited again with no return of symptoms.

Authenticity of Cure

CD Reference: P001-ANXIETY-NEUROSIS-FK

11 Respiratory Diseases - Cured Cases

CHAPTER

1. A CASE OF PLEURAL EFFUSION: DR. S.K.C.

Case No. RE001

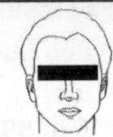

Photo of the patient,
DR. S.K.C.

Presenting Complaints

Dr.S.K.C., 53 years, an allopathic physician visited me on 27th May 1989 with the following complaints:

- In the first week of February 1989, the problem began with a high rise in temperature. Severe dyspnoea and pain in the left lateral side of the chest, aggravated by respiratory movements, ameliorated by lying on the left side.
- Physical signs were: movement of the left chest wall reduced, with stony dullness on percussion. Breathing sounds diminished. Pleural rub present.
- Pain felt on taking a deep breath and yawning. Pain more on the left lower and lateral part of the chest and a little towards the back.
- Feverish always with frequent high-rise of temperature, cough followed by dyspnoea, aggravated in the evening.
- Sense of heaviness in the left part of the chest.
- Dry lips.
- Cough: has to sit up and aggravated after eating.
- Likes to expand his chest, but cannot.
- Mild temperament. Likes to be neat and clean. No fears.
- Likes fresh foods.
- Thirst: Profuse (+++)
- Sweat: Average (++)
- Hot-Chilly: Hot Patient.

- Sleep: Normal.
- Dreams: Dreams of incurable disease and of work.
- Stool: More towards constipation.
- Tongue: Dry.
- Cough – Expectoration: Occasional dry cough with no expectoration.

Investigations Carried Out before After Dr Banerjea's Treatment

5th Feb'89: Haemoglobin %:- 78%, Erythrocyte Sedimentation Rate - 65, X-ray Chest - Consolidation with collapse of left lower zone with Pleural Effusion.

16th Feb'89: B.S.P.P. (Blood Sugar Post Prandial): 135.

24th Feb'89: Chest X-ray - Translucent cresentric outline is seen above the dome.

30th Jun'89: X-ray chest - No pleural thickening at the left. Costo-phrenic angles are clear. Provisional diagnosis:- Pleural Effusion.

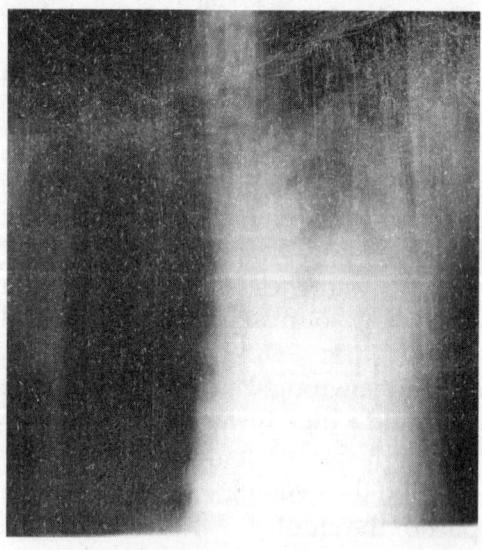 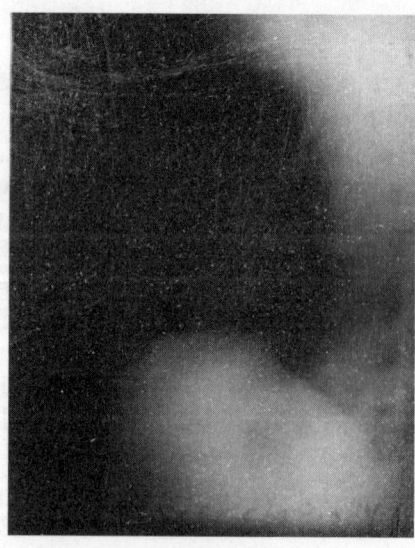

Chest X-Ray (Complete Collapse of Left Lung) of Dr. SKC, a case of Pleural effusion, before treatment

Chest X-Ray, before treatment

Respiratory Diseases - Cured Cases

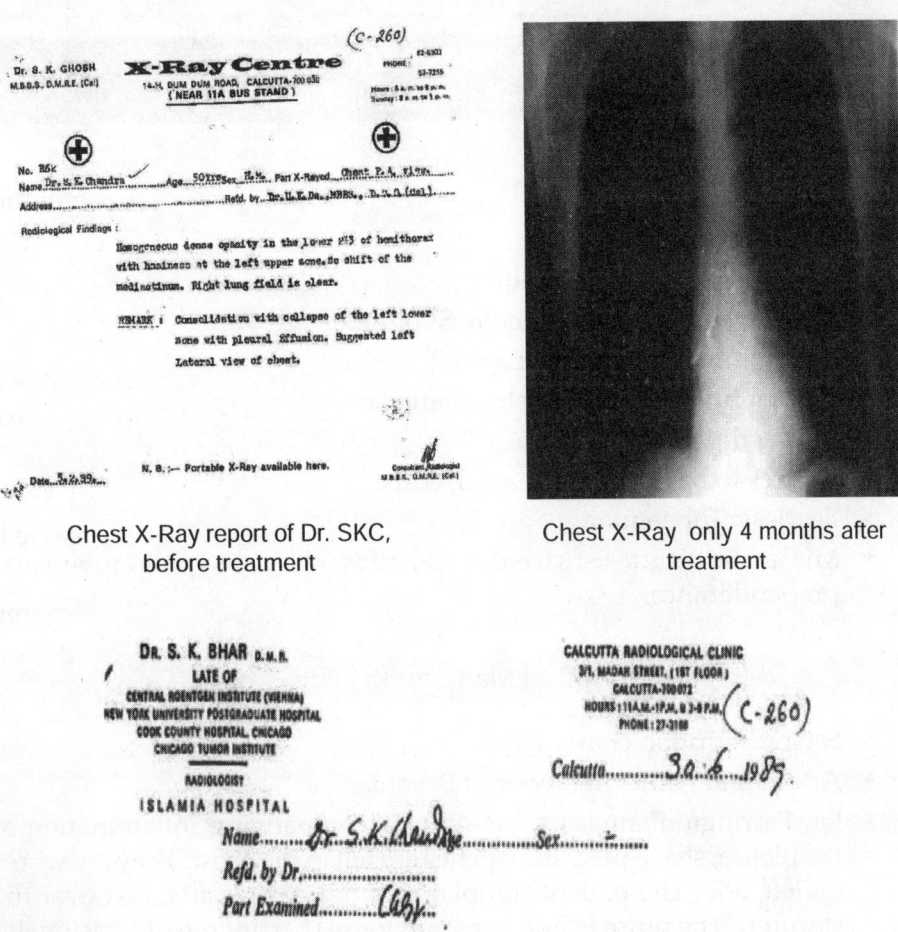

Chest X-Ray report of Dr. SKC, before treatment

Chest X-Ray only 4 months after treatment

Chest X-Ray report only 4 months after treatment

CASE ANALYSIS, MIASMATIC DIAGNOSIS AND FINAL PRESCRIPTION

Miasmatic Analysis

- Pleural effusion: Sycotic.
- Painful dyspnoea: Syphilitic.
- Aggravation from movement: Syphilitic.
- Painful respiration: Tubercular.
- Cannot fully expand chest: Tubercular.
- Mild temperament: Psora.
- Desires to be neat and clean: Sycosis.
- Fearless: Tubercular.
- Miasmatic diagnosis: Mixed miasmatic with syco-syphilo-tubercular preponderance.

Prescription Made on the Basis of

- See prescription chart below.
- Additional Points in favour of Bryonia:
- Dr. Farrington suggests, owing to accompanying inflammation of the pleura, sharp pleuritic stitches are felt in the chest. They are worse on left side. The patient complains of heavy pressure, just over the sternum. The pulse is full, hard and tense (Farrington). Occasionally in Bryonia you may find in cases of pleurisy or pneumonia, there is heat in the chest (Clarke). Continued inclination to draw a long breath (Clarke). Dr. Clarke says "must expand the chest" is a characteristic.
- The miasmatic breakdown of Bryonia is Psora ++, Sycosis +++, Syphilis +, Tubercular++.

Bryonia covers the case miasmatically as well.

Short Comparison: Effusion in Serous Cavities

(i) BRYONIA:- Effusions characterised with stitching pains < motion > rest, lying on painful side. (ii) APIS:- Effusion with stinging pains. (iii) KALI CARB:- Effusion with stitching pain, irrespective of motion.

Final Prescription and Remedy Reaction

The case was begun with Bryonia 12 C. In this case there was a complete collapse of the lung; the potency of 12 C was therefore used to proceed very cautiously. The patient was cured in less than 2 months, finishing with a potency of 200 C to prevent further relapses.

Prescription Chart

Date	Report after Last Medication	Prescription Done on the Basis of	Treatment
27th May'89		• Warmer days after winter. • Pain aggravated by movement, better by pressure. • Pain ameliorated by lying on painful side. • Synovial effusion. • Dry lips. • Sense of heaviness in the chest, around sternum, more on the left. • Thirst: Profuse (+++) • Hot Patient. • Dreams of work. • Stool: More towards constipation. • Tongue: Dry. • Occasional dry cough with no expectoration.	Bryonia 12 C: 2 doses: each dose given in water, to sip throughout the day. [2 doses: Alternate days].
14th Jun'89	Feeling better: fever, cough, dyspnoea improved.	Wait and watch	Sac lac.
24th Jun'89	As a whole improving.	Wait and watch	Sac lac.
15th Jul'89	Much better, cured of his complaints (clear chest x-ray 30.6.89).	Go higher in potency to prevent any relapse.	Bryonia 200C, 1 dose.

Authenticity of Cure

CD Reference: RE001-PLEURAL EFFUSION-SKC

2. A CASE OF EMPHYSEMA WITH BRONCHOSPASM: MR N.C.D.

Case No. RE002

64 year-old, Hindu male, brought to me first on 9th of October 1987.

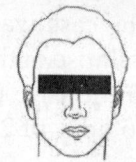

Photo of the patient, Mr. N.C.D.

Presenting Complaints

- Dry cough: aggravated at night. On prolonged coughing, a little expectoration of whitish-yellow colour and stringy character.
- Sometimes a small clump of mucus forcibly ejects out with violent coughing.
- Throat dry and a sensation of rawness.
- Bronchospasm since 14 years old, not very severe. Aggravates during change of weather, rainy, damp, and in winter season. Aggravates in the early morning, on waking with panting.
- Cannot expand chest: desire to take a deep full respiration, but a sensation of oppression in chest; more in the morning on waking, clears up during day, but again aggravates on exertion, ascending stairs etc.
- Bronchospasm aggravation: 3-7 a.m. Cough aggravation: 7-10 p.m. and also on waking.
- Sensation of oppression of chest, aggravation: on motion.
- Rainy weather and winter aggravation.
- Likes to bath in luke warm water.
- Better by bending forward.
- Aggravation from spicy foods.
- Aggravation from sweet.
- Spasm and oppression aggravation from anger.
- Gouty pain aggravates occasionally.
- Head - Occasional headache: aggravation in the sun; damp.
- Ear – History of C.S.O.M (Chronic Suppurative Otitis Media) in childhood -> homoeopathically treated.
- Nose- Nasal blockage and sneezing, aggravation during change of weather.
- Mouth- Bad odour, aggravation on waking (could be due to nose block).
- Teeth- History of Pyorrhoea.

- Tongue- Moist, flabby.
- Throat (Internal)-History of recurrent tonsillitis during childhood. Susceptible to cold. Cold settles in tonsils. Many medications (allopathic and homoeopathic). Now better.
- Lungs- Dry cough with pain in chest, more at night. Stringy expectoration can be drawn into threads.
- Heart- Palpitation on movement, exertion.
- Chest- Pain in chest from excessive coughing.
- Abdomen -Gas and distension. No eructation.
- Stomach - Appetite: Average.
- Sweat- Perspiration ++, offensive +.
- Urine - Regular.
- Stool- Previously constipated, now okay. Mucus in stool occasionally.
- Lower Extremities - Occasional pain in ankle.
- Male Genital Organs - Previous history of Spermatorrhoea. Sexual desire ++.
- Skin Disease - Itching in the groin for many years. Has applied many creams (ointments). No lasting improvement. Itching, aggravates from undressing, cold weather, at night in bed.
- Mind- Mild; occasional suicidal tendency. Silent habit, timid.
- Desires to be neat and clean. Wants to be alone. Disgusted with life.
- Memory: weak. Involuntary sighing. Cries when reprimanded or gets more angry. Averagely sympathetic. Cannot tolerate blood letting.
- Fear of darkness, dogs, incurable disease, and failure.
- History of :Mental worry, grief, financial loss.
- History of: Masturbation, night watching: occasionally.
- History of: Skin disease: during youth: allopathically treated.
- History of: Bronchospasm: taken inhaler and steroids: no lasting improvement.
- History of: Pneumonia: 1970, 1971, 1973, 1979 and 1987 (Recurrent).
- Allopathically treated, had lots of antibiotics, injections. Slow and delayed resolution. Weakness since.
- Had Pneumonia 5 times: N.B.W.S.(Never Been Well Since).
- Chilly. Does not like the open air.
- Catches cold easily (++).
- Desire:- (i) Sweet + (ii) Sour + (iii) Pungent and hot ++ (iv) Salt ++ (v) Salty ++ (vi) Bitter: No (vii) Vegetables & Spinach : aversion (viii)

Fruits + (ix) Meat + (x) Cold food + (xi) Cold drinks +.
- Thirsty: ++.
- Sleep - Disturbed.
- Married: 5 children.
- Family History - Mother - Cholera, Father - Pleurisy (? Tb).

Investigations Carried Out Before and After Dr. Banerjea's Treatment

9th Oct'87: Xray chest: Lower zonal emphysematous translucency, both lungs, especially on right-side.

8th May'89: Xray chest: Scarring both apical regions with mild accentuation of pulmonary markings in both lung fields. Blood: Haemoglobin: 11.1 gm %, Total Count: 5400, Erythrocyte Sedimentation Rate: 23mm/1st hour Urine: Albumen - faint trace. Epithelial cells: a few.

12th Feb''90: Xray Chest: No lung infiltration seen. Good improvement noted. Blood: Haemoglobin: 11.6 gm %. Total Count 7600 Erythrocyte Sedimentation Rate: 24. Urine: Albumen: nil.

CASE ANALYSIS, MIASMATIC DIAGNOSIS AND FINAL PRESCRIPTION

- Clinical findings:- Dullness of percussion note and restricted movement of chest wall of lower zone of right lung was previously noted, which improved considerably after treatment.
- Provisional diagnosis:- Bronchospasm with emphysema of the lung.
- Miasmatic diagnosis:- Syco- Psora.
- Constitutional remedy:- Thuja.
- Satellite medicines:- Arsenicum, Kali carb., Pneumococcin.

Miasmatic Analysis

- Dry cough: Psora.
- Aggravation at night: Syphilis.
- Expectoration of whitish-yellow colour and stringy character: Syco-syphilis.
- Mucus forcibly ejects out with violent coughing: Sycosis.
- Throat dry and a sensation of rawness: Syphilitic.

Chest X-Ray report of Mr. N.C.D., Emphysema with Bronchospasm, before treatment of Dr. Banerjea

Normal X-Ray report after treatment

- Bronchospasm aggravates during change of weather, rainy, damp: Sycosis
- Aggravation in the early morning: Psora.
- Cannot expand chest: desire to take a deep full respiration: Tubercular.
- Bronchospasm aggravation: 3-7 a.m.: Psora.
- Sensation of oppression of chest: Tubercular.
- Rainy weather and winter aggravation: Sycosis.

- Gouty pain aggravates occasionally during rainy season: Sycosis.
- Head –headache: aggravation damp: Sycosis.
- Nose- Sneezing: aggravation during change of weather: Sycosis.
- Tongue- Moist, flabby: Sycosis.
- Susceptible to cold. Cold settles in tonsils: Tubercular.
- Lungs-Stringy expectoration can be drawn into threads: Syphilis.
- Heart- Palpitation on movement: Tubercular.
- Sweat- Perspiration ++: Sycosis.
- Male Genital Organs - Sexual desire ++: Sycosis.
- Skin Disease – Itching: aggravation from undressing, cold weather, at night in bed: Syphilis.
- Stool: Mucus: Sycosis.
- Mind- Mild: Psora.
- Occasional suicidal tendency: Syphilis.
- Disgusted with life: Syphilis.
- Cannot tolerate blood letting: Psora.
- Memory: weak: Psora.
- Desires: Pungent and hot: Sycosis. Salt and salty: Syco-tubercular. Cold food: Syco-tubercular. Cold drinks: Syphilitic. Aversion vegetables: Hydrogenoid: Sycosis.
- Had Pneumonia 5 times: Recurrent infection: Tubercular.
- Chilly. Catches cold easily (++): Psora-Tubercular.

It's a mixed miasmatic case with Psora- sycotic preponderance.

Prescription Made on the Basis of

- See prescription chart below.
- Dry hacking cough.
- Bronchospasm aggravation 3am –7am.
- Rainy damp weather aggravation.
- Aversion vegetable & spinach.
- History of pyorrhoea.
- Disturbed sleep.
- Chilly, but desires cold food and drinks.
- Mind- Mild; silent habit; wants to be alone; loathing of life. Occasional suicidal tendency.

The miasmatic breakdown of Thuja is Psora ++, Sycosis +++, Syphilis ++, Tubercular ++.

Thuja covers the case miasmatically as well.

Final Prescription and Remedy Reaction

I began treatment with Thuja 200 C, taking into account the vital energy of the patient and the nature of his condition. Patient was cured of his symptoms in just over 2 years of treatment; other remedies were used as new symptom pictures were uncovered (Badiaga, Kali carb., Natrum sulph. and Pneumococcin), but the case was finished with Thuja 1M.

PNEUMOCOCCIN

Preparation: Prepared from the culture of Diplococcus lanceolatus organism. Therapeutic field: (a) Pneumonia (especially recurrent). (b) Paresis & paralysis. (c) Pleuritic pain.

MATERIA MEDICA

- Never been well since pneumonia.
- Delayed resolution in pneumonia.
- In complicated pneumonias, when many infections intervene, a dose of pneumococcin arranges the symptoms.
- Recurrent attacks of broncho-pneumonia : it arrests further attacks.
- Cough, as if the sound is coming up from mucus loaded and consolidated lung with inability to expand the chest to take a full respiration.

Prescription Chart

Date	Prescription Done on the Basis of	Treatment
9th Oct'87	Considering chilly patient, desires cold food, salt, salty foods, repeated attacks of Pneumonia: Bronchospasm aggravates in damp, rainy weather.	Thuja 200/ 2 doses. (1 globule of poppy-seed size, dissolved in distilled water and divide into two doses).
7th Nov'87	No Appreciable change. Wait and watch	Sac lac.
18th Dec'87	No Appreciable change. Wait and watch	Sac lac. Date

Date	Prescription Done on the Basis of	Treatment
20th Jan'88	Severe bronchospasm. Cough also aggravated. Spasm better by bending forward. Complementary of Thuja given Patient is on inhaler, as well; asked to wean off gradually.	Ars. alb. 12C, 3 doses.
2nd Feb'88	A little better. Inhaler discontinued.	Sac lac.
27th Feb'88	Again cough severely aggravated. Dry cough aggravates at night. Small clumps of mucus fly out from mouth [keynote of Badiaga].	Badiaga 30, 2 doses.
26th Mar'88	A little better, but still heaviness in chest. Occasional pain in chest and spasm in the morning. Back to constitutional.	Thuja 1m, 2 doses.
30th Apr'88	Spasm persisting in the morning. Change in the plan of treatment, considering early morning aggravation. Mucus flies out from mouth. Tenacious, yellow expectoration: Wheeze ++.	Kali carb. 30, 2 doses.
27th May'88	No Appreciable change.	Kali carb. 200, 2 doses.
6th Jun'88	Pain in chest, must hold chest while coughing. Spasm again aggravated by the rainy weather, rattling, wheeze aggravated 4-7 a.m. Depressed ++, gloomy. Change in the plan of treatment.	Nat. sulph. 200, 2 doses.
14th Jul'88	Severe aggravation. Patient is again on inhaler. Wait	Sac lac.
6th Aug'88	Rainy season over. Patient at standstill. Spasm less. Put off the inhaler.	Nat. sulph. 0/1 (LM 1) 15 doses.
6th Sep'88	No Appreciable change.	Nat. sulph. 0/3 (LM 3) 15 doses.
10th Oct'88	Colder days are setting in, so heavy breathing, wheeze ++.	Nat. sulph. 1M, 2 doses.
7th Nov'88	Absolutely no change. Change in the plan of treatment. Has had 5 Pneumonias. To remove the bad effects, if any. Given as an intercurrent.	Pneumococcin 200, 2 doses.
19th Dec'88	Patient standstill, depression is somewhat better.	Sac lac.
29th Jan'89	Patient feels better. Though there is wheeze and ronchi in the chest, but spasm is under control this winter and he feels he can expand his chest a little more to take a long respiration.	Sac lac.
18th Feb'89	Wheeze, a little more for the colder days.	Pneumococcin 200, 2 doses. 1M: 1 dose.

Respiratory Diseases - Cured Cases

Date	Prescription Done on the Basis of	Treatment
15th Mar'89	Feeling much better. Wait and watch. I have advised for Xray and blood test.	Sac lac.
12th May'89	Xray reports are a little better. Patient is having occasional spasms in the early morning.	Pneumococcin 1M, 2 doses, 10M : 1 dose
29th Jun'89	Doing better. But wheeze and spasm occasionally occurring with the change of temperature and with the onset of rain.	Sac lac.
1st Aug'89	Again wheeze and spasm aggravated but patient can manage without inhaler. Re-assessed and on the basis of totality.	Nat. sulph. 200, 2 doses.
2nd Sep'89	Occasional wheeze, spasm much better. Better in every way.	Sac lac.
16th Oct'89	Standstill. Wait	Sac lac.
14th Nov'89	Standstill. Changed the plan of treatment. Deep acting anti-sycotic to finish the problem.	Thuja 200, 2 doses.
20th Dec'89	Doing better. Wait	Sac lac.
11th Jan'90	Doing better. Only occasional wheeze (once a week in the morning in an apparently cold day of the present winter). Asked to re-assess his chest X-ray & Blood.	Thuja 1m, 2 doses.
14th Feb'90	X-ray report shows much better. No fresh attack in this winter. Pneumonic consolidation, wheeze, ronchi are all clear on auscultation.	Sac lac.

Note: Patient has stopped treatment, as he does not have any further symptoms to complain about. Recently (in March 1992) assessed, doing okay.

Authenticity of Cure

CD Reference: RE002-EMPHYSEMA WITH BRONCHOSPASM-NCD

3. A CASE OF EMPHYSEMA OF BOTH LUNGS

Case No. RE003

Mr. M.K.N., 39 year old male.

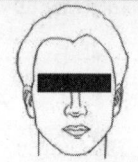

Photo of the patient, Mr. M.K.N

Presenting Complaints

- Stool with blood → Piles for 15 years, recurrent.
- Ayurvedic treatment and then operation done. But after operation a marble like out growth appeared in Rectum.
- Cough profuse, 3-4 times per minute, sometimes stitching pain inside left chest. °
- Tingling sensation in chest and back.
- Sticky expectoration during coughing.
- History of pain in throat and slight bleeding through the mouth.
- Gums bleed.
- Stool with mucous.
- Complaints < in very hot and very cold weather.
- Likes luke warm water for bathing.
- Head:- Occasional vertigo.
- Eye:- Slight dim vision at night.
- Stoppage of both nostrils.
- Occassional foetor oris.
- Tongue:- Thick yellow coating.
- Throat:- 2-3 years ago pain inside throat, blood comes out.
- Tonsillitis: Recurrent swelling of tonsil.
- Lungs:- Dry cough, expectoration drawn in long threads.
- Occassional breathing problem.
- Occassional palpitation - < walking, running.
- Chest:- Stitching pain. Occ. burning chest.
- Weakness in left side of chest.
- Abdomen:- Gas in whole abdomen. Occ. eructation. Feels better after passing gas. Feels pain in ribs.
- Stomach:- Appetite – sometimes increased, sometimes less. Hungry in the morning.
- Perspiration with odour. Sweat in neck, chest and back.

- Urine:- Yellowish. No odour.
- Stool:- Constipated – stool with white mucous.
- Sweat +++ on palm during summer.
- Pain in knee joint. History of trauma in knee joint.
- He has pain in right knee joint.
- Anus:- Piles. Sensation in anus.
- Mental:- Mild obstinate, suspicious, silent habit.
- Likes to be neat and clean.
- Memory – Weak, gradual loss memory.
- Sympathetic, can not tolerate blood letting.
- He wants to do everything in a hurry.
- He is active.
- Fear of thunderstorm, incurable diseases.
- Past History:- Typhoid, measles. Chicken pox – 2-3 times.
- First cause of break down of health is – history of piles operation by quack Ayurvedic Doctor.
- Hot patient; likes open air.
- Easily catches cold.
- Desire:- Pungent and hot food, Salt+, Salty, Bitter, Milk, Vegetables & Spinach, Chicken, Boiled Egg. Warm Food. Thirst – Average.
- Sleep – Sound. No particular dream.
- He is married with four children.
- Family History:- Father – urinary trouble. Mother – Paralysis. Maternal side – Piles.

Investigations Carried Out Before/After Dr. Banerjea's Treatment

24th Aug'86: Chest X-Ray – Early emphysema.

17th Nov'89: Chest X-Ray – No Radiological evidence of active parenchymal lesion seen.

CASE ANALYSIS, MIASMATIC DIAGNOSIS AND FINAL PRESCRIPTION

This is an interesting case of emphysema (which is miasmatically Sycotic because of thickening of lung alveoli) and Bryonia has been prescribed which is one of our leading anti-sycotic medicine.

X-RAY REPORT
NEW DEBENDRA X-RAY CLINIC
BARUIPUR, KACHARI BAZAR
KULPI ROAD, (BISWALAXMITALA),
24-PARGANAS

Dr. S. K. GHOSH
M.B.B.S., D.M.R.E.
EX-LECT. MEDICAL COLLEGE CALCUTTA
EX-HEAD OF DEPT. B. S. MEDICAL COLLEGE HOSPITAL, BANKURA
EX-CONSULTANT MULAGO HOSPITAL, KAMPALA, UGANDA (E. AFR.)
EX. MEDICAL SUPDT. E. S. I. HOSPITAL ASANSOL

Name: Mihir Kanta Naskar   Age: 35   Date: 24.8.86

Part Examined: 1) Chest PA View (Erect) 11) Soft tissue of neck   Ref. by Dr. B. B. Ghosh, MBBS

1) Both hila heavy with early emphysema in both lungs.
   Adv. Lab. investigation.
11) No abnormality is detected.

(Radiologist)

PORTABLE X-RAY AVAILABLE

Chest X-Ray report of Mr. M.K.N., Emphysema in both lungs, before treatment

Dr. N. KARMAKAR
M.B.B.S., D.M.R.D.
DOCTOR-IN-CHARGE
9-30 A. M. to 1. P. M.
7-30 P. M. to 8-30 P. M.
Sundays—by appointment.
Thursday Evening-by appointment

Residence : 35-0475
Chamber : 27-1675
Branch : 35-0476
2 (Lines)
(Personal : 27-8176
only by appointment)

*Laboratory & X-Ray Hours :-9 a. m. to 8 p. m.
Sundays—10 a. m. to 12 Noon

"X-RAY RELIEF"
Portable X-Rays, Electro-therapy, Blood Exam, etc.
213/8, BEPIN BEHARI GANGULY STREET, (1st Floor) CAL-12
(COLLEGE STREET & BOWBAZAR STREET, JUNCTION)
BRANCH :—26/8/1A. M. G. ROAD.

X-RAY REPORT

Name of Patient: Mr. Mihir Kanta Naskar.   Date: 17.11.89.
Referred by Physician/Surgeon: Dr. Subrata Kr. Banerjea.

Radiogram of: Chest (P-A-V——Erect).

No radiological evidence of active parenchymal lesion seen; lung-field shows catarrhal changes.

Radiologist

Cured Chest X-Ray report 9 months after treatment

Miasmatic Analysis

- Bleeding gums, bleeding through mouth, stool with blood: Tubercular (haemorrhagic).
- Stool with mucous: Sycotic. Constipation: Psora.
- Stoppage of both nostrils: Sycotic.
- Tongue – yellow thick coating, occassional foetor oris: Syco-Tubercular.
- Lungs - dry cough: Psora, sticky expectoration: Tubercular.
- Palpitation: Tubercular.
- Chest-stitching pain: Sycotic, occassional burning: Syphilitic, weakness in left chest: Tubercular.
- Stomach-appetite increased: Sycotic.
- Abdomen-gas: Psora.
- Anus – bleeding piles: Syco-Tubercular.
- Mind-mild, silent habit: Psora, obstinate: Tubercular, suspicious: Sycotic.
- Memory - weak gradual loss: Psora-Sycotic, wants to do everything in a hurry: Sycotic.
- Joint Pains: Sycotic.
- Cannot tolerate blood letting: Psora.
- Fears - thunderstorm, incurable diseases: Psora.
- Easily catches cold, but likes open air: Tubercular.
- Desires - Pungent, hot: Psora-ubercular, Salt salty: Syco-Tubercular, Warm food: Sycotic.

It's a mixed miasmatic case with Psora- sycotic preponderance.

Final Prescription Made on the Basis of

- Cough ++ profuse 3-4 times minute-stitching pain (aggravation: motion).
- Tingling, weakness inside left chest-occassional burning, Dry cough (sticky expectoration drawn into long threads).
- Stoppage of both nostrils.
- Constipation.
- Sweat ++.
- Knee joint pain (right sided).
- Memory-weak-gradual loss.
- Hot patient.

- Suspicious; obstinate.
- Desire Salt and salty.
- Sycotic preponderance.

The miasmatic breakdown of Bryonia is: Psora++, Sycotic +++, Syphilitic +, Tubercular ++ Hot ++. Sycosis is the predominant miasm in this case, which Bryonia covers.

Bryonia covers the case miasmatically as well.

Final Prescription

BRYONIA: 30C, 2 doses: later on 200C, 1 dose.

Remedy Reaction

Bryonia 30C is a good potency to start for respiratory complaints and to avoid aggravation. I have also chosen 30C considering the low vitality of the patient.

Prescription Chart

Date	Prescription Done on the Basis of	Treatment
11th Nov'88		Bryonia, 30C, 2 doses.
19th Jan'89		Sac lac.
2nd Apr'89	Standstill. Repeated	Bryonia 30C, 2 doses.
19th Jul'89	No appreciable change. Wait and Watch.	Sac lac.
4th Sep'89		Bryonia 200C, 1 dose.
20th Nov'89	Much better. According to radiological diagnosis (17th November 1989): Chest is clear.	
23rd Mar'90	Occasional Gas abdomen > eructation.	Carbo Veg, 200C, 2 doses.

Authenticity of Cure

CD Reference: RE003-EMPHYSEMA-MKN

4. A CASE OF EOSINOPHILIA: MR. S.H.M.

Case No. RE004

Age : 19 years as on 17th February, 1992
Sex : Male
Height : 5'5"
Weight : 48 kg.

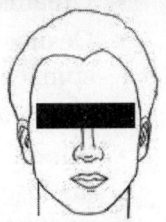

Photo of the patient, Mr. S.H.M

Presenting Complaints

- Bronchospasm aggravated by change of weather.
- Catches cold easily; sneezing++.
- Stoppage of nose alternately, aggravates during early morning.
- Moist cough aggravated at night, ameliorated by scanty whitish expectoration.
- Wheezing sound in chest; bronchospasm aggravates at midnight, ameliorates during early morning (sunrise). Better by bending forward.
- Pain in chest & back: better by hot oil massaging.
- Frontal headache: throbbing pain: better by massaging.
- Profuse perspiration on forehead & nose.
- Bronchospasm and recurrent respiratory infections: aggravation during the entire winter season. Better during the summer.
- Hereditary cause: Mother and maternal uncle have asthma.
- Weakness++. Physically feels restless and wants to move, but physically too
- weak to move (prostration with desire to move). Exhaustion after slightest exertion.
- Stool: Regular; Okay.
- Urine: Okay.
- Appetite: Average.
- Thirsty++ generally luke warm water (not very cold water, never from fridge).
- Chilly patient.
- Profuse perspiration all over the body in summer season. Bad smell in sweat.

- Sleep – disturbed.
- Dreams of various things.
- Desires: Salty food (++); sweet (+); bitter; milk; potato (++); veg. & spinach; meat;
- Warm food. Aversion to sour.
- Mind: Angry; talkative; desires company. Very anxious (+++) about his diseases [anxiety is almost out of proportion considering his age and disease] with occasional fear of death. Occasionally depressed.
- Memory – weak++.
- Possessive and selfish. Keeps his own things in order and tidy; does not allow anyone to touch or move them.
- Patient gets angry when reprimanded.
- Past History: Skin disease (itching) – 3 yrs. back. Treated allopathically.
- Family History: Mother – Low blood pressure; asthma. Father – Blood sugar.
- Maternal uncle - Asthma.

Investigations Carried Out Before/After Dr. Banerjea's Treatment

20th Apr'91: Haemoglobin: 96% Erythrocyte Sedimentation Rate =14 Red Blood Cell : 4.8×10^6.

25th Sep'91: Chest X-Ray: Non-specific pneumonitis.

15th Jun'92: White Blood Cell 6,200 Neutrophil$_{52}$ Lymphocyte$_{43}$ Monocyte$_1$ Eosinophil$_4$ Basophil$_0$.

18th Jul'92: Chest X-Ray – Mild non-specific pneumonitis, Left lung.

6th Apr'93: Chest X-Ray – No active parenchymal lesion seen.

2nd Apr'94: Haemoglobin: 13.9% Neutrophil$_{69}$ Lymphocyte$_{28}$ Monocyte$_1$ Eosinophil$_2$ Basophil$_0$.

23rd Nov'94: Haemoglobin: 14.1 % White Blood Cell 4,500, Neutrophil$_{56}$ Lymphocyte$_{36}$ Monocyte$_1$ Eosinophil$_7$ Basophil$_0$ Erythrocyte Sedimentation Rate – 2mm. Chest X-Ray: No active parenchymal lesion.

8th Nov'97: Haemoglobin: 14.5. Neutrophil$_{60}$ Lymphocyte$_{33}$ Monocyte$_1$ Eosinophil$_6$ Basophil$_0$.

7th Aug'98: Haemoglobin: 14.4% White Blood Cell 7,800, Neutrophil$_{58}$ Lymphocyte$_{40}$ Monocyte$_1$ Eosinophil$_1$ Basophil$_0$ Erythrocyte Sedimentation Rate – 9mm

Respiratory Diseases - Cured Cases

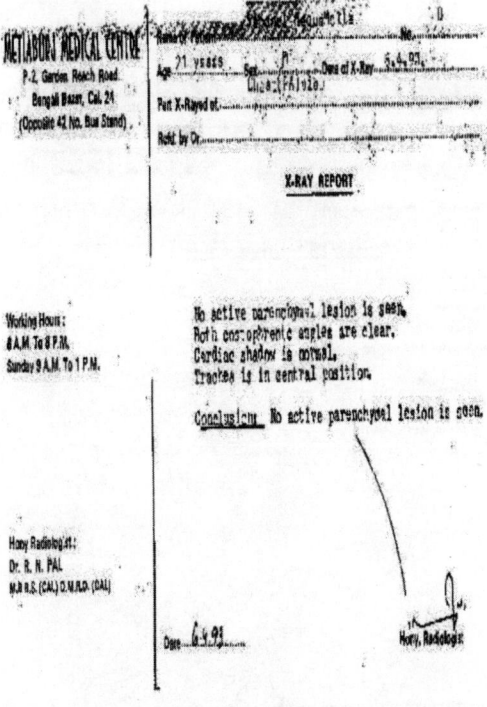

Blood report of Mr. S.H.M, before treatment

X-Ray report Mr. S.H.M, before treatment

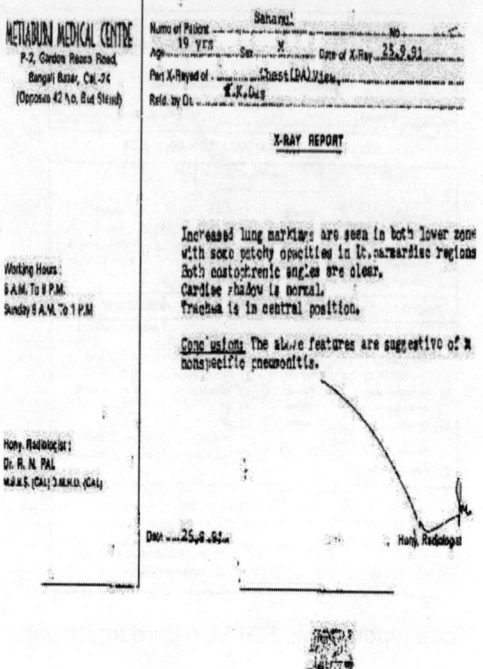

X-Ray report, 8 months after treatment

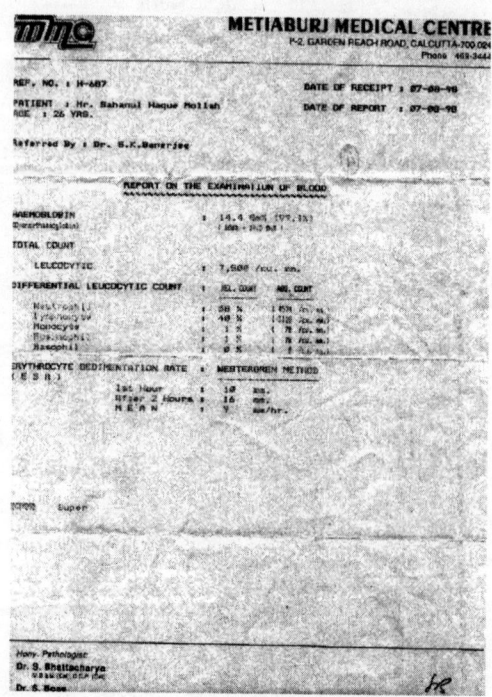

Blood report after treatment

CASE ANALYSIS, MIASMATIC DIAGNOSIS AND FINAL PRESCRIPTION

Miasmatic Analysis

- Bronchospasm aggravated by change of weather: Sycosis.
- Catches cold easily: Psora.
- Stoppage of nose alternately: Tubercular.
- Moist cough aggravates at night: Syphilis.
- Scanty expectoration: Psora.
- Broncho-spasm aggravates at midnight: Syphilis.
- Profuse perspiration: Sycosis.
- Recurrent respiratory infections: Tubercular.
- Bronchospasm and recurrent respiratory infections aggravated in winter, amelioration summer: Psora.
- Hereditary broncho-spasm: Sycosis.
- Frontal headache: Sycosis. Throbbing pain: Psora.
- Weakness++: Psora.
- Physically restless: Sycosis.
- Bad smell to sweat: Syphilis.
- Desires: Salty food: Syco-tubercular. Sweet: Psora. Potatoes: Tubercular. Warm food: Sycosis.
- Very anxious (+++): Psora.
- Fear of death: Psora.
- Talkative: Sycosis.
- Occasionally depressed: Syphilis.
- Memory – weak++: Psora.
- Possessive and selfish: Sycosis.
- Keeps his own things in order and tidy: Sycosis.

It's a mixed miasmatic case with Psora- sycotic preponderance.

Prescription Made on the Basis of

- Bronchospasm aggravated by change of weather.
- Catches cold easily; sneezing++.
- Stoppage of nose alternately, aggravates during early morning.
- Moist cough aggravates at night.

- Wheezing sound in chest.
- Broncho-spasm aggravates at midnight. Better by bending forward.
- Broncho-spasm and recurrent respiratory infections: Aggravates during the entire winter season. Better during the summer.
- Weakness++. Physically feels restless and wants to move, but physically too
- weak to move (prostration with desire to move). Exhaustion after slightest exertion.
- Thirsty++ generally luke warm water (not very cold water, never from fridge).
- Chilly patient
- Desire: Warm food.
- Mind: Desires for company. Very anxious (+++) about his diseases [anxiety is almost out of proportion considering his age and disease] with occasional fear of death. Occasionally depressed.
- Memory – weak++.
- Possessive and selfish. Keeps his own things in order and tidy; does not allow anyone to touch or move them.
- Past History: Skin disease (itching) – 3 yrs. back. Treated allopathically.

The miasmatic breakdown of Arsenicum is Psora +++, Sycosis +++, Syphilis +, Tubercular ++.

Arsenicum covers the case miasmatically as well.

Final Prescription and Remedy Reaction

Considering the above totality I treated the case with Arsenicum Alb. starting with 30 C and finishing the case with 1M. The 30 C potency was chosen because of the nature of the case and the vital energy of the patient, 30 C is also a good potency for bronchospasm. I wondered that I might need Thuja or Tuberculinum as a complementary to end the case, but the patient beautifully improved and was cured by Arsenicum alone. Unfortunately a detailed prescription chart is not available for this case; improvement was seen after 8 months of treatment.

Authenticity of Cure

CD Reference: RE004-EOSINOPHILIA WITH NON-SPECIFIC PNEUMONITIS-SHM

5. A CASE OF TUBERCULOSIS WITH BRONCHOSPASM: MISS B.K.

Case No. RE005

Age : 10+ years at 27th July, 1989.
Weight: 25 kgs.

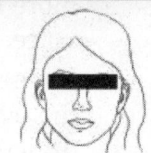

Photo of the patient,
Miss. B.K.

Presenting Complaints

- The young girl complained of breathing trouble, which had gradually built up over the last three years. Wheezing sound, aggravated in the evening over the whole night; ameliorated by bending forward, and in the open air.
- Tendency to catch cold very easily.
- Feverish feeling throughout the day with evening rise of temperature, occasionally it increases to 104 degrees Fahrenheit (almost 40 degree Centigrade).
- Dry, hacking cough with tickling in throat and thick greyish-yellow expectoration occasionally mixed or tinged with blood.
- Cough: Aggravates in the evening, towards night, occasionally aggravates in the early morning. Aggravates from ascending stairs, ameliorated by rest. Aggravated from cold, but she likes to be in the open air. Ameliorated by lying down.
- Aggravated by pressure over chest.
- Milk disagrees (makes her nauseated). No other particular desires or aversions to food.
- Profuse sweat especially in the upper part of the body, can be more in the back part of the head with strong sourish-pungent smell. Fever ameliorates after sweat.
- Cough, asthmatic oppression and fever: aggravates during new moon & full moon.
- Head:- Occasional headache ameliorated by lying down and closing the eyes.
- Ear:- Occasional discharge from nose, generally after severe chest congestion.
- Nose:- Takes cold and ends up in coryza. Bleeding twice.
- Mouth:- Mouth fills with sour water & water brash.
- Tongue:- Thickly coated, unclean.

- Throat:- (i) Recurrent sore-throat; (ii) Difficult to swallow; (iii) Pain more in the right and then left is also affected; (iv) Occasional husky voice.
- Lungs:- (i) Cough excited by tickling in larynx aggravated during the evening, in bed, when sleeping. (ii) Suffocation and breathing difficulty.
- Chest- Sharp stitches in chest aggravated by pressure.
- Abdomen:- (i) Pain in right hypochondriac region, after meals– liver tender, palpable. (ii) Cannot tighten the garments around the waist.
- Stomach:- (i) Poor Appetite. (ii) Sour taste. Acidity++. (iii) Milk disagrees
- Sweat:- (i) Profuse sweat (+++). Pungent –sourish smell. (ii) Especially in the upper part of the body.
- Urine:- (i) Nocturnal enuresis. (ii) Dark urine.
- Stool:- Constipation, but occasionally alternates with loose stool.
- Upper Extremities:- Occasional aches and stitches in the right shoulder and back of the neck, with the rise of fever (pyrexia).
- Palm:- Coldness of palms, can be clammy, occasionally get moist with high pyrexia.
- Joints:- Stiffness and aching in the joints especially during fever.
- Lower Extremities:- Cold feeling in the soles. Can get clammy.
- Menses:- Not started yet.
- Anus:- Occasional burning after dry, hard stool. Bleeding twice.
- Skin Disease:- Drug rash after previous intake of allopathic medicines, discontinued allopathy - better since.
- Mind:- Angry; irritable; quarrelsome; fault-finding. Silent habit; gloomy. Dirty habits. Fear of death; disgusted with life. Fear of animals (including dogs); insects and spiders. Memory weak. Can be dull and lose memory. Weeping mood. Intensely sympathetic. Reliable, responsible and duty bound. Fear of ghosts, darkness (+++), animals, incurable diseases, failures.
- Past History: (i) Tb. (ii) Asthma. (iii) Pulmonary Koch's [Tb] (now suffering). (iv) Bronchospasm (now suffering). (v) History of Measles in 1984. (vi) Milestones – regular.

What was The First Cause of Breakdown in Health

- Parents related that the patient was in a habit of 2-3 swims per day; cough & cold settled in chest: Never been well since.

- Chilly. Does catch cold very easily (+++) now.
- Desires: [I] Sweet ++ [ii] Sour ++ [iii] Pungent + [iv] Salt ++ [v] Salty ++ [vi] Bitter: no [vii] Bread: no [viii] Milk: no [ix] Potato: no [x] Vegetables & spinach: no [xi] Onion: no [xii] Fruits: no [xiii] Fish ++ [xiv] Meat/Chicken: no [xv] Egg ++ [xvi] Rich, spicy & fat food + [xvii] Warm food: no [xviii] Cold food + [xix] Warm drinks: no [xx] Cold drinks ++ [xxi] Ice cream +++.
- Thirsty +.
- Sleep – Disturbed sleep.
- Dreams- Dreams of daily works, robbers, horrors.
- Family History – Father had Tuberculosis in 1982 treated with Streptomycin shots. Family History of asthma, diabetes, pleurisy, rheumatism and cancer.

Previous Homoeopathic Treatment

- Acalypha indica 6 (no permanent result).
- Arsenicum iodatum 6 (no permanent result).
- Tuberculinum 30 (no effect).
- Phosphorus 30 (cough was better, but after the course was over it relapsed again).
- Calcarea Phosphorica (cough and dyspnoea was severely aggravated).

Investigations Carried Out Before and During Dr. Banerjea's Treatment

13th Jul'89: Blood: Haemoglobin% 11.6, Red Blood Cell – 3.9×10^6 White Blood Cell. 11.450. Neutrophil – 70, Eosinophil – 1. Basophil – 0. Lymphocyte – 27. Monocyte – 2. Erythrocyte Sedimentation Rate: 86 mm.

15th Jul'89: Chest X-ray: Coarse lung marking with fine mottled shadows, both sides.

15th Jul'89: Mantoux Test: Strongly Positive: (25 mm with blister formation).

20th Dec'89: Chest X-ray: No active lung lesion is seen. Cardiac contour is normal.

8th Sep'90: Blood: Haemoglobin % - 13.9. White Blood Cell – 6,100. Eosinophil – 3. Erythrocyte Sedimentation Rate – 11.

8th Sep'90: Chest X-ray: Nothing abnormal is detected.

Blood report of Miss B.K., before treatment

Chest X-Ray report, before treatment

Respiratory Diseases - Cured Cases

Chest X-Ray report, 5 months after treatment

Blood report, 12 months after treatment

CASE ANALYSIS, MIASMATIC DIAGNOSIS AND FINAL PRESCRIPTION

- Clinical findings: Lung congestion ++
- Provisional diagnosis: A known case of PULMONARY TUBERCULOSIS.
- Miasmatic diagnosis: PSORA-TUBERCULAR
- Constitutional remedy: Calc. Carb.

Miasmatic Analysis

- Breathing trouble (family history): Sycosis.
- Tendency to catch cold very easily: Psora-tubercular.
- Feverish feeling throughout the day with evening rise of temperature: Tubercular.
- Dry, hacking cough with tickling in throat: Tubercular.
- Expectoration: thick greyish-yellow: Sycosis.
- Occasionally mixed or tinged with blood: Tubercular.
- Cough: Aggravated by cold, but she likes to be in the open air: Tubercular.
- Profuse sweat: Sycosis.
- Cough, asthmatic oppression and fever: Aggravated during new moon & full moon: Tubercular.
- Nose - Takes cold and ends up in coryza. Bleeding twice: Tubercular.
- Mouth - Mouth fills with sour water & water brash: Psora.
- Recurrent sore throat: Tubercular.
- Stomach – Sour taste. Acidity++: Psora.
- Sweat – Profuse sweat (+++): Sycosis.
- Urine – Nocturnal enuresis: Tubercular.
- Stool – Constipation: Psora.
- Alternates with loose stool: Tubercular.
- Palm – Coldness of palms, can be clammy: Psora.
- Joints – Stiffness and aching in the joints: Sycosis.
- Lower Extremities – Cold feeling in the soles: Psora.

- Desires: Salt / salty: Syco-tubercular. Pungent: Sycosis. Sweet: Psora. Cold food: Syco-tubercular. Cold drinks: Syphilitic.
- Aversion: Milk: Psora-sycotic. Vegetables: Sycosis.
- Mind – Quarrelsome: Sycosis.
- Fault-finding: Tubercular.
- Silent habit: Psora.
- Fear of death: Psora.
- Disgusted with life: Syphilis.
- Fear of animals (including dogs); Tubercular.
- Fear of insects & spiders: Tubercular.
- Memory weak: Psora.
- Intensely sympathetic: Sycosis.
- Fear of ghost, darkness (+++): Psora.
- Past History: Tb.: Tubercular.
- Chilly. Does catch cold very easily (+++): Psora-tubercular.
- Family History – Father had Tuberculosis: Tubercular. Family History of asthma: Sycosis. Pleurisy: Tubercular. Rheumatism: Sycosis.

It's a mixed miasmatic case with Psora- syco-tubercular preponderance.

Final Prescription and Remedy Reaction

Calc. carb. was chosen for the reasons given in the prescription chart below. The case was begun with the 30 C potency as, in Calc. Carb., this is a particularly good potency for respiratory ailments and in addition there is a family history of tuberculosis; it is therefore necessary to be prudent when giving a remedy with a strong tubercular element as in this case. The patient was cured of her symptoms in just over a year of treatment.

Calcarea Carb covers the case miasmatically as well.

Prescription Chart

Date	Prescription Made on the Basis of	Treatment
27th Jul'89	Breathing trouble with wheezing sound, aggravated in the evening for whole night; ameliorated in open air. Tendency to catch cold very easily. Evening feverishness – Tubercular diathesis Dry, hacking cough with tickling. Expectoration: Thick greyish-yellow expectoration, tinged with blood. Profuse sweat especially in the upper part of the body, can be more in the back part of the head with strong sourish-pungent smell. Cough, asthmatic oppression and fever: aggravated during new moon & full moon. Stomach:- (i) Poor appetite; (ii) Sour taste. Acidity++; (iii) Milk disagrees Sweat:- (i) Profuse sweat (+++). Pungent –sourish smell. (ii) Especially in the upper part of the body. Urine:- (i) Nocturnal enuresis. Stool:- Constipation, but occasionally alternates with loose stool. Palm:- Coldness of palms, can be clammy, occasionally get moist with high pyrexia. Lower Extremities:- Cold feeling in the soles. Can get clammy. Mind:- Fault-finding. Silent habit; gloomy. Fear of death; disgusted with life. Fear of animals (including dogs), insects and spiders. Memory weak. Reliable, responsible and duty bound. Fear of ghosts, darkness (+++), animals, incurable diseases, failures. Chilly. Does catch cold very easily (+++) now. Desires: Sweet++; sour++; salt++; salty++; egg++; cold food+; ice cream+++. Aversion: Meat. Thirsty+. Miasmatic coverage [Psora-Tubercular]. Miasmatic breakdown of Calc carb. is Psora+++, Sycosis+++, Syphilis++, Tubercular+++.	Calc. carb. 30 [1 globule of No. X size, dissolved in distilled water and divided into 2 doses
16th Aug'89	Cough has aggravated and expectoration increased. Wait and watch.	Sac lac.

Respiratory Diseases - Cured Cases

Date	Prescription Made on the Basis of	Treatment
3rd Sep'89	Standstill. (Ancestral tip – longer you wait, more you gain, after a right prescription!]	Sac lac.
25th Sep'89	Cough is much better, dyspnoea is less, but the girl is complaining of tickling in throat and pain in chest. Wait.	Sac lac.
12th Oct'.89	As colder days setting-in; cough is again aggravated along with the dyspnoea. Repeat.	Calc. carb. 30; 2 doses (1 globule divided into 2 doses).
28th Oct'.89	No change in cough. Once she had blood mixed sputa. Go to higher potency, as the former is not holding the case properly.	Cal. carb. 200 (2 doses) alternate mornings.
14th Nov'89	Dramatically better, cough and dyspnoea much reduced even in the cold weather.	Sac lac.
3rd Dec'89	Doing better; cough, respiratory discomfort, fever even indigestion: all are better. Asked to review the X-Ray of the chest.	Sac lac.
23rd Dec'89	X-Ray (20.12.89) shows much improvement: previous mottled shadows have disappeared.	Sac lac.
28th Jan'90	Was doing okay, but with the exposure to cold air, sore throat has again appeared. Acute of Calcarea being given (A Syphilo-tubercular manifestation)	Belladonna 30, 2 doses daily in the morning.
18th Feb'90	Sore throat better.	Sac lac.
27th Mar'90	After the sore throat got better; the tingling throat has again increased with dry cough (occasional)	Calc. carb. 1M, 2 doses alternate morning
2nd May'90	Tickling better and cough disappeared. Wait & watch.	Sac lac.
2nd Jun'90	With the onset of rain, patient is complaining of some joint aches. Wait for more movement and surfacing of symptoms	Sac lac.
22nd Jun'90	Joint aches have aggravated with occasional dry cough. Repeat again (As high potency, asked the patient to review after one month).	Calc. Carb. 1M, 2 doses.
14th Jul'90	No change in the joint pains. Possibly suppressed/dormant/latent inherited sycosis is coming to the surface. Change in the plan of treatment (complementary prescribing).	Rhus tox. 200, 2 doses alternate mornings.
1st Aug'90	Much better, wait & watch	Sac lac.

Date	Prescription Made on the Basis of	Treatment
21st Aug'90	Patent is better in every regard. Developing (growing) rapidly, mentally calmer, amiable, intellect has much improved, but fears are still present. Go higher in potency and asked to review X-Ray chest and blood test.	Calc. carb. 10M, 2 doses alternate mornings.
22nd Sep'90	X-Ray shows absolutely normal, E.S.R. has come down to 11(8.9.90) from previous 86 (13.7.89) better in every respect; fears are less.	Sac lac.
	STOPPED TREATMENT AS THE PATIENT SAYS THOROUGHLY CURED OF HER PROBLEM.	

Authenticity of Cure

CD Reference: RE005-PRIMARY KOCH'S WITH BRONCHOSPASM-BK

6. A CASE OF PULMONARY KOCH'S (TUBERCULOSIS) WITH BRONCHOSPASM IN 30 YEAR OLD FEMALE

Case No. RE006

MRS. D.M:

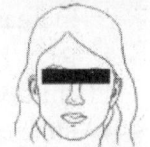

Photo of the patient, Mrs. D.M.

Presenting Complaints

- Breathing problems 4 years back, < Summer, < checked perspiration. > by sitting, winter, open air.
- Moist cough, whitish, thin expectoration.
- Burning vertex, does not tolerate any covering on her body. Easily catches cold.
- Sneezing – thin, watery discharge, moist cough < night (bed time).
- Habit of bathing early morning.
- Previously had Allopathic treatment.
- Breathing troubles appear after suppression of eczema on both legs.
- Complaints < perspiration.
- Head – Hot vertex, perspiration back part of head.
- Tongue – Dry.
- Breathing trouble, rattling cough.
- Stomach:- Appetite – poor.
- Profuse sweating all over the body, offensive odour ++.
- Stool – Regular.
- Menses:- 1st started 13 years of age. No pain. 27 – 28 days interval.
- Contraceptive pills for 3 years – after 1st issue.
- Scanty menses – duration 3 days; blackish, 1st day more bleeding – small clots.
- Skin:- Delayed healing.
- Eczema on both legs, 6 years back, excessive itching < late night. Thick, whitish, sticky discharge. Burning after itching, > cold water.
- Mental:- Angry. Talkative, desire to be neat and clean, wants to be alone.
- Desire for death, disgusted with life.
- Memory – Medium.
- Gets more angry when reprimanded.

- Sympathetic, can tolerate blood letting.
- She does everything slowly.
- History of taking Allopathic medicine for 3 years – sometimes increase/decrease.
- Past History:- Typhoid. Asthma. Skin diseases, chicken pox in childhood. Tumour operation on right breast.
- Hot patient, likes open air.
- Desire – Pungent and hot++, Salt+, Salty+, Sweet +, Milk+, Onion, Fruits, Fish++, Warm food.
- Thirst – Average.
- Sleep – Sound.
- She is married – 1 son; 7 years.
- Family History:- Father – suffered from Eczema.

Investigations Carried Out Before/After Dr. Banerjea's Treatment

1st May'90: Chest X-Ray:- Irregular areas of patchy consolidation. Koch's.

1st May'90: Blood report:- Hb% - 13.2, W.B.C. = 8,400. Neutrophil- 66, Eosinophil – 6, Basophil – 0; Lymphocyte – 24, Monocyte-4, Erythrocyte Sedimentation Rate – 46 mm.

28th Jul'90: Chest X-Ray:- Nothing abnormal detected.

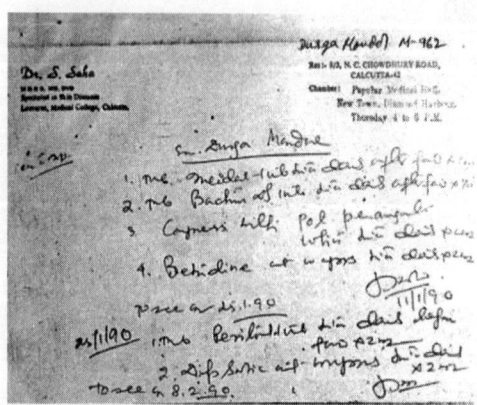

Allopathic (conventional) prescription of Mrs. D. M. before treatment

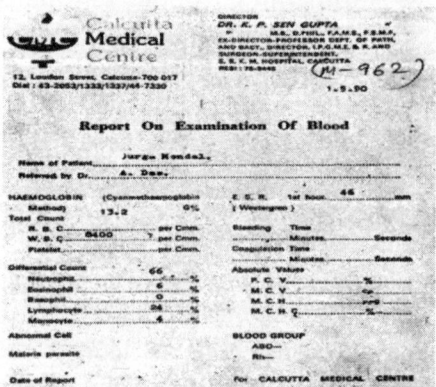

Blood report before treatment

Respiratory Diseases - Cured Cases

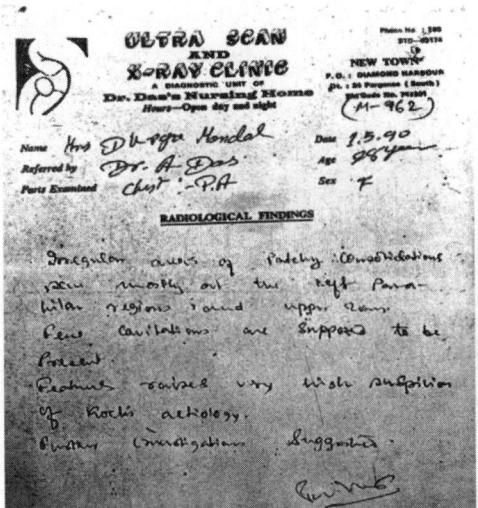
Chest X-Ray report, before treatment

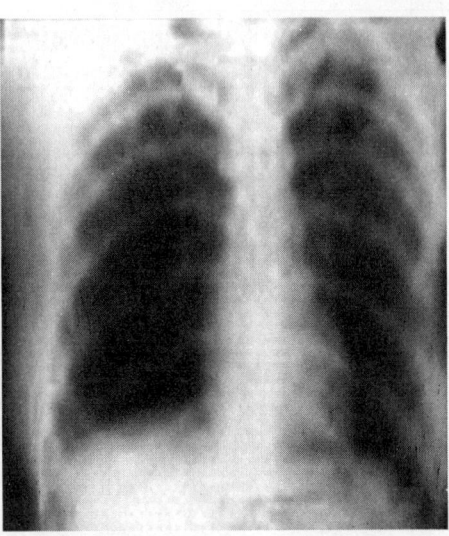
Chest X-ray skiagram, before treatment

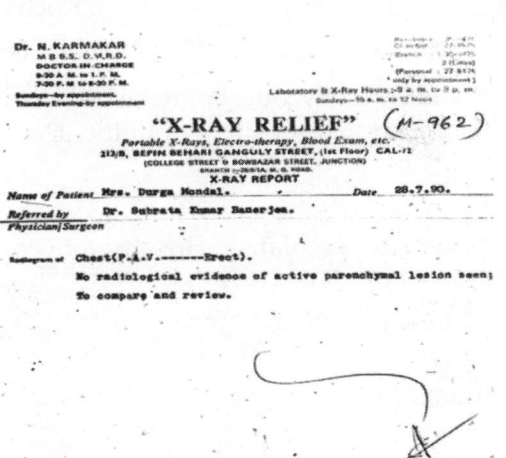
Chest X-ray report, 5 months after treatment

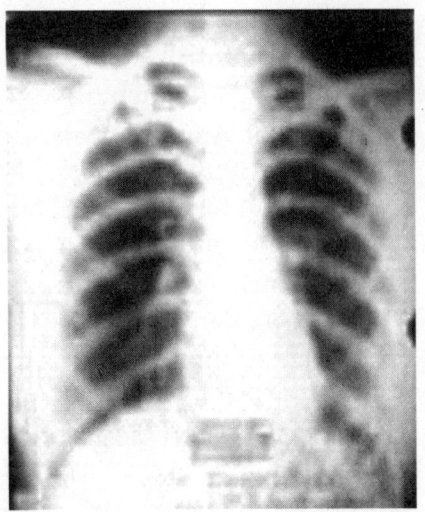
Chest X-ray after treatment

CASE ANALYSIS, MIASMATIC DIAGNOSIS AND FINAL PRESCRIPTION

This is an interesting case of tuberculosis of the chest associated with bronchospasm and even in a situation like this, the prescription was made on the basis of entire totality of the case, rather than prescribing for the pathology. This is once again a good learning for all of us, that if we prescribe on the basis of the totality; pathology will cease to exist.

Miasmatic Analysis

- Breathing problems - < summer > winter: Syphilitic, > sitting: Psora, > open air: Tubercular.
- Moist cough-whitish expect: Sycotic < night – Syphilo-Tubercular.
- Burning vertex: Syphilitic.
- ECC – likes open air: Tubercular.
- Sneezing thin watery discharge: Psora.
- Profuse sweat: Sycotic, complaints < perspiration: Syphilitic.
- Rattling cough: Sycotic.
- Appetite poor: Psora.
- Scanty menses, clots: Psora-Tubercular.
- Skin – Delayed healing: Syphilitic.
- Eczema – Excessive itching: Psora-Sycotic, < night-Syphilitic.
- Thick whitish sticky discharge: Sycotic.
- Burning after itching > by cold: Syphilitic.
- Mental: Angry, Talkative, Neat and clean: Sycotic, Wants to be alone: Psora-Syphilitic, Desire for death, disgust for life: Syphilitic, Does everything slowly: Psora.
- Past history – Tumour: Sycotic.
- Desires – Pungent, hot: Psora-Tubercular, Salt/salty: Syco-Tubercular, Warm food: Sycotic.

It's a mixed miasmatic case with Psora- syco-tubercular preponderance.

Final Prescription Made on the Basis of
SULPHUR

- Tuberculosis with Bronchospasm.
- Breathing problems < checked perspiration. Breathing troubles appear after suppression of eczema.
- Rattling cough, moist cough < night.
- Habit of bathing early morning.
- Hot and burning vertex, cannot tolerate any covering on her body.
- Skin – Excessive itching, burning after scratching < night, < scratching, < perspiration.

- Profuse sweat with offensive odour.
- Delayed healing.
- Hot patient.
- ECC (easily catches cold) – likes open air.
- Desire Salt, salty and sweet.
- Warm food.
- Appetite poor.
- Mental – Angry, Talkative, does everything slowly. Desire for death, disgust for life, wants to be alone.

The miasmatic breakdown of Sulphur is Psora +++, Sycosis ++, Syphilis +++, Tubercular +++

Mixed miasmatic case; Sulphur is a leading Tri-miasmatic medicine. Sulphur covers the case miasmatically as well.

Final Prescription And Remedy Reaction

Sulphur was given only in 30C potency because of the lung pathology and to avoid any aggravation whatsoever, considering first observation of Kent. Later on 200C was given as the patient's reactive capability has been established and it dramatically improved the case.

Prescription Chart

Date	Prescription Done on the Basis of	Treatment
3rd May'90		Sulphur 30C, 2 doses.
1st Jun'90	Breathing problem little better; cough standstill. Wait and watch.	Sac lac.
2nd Jul'90	Patient feels standstill.	Sulphur, 200C, 1 dose.
26th Jul'90	Patient returned with excitement. Breathing trouble, cough, 95% better. Advised to repeat chest x-ray.	
5th Aug'90	Chest x-ray clear (as on 28th July 1990); no medicine given.	

Authenticity of Cure

CD Reference: RE006-PULMONARY KOCH'S WITH BRONCHOSPASM-DM

12 Rheumatological Diseases - Cured Cases

CHAPTER

1. A CASE OF SHOULDER JOINT DISLOCATION: MISS O. S.

Case No. RH001

Age : 12 years 11 months as on 27th August, 1993
Height : 5 ft. 3 inches

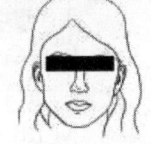

Photo of the patient, Miss. O.S.

Presenting Complaints

- Recurrent dislocation of right shoulder joint, originally occurring whilst playing tennis.
- Occurred 20 days previously, aggravated during playing (tennis).
- Slight swelling with pain.
- No treatment.
- Intra-uterine incidence: History of jaundice of mother.
- Normal delivery.
- Recurrent common cold with dyspnoea, aggravated by exposure to cold, after allopathy symptoms disappear.
- Pain in the right hand, drawing tensive pain.
- Pain in the limbs. Shifting rapidly.
- Vomiting tendency.
- Vomiting during fever, after taking rich food.
- Trembling of hands during fever.
- Acne – on the forehead on both cheeks. Nape, back, occasional itching.
- Skin: Itching on the soles (both legs) after scratching bleeds slightly.
- Allergy – Brinjal (aubergine).

- Homoeopathic generalities: Chilly patient.
- Amelioration of symptoms in open air.
- Desires: Meat+++, egg+++, salty+++, sour, cold food.
- Aversions – fish; milk.
- Aggravation: Brinjal.
- Thirst: Average.
- Sleep: Sound.
- Appetite: Increased.
- Stool: Irregular not clear, hard stool.
- Urine: Clear.
- Sweat: Profuse sweat throughout the body, offensive odour.
- Menstruation: Time - regular. Quantity – average. Duration – about 4 days.
- Character of pain – Onset of menses: pain in lower abdomen.
- Character of blood – Bright blood with black clots.
- Mind: Anger+++. Restless, dirty habit, timid, sympathetic, fear of failure.
- Weeps easily.
- Chilly patient.
- Past History: Skin disease, malaria, measles, burns, accident, and chickenpox.
- Paternal Grand Father:- TB, Cancer.
- Grand Mother:- Asthma.

Investigations Carried Out Before/After Dr. Banerjea's Treatment

10th Aug'93 X-ray Shoulder :- Although skiagram of right humeral head taken in different degrees of internal rotation, it failed to identify any significant congenital defect; that taken in the axillary view showed the characteristic medial slope usually seen with the recurrent dislocation of shoulder joint.

11th May'94 X-ray right shoulder – Nothing abnormal detected.

Rheumatological Diseases - Cured Cases

X-Ray of both shoulder of Miss O.S., before treatment

X-Ray of Right shoulder, 9 months after treatment

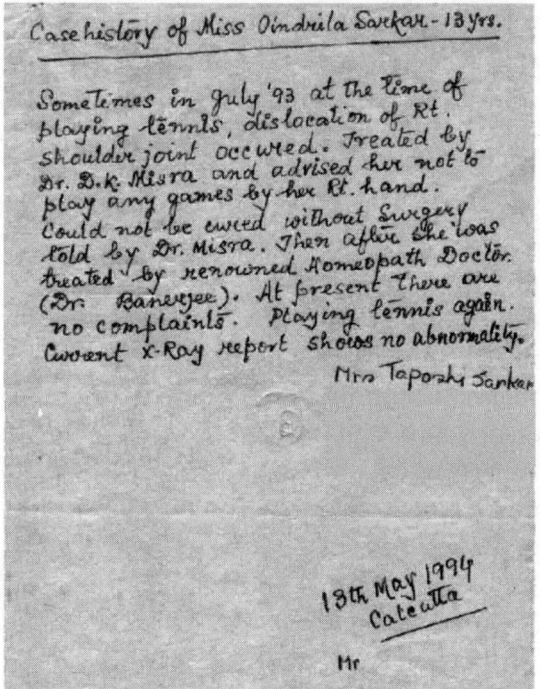

Comments of the patients, after treatment

CASE ANALYSIS, MIASMATIC DIAGNOSIS AND FINAL PRESCRIPTION

Miasmatic Analysis

- Joint problems: Sycosis.
- Swelling: Sycosis.
- Aggravation motion: Syco-Syphilis.
- Cold symptoms aggravated by cold exposure: Psora.
- Vomiting: Psora.
- Acne: Sycosis.
- Itching skin (soles of both legs): Psora.
- Allergy – Brinjal (aubergine): Tubercular.
- Desires salty+++: Syco- tubercular.
- Desires meat: Tubercular
- Desires sour: Psora-syphilitic.
- Desires cold food: Syco – tubercular.
- Profuse sweat: Sycotic.
- Offensive odour to sweat: Syphilitic.
- Mental restlessness: Psora.
- Timid: Psora.
- Fear of failure: Psora.

It's a mixed miasmatic case with Psora- sycotic preponderance.

Reasoning for Prescription

- The initial prescription made was **Pulsatilla 200c.** This was based on:
- Aggravation from rich food;
- Amelioration from open air;
- Pain in the right hand, drawing tensive pain.
- Pain in the limbs. Shifting rapidly.
- Sycotic remedy as a joint problem;
- Acne at puberty;
- Clotted menses;
- Sound sleep when time to get up;
- Shy and timid. Weepy.
- Chilly, better open air.
- Desire cold food.
- Thirst: average.
- Sympathetic (but gives to receive consolation)

The miasmatic breakdown of this remedy is: Psora ++, Sycosis +++, Syphilis +, Tubercular ++.

Pulsatilla covers the case miasmatically as well.

Appearance and Personality

Pulsatilla is particularly suited to those who are fair and beautiful-looking, but inclined to be fleshy with fine hair and blue eyes, soft and lax muscles, anaemic and chlorotic with pale face at puberty. It is particularly suitable for females when they have delayed onset of menstruation.

Pulsatilla is full of tears and has sluggish activity of body and mind. Easily moved to laughter or tears. Affectionate, yielding disposition – the woman's remedy. Slow, phlegmatic and indecisive. Mild, gentle, Pulsatilla is the mildest patient in Materia Medica (opposite to Nux, where patient is irritable). A timid, lachrymose disposition with a tendency to inward grief and silent peevishness. Especially suited when the patient must be a long time in bed at night before he can get to sleep and is worse in the evening.

Dr. Hering denotes the Pulsatilla patient – sandy hair, blue eyes, pale face, easily moved to laughter or tears, affectionate, gentle, women inclined to be fleshy. Tearfulness (Sepia –weeps when questioned about her symptoms, but Puls. cries when telling her symptom). Sometimes, silent peevishness, sometimes dormant irritability.

Prescription Chart

Date	Prescription Done on the Basis of	Treatment
27th Aug'93	Reasoning for prescription of Pulsatilla given above.	Pulsatilla, 200 C, 2 doses.
24th Sep'93		Sac lac
19th Nov'93		Pulsatilla, 200C, 2 doses.
15th Dec'93		Sac Lac
4th Feb'94	Dislocation of shoulder better. Chilly. Offensive stool and urine. Eczema.	Pulsatilla, 1M, 2 doses.
7th Mar'94		Sac lac.
13th Apr'94		Sac Lac

Authenticity of Cure

CD Reference: RH001-RECURRENT SHOULDER JOINT DISLOCATION-OS

2. A CASE OF RHEUMATOID ARTHRITIS IN A 18 YEARS OLD FEMALE, ARNICA MONTANA GIVEN

Case No. RH002

Age : 17 years old as on 11th January, 1995
Sex : Female

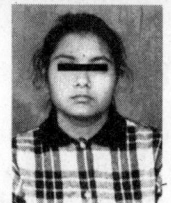

Photo of the patient Miss D. B.

Presenting Complaints

- Pain in the lower extremities with heaviness and numbness. Pain on both legs (loin to ankle) → more in left leg previous, pain ascends upwards (ankle to loin).
- Pain more in left leg than the right leg.
- Commence from ankle and ascends upwards to the lip and then it settles in the lumbo-sacral region. Now back pain as well. Sore, bruised and sensitive (+++) to touch.
- Now the pain in the lumbo-sacral region and also legs and ankle.
- Both legs are sore and tender (+++) to touch, as well.
- Patient have had fracture of the shaft of the tibia & fibula: 3 months after pain started.
- Aggravation of pain: from walking, sitting, new and full moon. Aggravation from cold weather.
- Amelioration by rest and lying down.
- Pain along with numbness & heaviness < walking, < touch (+++); sitting. > lying, > hot application. Lack of strength in both legs. Pain comes gradually after walking with short steps.
- Hot water relieves the pain for a short time.
- Pain increases on standing and sitting position.
- Occasional acidity with heaviness of abdomen.
- Frontal headache better lying down with head low.
- Heat on the vertex.
- Stoppage of left nose.
- Occasional throat pain. > gurgling.
- Breathing trouble. < Change of weather → since 3 years back. < inhaling dust, fumes & smoke. Brochospasm since the age of 14 years. Hereditory cause → Maternal side had these problems → <

change of weather. Catches cold easily → Sneezing+++ → running nose (watery)++, cough < night. Occasional whitish-yellowish phlegm expel out → heaviness feels in the chest → wheezing sound in chest → spasm < mid-night, > head bends backwards. H/O cold allergy - < dust, fumes, smoke, < when washing the face. Sneezing++, Running nose++, Tickling in throat. Spasm and cold allergy started after the fracture of her leg → N.B.W.S.

- Spasm < evening and 2 a.m. Susceptible to cold.
- Cough dry in day time.
- Sweat in the axilla region. Sweating → bad odour in sweat.
- Patient is constipated. Stool hard. Knotty.
- Menses – Time – regular. Pain in lower abdomen (1st days). Duration – 4 days. Colour- Red. Dysmenorrhoea (occasional pain during menses).
- Angry. Obstinate. Silent habit. Absent-minded. Desires for company. Disgusted with life for pain. Weeping mood. Consolation >. Wants to do everything slowly. Fear of noise, accidents, failures.
- Skin eruptions on right palm.
- Hot patient. Likes winter and open air.
- Food Preferences:- Sweet+, Sour++, Salty++, Fish++, Bitter++, Milk++, Vegetables++, Cold drinks++, Ice cream++, Meat+, Egg+.
- Sleep – Sound.
- Family Medical History – Skin diseases. Measles. Jaundice. Father and mother alive. Paternal side:- High Blood pressure, Piles, Asthma. Maternal side:- Asthma, Rheumatism.
- Dreams of various kinds.
- At the end of Oct'94 a little bit of pain started on her left foot and started ascending upwards upto her waist.
- At that time she had very feeble feeling on both the legs and could not walk properly and she had to walk with other's help. Thereafter the pain also started in her "Spinal Cord" and the upper portion of her body which made her bending forward from waist. That time giddiness also started. Allopathic doctor was consulted on 26th Oct'94. Investigations were done. But the matter of fact there was no improvement.
- She was taken to Dr. D. M. Choudhury with severe pain on 29th Oct'94 at his chamber for consultation.
- Dr. A. K. Basu was also consulted on 7th Nov'94 at his Nursing Home.
- The following day she was again taken to Dr. Choudhury. Both the

Surgeons were of the same opinion and she had to be admitted to the Nursing Home for traction and associated treatments for about 10 days. She felt a little better and was discharged from Nursing Home and was advised to be under traction at home for 40 days. Pain was still there and Dr. Choudhury advised her for CT scan. Before going for scanning I was taken to Dr. D. Mishra. He was not of the opinion of scaning and prescribed some medicine on 10th Jan'95. But overall no lasting improvement happened and then she was totally frustrated and brought to me for homoeopathic treatment.

Investigations Carried Out Before/After Dr. Banerjea's Treatment

31st Oct'94: X-Ray Lumbar spine:- Sacralisation of L5 with diminish of disc space.

14th Jan'95: Mantoux test:- Area of induration 8 x 8 mm.

11th Jan'95: Haemoglobin 12 gm%. White Blood Cell (W.B.C.) 8.600, Neutrophil 52 Lymphocyte 28 Monocyte 3 Eosinophyl 17.

14th Jan'95: Uric acid 4.3 mg%.

14th Jan'95: Later fixation test negative.

30th Apr'96: X-Ray Lumbar spine: Sacralisation. L5 with diminution of disc space between L5 S1. Sacro-iliac joint Normal.

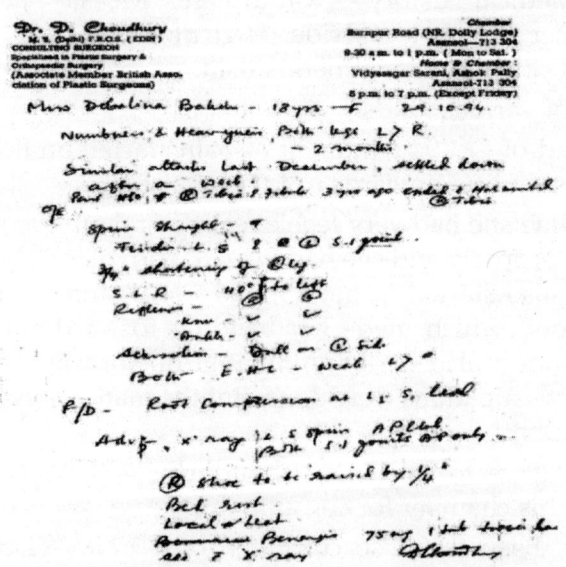

Allopathic prescription of Miss D. B. before treatment

Rheumatological Diseases - Cured Cases

X-Ray report before treatment

X-Ray report before treatment

Patient's comments 8 months after treatment

CASE ANALYSIS, MIASMATIC DIAGNOSIS AND FINAL PRESCRIPTION

Miasmatic Analysis

- Pain in the lower extremities: Sycotic.
- Pain on both legs: Sycotic.
- Sore, bruised and sensitive to touch: Psora.
- Aggravation of pain: new and full moon: Tubercular.
- Amelioration by rest and lying down: Psora.
- Pain along with numbness & heaviness: Psora.
- Lack of strength in both legs: Psora.
- Pain comes gradually after walking with short steps: Sycotic.
- Occasional acidity with heaviness of abdomen: Psora.
- Frontal headache better lying down: Psora.
- Breathing trouble. < Change of weather: Sycotic. < inhale dust, fumes & smoke: Tubercular.
- Cold allergy: Tubercular.

Final Prescription Made on the Basis of

- Pain in the lower extremities with heaviness and numbness. Pain on both legs (loin to ankle) → more in left leg previous, pain ascends upwards (ankle to loin). Ascending type.
- Commence from ankle and ascends upwards to the lip and then it settles in the lumbo-sacral region. Now back pain as well. Sore, bruised and sensitive to touch.
- Both legs are sore and tender (+++) to touch, as well.
- Patient have had fracture of shaft of the tibia & fibula: 3 months after pain started: NBWS (Never Been Well Since).
- Aggravation of pain: from walking, sitting, new and full moon. Aggravation from cold weather.
- Amelioration by rest and lying down.
- Pain along with numbness & heaviness < walking, < touch (+++); sitting. > lying, > hot application. Lack of strength in both legs. Pain comes gradually after walking with short steps.
- Occasional acidity with heaviness of abdomen.

- Frontal headache better lying down with head low.
- Breathing trouble. < Change of weather → since 3 years back. < inhale dust, fumes & smoke. Tubercular miasm which is covered by Arnica. H/O cold allergy - < dust, fumes, smoke, < when washing the face. Sneezing++, Running nose++, Tickling in throat.

Final Prescription and Remedy Reaction

- Patient's comment's after homoeopathic treatment: can be viwed in the CD & Web:
- Dr. Banerjea was first consulted on 11th Jan'95.
- Much improved felt and started walking slowly with others help after seven days.
- Then I started recovering steadily and the pain on my waist was also started reducing.
- I was able to walk slowly without any help and the upper portion of my body started to be on the normal position.
- At present I can cycle a lot and feel no difficulty.
- Now a days the incidences of Asthma and associated symptoms have been reduced.

Prescription Chart

Dates	Points in Favour of the Prescription	Prescribed Medicine
11th Jan'95		Arnica 200C: 1 dose; Arnica 1M: 1 dose
27th Jan'95	As a whole >>. Pain < from cold. Vertigo >. Acidity >.	PL15 (Sac Lac)
28th Feb'95	As a whole feeling better.	PL15
19th Apr'95	Occasional leg pain on standing long time. Dysmenorrhoea. As a whole 50% better.	PL15 (Sac Lac)
8th May'95	Doing better. Leg pain < walking. As a whole better.	PL15
13th Jun'95	Leg pain < long walking. As a whole feels standstill.	Arnica 1M: 1 dose. Arnica 10M: 1 dose
2nd Aug'95	Doing better.	PL15
26th sep'95	Doing much better. Reported as 100% improvement of pain. Patient likes to continue treatment later on for Asthma.	Cured

Authenticity of Cure

CD Reference: RH002-RHEUMATOID ARTHRITIS-DB

13

CHAPTER

Urological Diseases - Cured Cases

1. A CASE OF RENAL CALCULI: MR. R.C.

Case No. U001

Age : 65 years as on 7th August, 1992
Height : 5 ft. 6 inches.
Weight : 60 kgs.

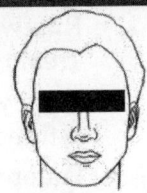

Photo of the patient, Mr. R.C.

Presenting Complaints

- Pain in loin region, shifting in nature, mostly in the right side, occasionally in the left side. Pain stays 1-2 minutes, 8-10 times in a day. Sometimes pain radiates to the right side of the testis, began 5 months ago. Pain better by hot application.
- Urine: Frequent urination ½ / 1 hr. intervals, urging to urinate. Occasional reddish sediment.
- Tumour on left hand → began 12 years back. Pain aggravates by pressure.
- Stool: Regular: Stool is not clear: muddy / yellow in colour, occasionally offensive odour, soft stool, white mucus in stool. Pin worms ++ in stool, itching in rectum both day & night.
- Reeling of head, aggravated from journey & excessive talking.
- Hardness of hearing in right ear, occasional violent itching.
- Appetite: Normal.
- Thirst: Normal.
- Hot patient.
- Sweat on back & chest: Bad odour to sweat.

- Heals ok.
- Sleep: disturbed.
- Dreams of various things.
- Hoarseness of voice, aggravated by loud talking.
- Desires: Sweet; vegetables & spinach (++); salt; bitter (++); curds; fish; warm food; cold drinks.
- Sun aggravates in general, makes him weak.
- Mind: Angry. Talkative. Absent minded. Desire for company. Fear of death. Involuntary sighing. Patient gets angry when reprimanded. Sympathetic. Cannot tolerate blood letting.
- Fear of darkness, snakes, thunderstorm++, accidents.
- Past History:- Kala-azar in childhood – Treated with allopathy. Ringworm – used ointment. Now OK. Dog bite at the age of 12 – Treatment: Ayurvedic.
- Family History:- Father died of pneumonia. Mother – Insanity; asthma, died of heart attack.
- Patient was treated by another homoeopath with Natrum Mur from 200 C to 10M for 6 months, no lasting improvement.

Investigations Carried Out Before/After Dr. Banerjea's Treatment

1st Jul'92:	X-ray KUB (Kidney, Ureter, Bladder): Radio Opaque Calculi (Right) Kidney. BSPP (Blood Sugar Post Prandial): 60. Urine: RBC (Red Blood Cells) 25 – 30 HPF (High Power Field)
3rd Feb'93:	Ultrasonography Kidney, Ureter, Bladder: No calculus.
20th Jul'93:	X-ray Kidney, Ureter, Bladder: No calculus on Kidney, Ureter, Bladder. Normal.

CASE ANALYSIS, MIASMATIC DIAGNOSIS AND FINAL PRESCRIPTION

Miasmatic Analysis

- Wandering pains – Sycosis.
- Pains better by hot application – Psora.
- Calculi, renal – Sycosis.
- Pain (in hand) aggravated by pressure – Tubercular.

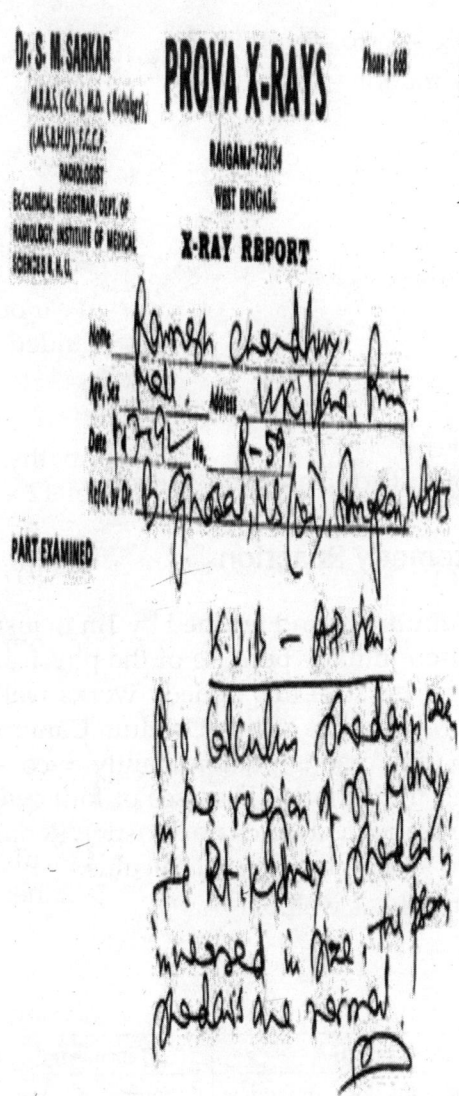

- Frequent micturation – Psora – sycosis,
- Reddish sediment in urine – Tubercular.
- Stool, yellowish – Sycosis.
- Pinworms – Tubercular.
- Aggravation from sun – Psora

- Sweat on back & chest, offensive – Syco – syphilitic.
- Reeling of head, aggravated by motion – Psora.
- Itching in ear – Psora.
- Absent minded – Sycosis
- Fear of death – Psora.
- Cannot tolerate blood letting – Psora.
- Angry when reprimanded – Sycosis.
- Desires warm food – Sycosis.
- Desires bitter – Psora.
- Desires cold drinks – Syphilis.
- Fear of thunderstorms - Psora

It's a mixed miasmatic case with Syco-Psoric preponderance.

Reasoning for Prescription and Remedy Reaction

The case was started with **Ocimum Canum 30c** and finished by 1m in just over a year. The 30c potency was chosen initially because of the physical nature of the presenting complaint and because this remedy works well for urinary problems in this potency. Miasmatics of this Ocimum Canum are: Psora ++, Sycosis +++, Syphilis +, this case is predominantly Syco – psoric. This remedy has the following indications:- Diseases of kidneys, bladder and urethra; Red sand in the urine (a chief characteristic); Renal colic, especially right side. Pronounced symptoms of renal calculus.

Ocimum Can covers the case miasmatically as well.

Prescription Chart

Date	Prescription Done on the Basis of	Treatment
7th Aug'92	Pain in loin region → mostly in the right side. Sometimes pain radiates to the right side of the testis. Pain better by hot application. Occasional reddish sediment.	Ocimum Canum, 30, in 2 doses, sipping each dose over 7 days.
27th Aug'92	No appreciable change.	Sac lac
19th Oct'92	Stand still	Ocimum Can., 30, in 2 doses
18th Dec'92	No appreciable change.	Ocimum Can. 200 in 2 doses.

Date	Prescription Done on the Basis of	Treatment
5th Feb'93	Much better. No stone showing on ultrasonography report.	Sac lac
7th Apr'93	Better. No pain.	Sac lac
11th Aug'93	Occasional pain in renal angle. Amoebiasis. Stool not clear. Felt like 200 C is not holding long enough.	Ocimum Can. 1M in 1 dose.
13th Dec'93	Stone cleared. Cured.	Cured.

Authenticity of Cure

CD Reference: U001-RENAL CALCULI-RC

2. A CASE OF RENAL CALCULI: MR. P.G.

Case No. U002

Age : 23 years as on 25/6/93
Weight : 60 kgs.

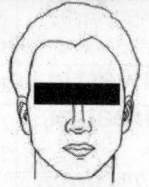

Photo of the patient, Mr. P.G.

Presenting Complaints

- Pain in the lower abdomen.
- Location: Onset of pain in left testis and goes upwards through left side and then goes medially to umbilicus – settles in the whole left side and upper abdomen.
- Sensation: Cramping, gripping pain.
- Duration: Suffering about 15 days.
- Concomitant: Nausea and vomiting during acute attack of pain.
- Onset: Onset gradual and goes gradually.
- Aggravation: After eating.
- Amelioration: By hard pressure and by bending double.
- Blurred vision.
- Duration: about 4 years.
- Burning sensation of the eyes, redness of the conjunctiva (both eyes).
- H/O: Swelling of the left lower gum (molar teeth).
- Relation to heat and cold: Chilly patient.
- Desires: Egg +++, sour++, salt++, vegetable, milk, cold food+++.
- Aversion: Sweet, meat, warm food.
- Thirst: Profuse. Takes a large quantity of water at a time.
- Sleep: Disturbed.
- Dream: Serpents, dead persons.
- Appetite: Average.
- Stool: Regular, but ineffectual urging to stool.
- Urine: Yellow colour, strong, offensive and burning sensation.
- Sweat: Perspiration on the forehead and back. Sour +++ smelling.
- Mental: Anger, irritable, absent minded. Desire for company, memory weak, weeping disposition, when reprimanded gets angrier, sympathetic, does everything very slowly ++ (takes his own time).

- Indolence. Likes to lie and watch TV.
- Fear of darkness, thunderstorm.

Investigations Carried Out Before/After Dr. Banerjea's Treatment

17th Jun'93: Urine culture : No growth. Urine :- Albumin – Occult Blood Test = +Ve. Red Blood Corpuscles – 6 – 8 hpf. Pus cell: Trace +.

17th Jun'93: Blood : Haemoglobin 16.3, White Blood Cell – 9000, Neutrophils$_{68}$ Lymphocytes$_{26}$ Monocyte$_{0.5}$ 5$_5$ Basophil$_0$ Red Blood Corpuscles – 5.3 X10^6

X-Ray Kidney - Ureter-Bladder of Mr. P.G. before treatment

X-Ray Kidney-Ureter-Bladder, 3 months after treatment

Blood Sugar Random:- 77 mg%.

19th Jun'93: X-ray KUB (Kidney, Ureter, Bladder) : Calculus in lower end of left ureter.

1st Sep'93: X-ray KUB (Kidney, Ureter, Bladder): No evidence of any Radio Opaque calculus in KUB (Kidney, Ureter, Bladder) areas an in the poserior urethra. Comparison with last skiagram of 19/6/93 shows that the oval density within the pelvic cavity is not present.

CASE ANALYSIS, MIASMATIC DIAGNOSIS AND FINAL PRESCRIPTION

Miasmatic Analysis

- Pain: abdomen: cramping: Sycosis.
- Onset gradually and goes gradually: Sycosis.
- Amelioration: By hard pressure: Sycosis.
- Nausea and vomiting: Psora.
- Blurred vision: Psora.
- Burning sensation in eyes: Psora –syphilitic.
- Eyes: Redness with sensation of heat – Tubercular.
- Thirst: Profuse: Sycosis.
- Desires cold food: Syco –tubercular, or syphilitic.
- Desires salt: Syco-tubercular.
- Aversion meat: Syco –syphilitic.
- Urine: Yellow colour: Sycosis.
- Offensive and burning sensation: Syphilis.
- Sweat: Perspiration on the forehead and back. Sour +++ smelling – Syco – psoric.
- Anger, irritable: Sycosis.
- Absent minded: Sycosis.
- Memory weak: Psora.
- Does everything very slowly: Psora.
- Indolence. Likes to lie and watch TV: Psora.
- Fear of darkness, thunderstorm: Psora.
- Dreams of dead bodies: Syphilis.

It's a mixed miasmatic case with Psora-sycotic preponderance.

Final Prescription and Remedy Reaction

This case was started with **Calcarea Carbonica** for the reasons outlined in the prescription chart below. The 30c potency was selected, as this is a good potency for urinary complaints. The case was cured with just one prescription of Calc. Carb in less than 2 months.

The miasmatic breakdown of Calc. Carb. is Psora +++L, Sycosis +++, Syphilis ++, Tubercular +++L and this covered the predominantly Psoric-sycotic nature of this case.

Calcarea Carb the case miasmatically as well.

Prescription Chart

Date	Prescription Done on the Basis of	Treatment
25th Jun'93	Pain in the lower abdomen; cramping, gripping pain. Amelioration: by hard pressure, and by bending double. Chilly patient. Desires: Egg +++, sour ++, salt ++, cold food +++. Aversions: meat, warm food. Sweat: Perspiration on the forehead and back. Sour +++ smelling. Mentals: Absent minded. Desire for company, memory weak, weeping disposition, sympathetic, does everything very slowly ++ (takes his own time). Indolence. Likes to lie and watch TV. Dreams of the dead. Fear of darkness, thunderstorm.	Calc Carb 30c, 2 doses, sipped in water.
12th Jul'93	Doing a little better	Sac lac.
3rd Sep'93	Stone came out.	Cured.

Authenticity of Cure

CD Reference: U002-RENAL CALCULI-PG

3. A CASE OF RENAL CALCULI : MR. S.P.M.

Case No. U003

Age : 32 years as on 21st August, 1987

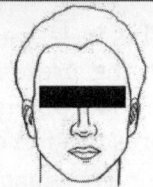

Photo of the patient,
Mr. S.P.M

Presenting Complaints

- Pain in chest due to carrying heavy weight on head, started 5 years ago. Pain aggravates during deep inspiration, heavy exertion and work.
- A sudden catch felt on the right side of abdomen during bathing 1 year ago, after that pain continued. Dribbling of urine with severe pain. Urine like thin thread sometimes accompanied with blood. Reddish sediment. Burning urination at that time. Urine – turbid, yellowish-red, with strong odour along with continuous pain in the right side of abdomen. Severe pain also felt in right waist.
- Violent cough for the last 25 days.
- Exposure to cold → cough started. Dry cough.
- Easily catches cold.
- Nasal coryza.
- Expectoration – scanty, thick yellowish mucus.
- Tingling sensation in throat.
- Aggravation in the evening and in the morning.
- Amelioration from profuse expectoration.
- Occasional pain in right lower abdomen, aggravates when stool is not clear.
- Dysenteric stool.
- Stool with white mucus.
- Frequent ineffectual urging.
- Loss of appetite.
- History of irregular eating habits.
- Allergic eruption throughout the body, aggravated from egg and aubergine.
- Chilly patient.
- Desires: Fish+++, egg+, sweet +++, pungent, bitter++, milk, vegetables, warm food ++.

- Aversions: Meat, sour.
- Aggravation from: Egg, aubergine.
- Thirstless.
- Sleep: sound sleep.
- Sweat: Profuse sweat throughout the body.
- Mind: Silent habit, mild. Low confidence and fears of failure, hesitation at the beginning, but can finish well. Fear of snakes, darkness.
- Past History: Typhoid, chickenpox.
- Family History: Father – piles, asthma.

Investigations Carried Out Before/After Dr. Banerjea's Treatment

21st Jan'87: Urine: Albumin – Faint Trace Crystals. Calcium – oxalate ++.

2nd Mar'87: X-ray KUB (Kidney, Ureter, Bladder): Radio opaque shadow in right side – possible calculus.

1st Dec'87: Pyelography – Nothing Abnormal Detected.

13th Aug'88: Ultra Sonography of KUB: Nothing Abnormal Detected.

12th Oct'88: Urine: Nothing Abnormal Detected.

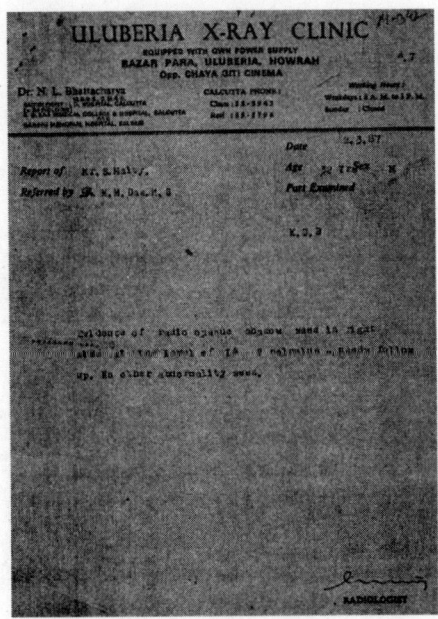

X-Ray report of Kidney-Ureter-Bladder of Mr. S.P.M., before treatment

DR. S. K. SHARMA
M.B., M.R.A.R., D.M.R.E. (HON)
MD (Radiology), F.R.C.A. (U.S.A.)
F.C.C.P. (USA), MEMBER, R.S.N.A. (U.S.A.)
Consultant Radiologist & Ultrasound Specialist

EKO X RAY
IMAGING & RESEARCH CENTRE
54, Jawaharlal Nehru Road
Calcutta-700 071

MR SANKARI PROSAD MAITY   34 yrs.   13-6-88

DR SUBRATA KUMAR BANERJEE

SONOGRAPHY OF K U B

KIDNEYS

Right kidney measures 9.1 cm.
Left kidney measures 9.2 cm.

Both kidneys are normal in size and shape. Renal parenchyma and central echo-complexes appear normal.

URINARY BLADDER

Urinary bladder is normal in size and shape. No residual urine noted in post voiding bladder.

DR S K SHARMA MD

Sonographic report, 12 months after treatment

D. Sircar
M.B.(Cal.) M.R.D., R.C.P. & R. (Engl), Hony. Professor of Radiology, Nilratan Sircar Medical College (formerly)

Sri Sankar Prasad Maity   (30)   1 Dec. 87.
   Dr. Subrata K. Banerjee, M.B.S., B.H.M.S (Hons).,
        F.A.H (Germany), FANM (Eng), MACH (USA).

Excretion pyelography

No urinary calculus, nor any abnormal calcified deposit present.

Shape, size, position & functional status of the kidneys, well within normal limits.

Intact pelvicalycine collecting system - no inflammatory fuzziness in the calyceal terminations.

Ureters average in calibre, course & peristalsis - no back pressure changes seen in them.

Bladder presents average capacity & smooth contour - small residual urine present in post-evac film.

Patient complaining of pain in the lower abdomen, more on the right side, with front to back radiation.

Normal osseous texture of the lumbar vertebrae - L.6 sacralised on the left side.

Normal pyelograms.

70, Ganesh Avenue, Calcutta-700 013 Phone: 27-1069, Res.: 44-5123

Pyelogram report, after treatment

CASE ANALYSIS, MIASMATIC DIAGNOSIS AND FINAL PRESCRIPTION

Miasmatic Analysis

- Pain in chest: aggravates during deep inspiration: Sycosis.
- Pain in right side of abdomen: Sycotic.
- Burning urination: Syphilis
- Sometimes accompanied with blood: Tubercular.
- Dry cough: Psora.
- Easily catches cold: Psora- tubercular.
- Nasal coryza: Sycosis.
- Expectoration: thick yellowish mucus: Sycosis.
- Amelioration from profuse expectoration: Un-natural discharge ameliorates: Sycosis.
- Dysenteric stool: Syphilis.
- Stool with mucus: Sycosis.
- Poor appetite: Psora.
- Aversion to meat: Syco – syphilitic.
- Desires sweet: Psora.
- Desires warm food: Sycosis.
- Allergic eruption: Tubercular.
- Sweat: Profuse: Sycosis.
- Mind: Silent habit: Psora.
- Low confidence: Psora.
- Fears of failure: Psora.

It's a mixed miasmatic case with Psora-sycotic preponderance.

Final Prescription and Remedy Reaction

Case was begun with **Lycopodium 200c** as this potency works well for urinary complaints. The case was finished with Lycopodium 1M within a year of treatment. The reasons for choosing this remedy are shown in the prescription chart below.

Lycopodium covers the case miasmatically as well.

Prescription Chart:

Date	Prescription Done on the Basis of	Treatment
21st Aug'87	Catch felt on the right side of abdomen. Reddish sediment. Burning urination along with continuous pain in the right side of abdomen. Severe pain also felt in right waist. Exposure to cold → cough started. Dry cough. Easily catches cold. Nasal coryza. Expectoration – scanty, thick yellowish mucus. Aggravation in the evening and in the morning. Occasional pain in right lower abdomen. Aggravation when stool is not clear. Frequent ineffectual urging. Loss of appetite. Chilly patient. Desires: Sweet +++, warm food ++. Mind: Silent habit, mild. Low confidence and fears of failure, hesitation at the beginning but can finish well. Fear of darkness. The miasmatics of Lycopodium are Psora +++L, Sycosis +++, Syphilis ++, Tubercular +++.	Lycopodium 200C, 2 doses, each dose sipped in water over 5 days.
10th Sep'87	No appreciable change.	Sac lac
12th Oct'87	Improved. As a whole feeling a little better.	Sac lac
11th Nov'87	Now stand still	Lycopodium 200C, 2 doses.
12th Dec'87	No appreciable change, but pyelography result is better.	Sac lac
12th Feb'88	Stand still status. Occasional pain in abdomen.	Lycopodium 1M, 1 dose (single dose as sensitive patient).
11th Apr'88	Wait & watch.	Sac lac
18th Jul'88	Doing a little better.	Sac lac
21st Aug'88	No pain. Repeat USG done. Cured.	Cured.

Authenticity of Cure

CD Reference: U003-RENAL CALCULI-SPM

4. A CASE OF RENAL CALCULI IN 48 YEARS OLD FEMALE

Case No. U004

Mrs. A.D.

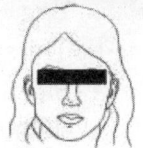

Photo of the patient, Mrs. A.D.

Presenting Complaints

- Renal Stone (left sided). Duration – 6 months. X-Ray shows – left ureteric stone, stagnant position. Off and on feels slight pain in lower abdomen.
- Muscular pain from waist to leg, feels at night.
- Acidity, < evening. Stool – loose generally.
- Catches cold easily. Dust allergy – produces sneezing.
- Hypertension, neck pain present.
- Headache < Sun heat, Sunlight disagrees. Pain, increases with excessive walking. Felt uneasy in pressure, jar, and noise.
- Head: Heat on vertex.
- Aphthae – in mouth, sometimes, but no specific season.
- Gum swollen – when catches cold.
- Palpitation - < during tension, especially when taken high dose medicine.
- Distention of abdomen, > by passing flatus.
- Appetite – decreased.
- Sweat – More than normal – no odour.
- Urine – Normal.
- Stool:- Bad odour, diarrhoea, regular.
- Sometimes joint pain in right arm.
- Lumbago, < after exertion.
- Menstrual cycle stopped at the age of 35 years. Menstruation first stated 15 years of age.
- Mental:- Mild. Desires to be neat and clean, desire for company. Fear of death. Memory active, weeping mood. Intensely sympathetic, cannot tolerate blood letting.
- Fear of ghost, darkness, and incurable diseases.
- Past History of Typhoid, Malaria, Falling injury 3 times – Cesarean section was done.
- First cause of break down of health – after the attacking Malignant Malaria.

- Chilly patient, likes open air. Easily catches cold.
- Desire:- Sweet++, Sour++, Pungent and Hot, Salty+, Bitter, Chicken, Egg ++, Warm food. Aversion to Vegetables.
- Thirst – Normal.
- Sleep – Disturbed – after 1.30 A.M. – Sleep is deeper. Married – 3 daughters.

Investigations Carried Out Before/After Dr. Banerjea's Treatment

28th Jun'00: Ultra Sonography (USG) – Kidney, Ureter, Bladder:- Solitary Calculus in Urinary Bladder.

Sonography report of Mrs. A. D. during treatment

Sonography report of Mrs. A. D., 5 months after treatment

7th Nov'00: X-Ray – KUB (Kidney, Ureter, Bladder):- Nothing Abnormal detected urinary bladder shows no calculus or growth.

CASE ANALYSIS, MIASMATIC DIAGNOSIS AND FINAL PRESCRIPTION

Miasmatic Analysis

- Renal Stone: Sycotic.
- Muscular pain (recurrent): < night: Syphilio-Tubercular.
- Acidity, distention of abdomen: Psora.
- Easily catches cold (ECC): Likes open air: Tubercular.
- Dust allergy: Tubercular.
- Hypertension: Sycotic.
- Apthae, bleeding gums: Syphilio-Tubercular.
- Palpitation: Tubercular.
- Decreased appetite: Psora.
- Sweat++: Sycotic.
- Stool-Diarrhoea: Sycotic.
- Joint Pain: Sycotic.
- Mentals: (a) Mild: Psora. Weeping mood: Psora-Sycotic. (b) Fears-Death, ghosts, darkness: Psora.
- Cannot tolerate blood letting: Psora.
- Desires-Sweet, sour-Psora. Pungent-hot-Syco-Tubercular. Warm food: Sycotic. Aversion vegetables: Sycotic.

It's a mixed miasmatic case with Syco-psoric preponderance.

Final Prescription Made on the Basis of

- Renal Stone: Sycotic.
- Occassional pain in knee joint (more left side). Muscular pain-waist to leg < night.
- Acidity aggravation evening.
- Occassional constipation.
- Appetite – Less.
- Desire-Sweet, Sour, spicy, egg ++. Aversion-vegetables.
- Takes cold easily: Chilly+.
- Perspiration++

- Mental Symptoms: (a) Mild, weeping mood. (b) Fears: Death, ghosts, darkness, incurable diseases. (c) Intensely sympathetic.
- Chilly patient, likes open air.
- Dust Allergy.
- Palpitation.
- Sleep disturbed.

The miasmatic analysis of Calc Carb is: Psora +++L, Sycosis +++, Syphilis ++, Tubercular +++L.

Calcarea Carb covers the case miasmatically as well.

Final Prescription

Calcarea carb.

Remedy Reaction

The medicine (Calc carb) was chosen on the basis of its multi-miasmatic preponderance including sycosis. Also it covers the totality, as stated above

Prescription Chart

Date	Prescription Done on the Basis of	Treatment
30th Jun'00		Calc- Carb 200C, 2 doses.
22nd Aug'00	Standstill. Pain in the lower abdomen persists. Blood pressure 170/90. Wait and watch.	Sac-lac.
24th Sep'00	BP- 190/98. 50 kgs+. Pain is less in the lower abdomen and also less pain after urination. Pain in left leg < after long walking. Stool – not clear, 2 times a day. Gas during stool.	Calc. Carb., 200C, 2 doses.
18th Oct'00	No appreciable change.	Calc-carb 1M, 1 dose.
6th Nov'00	Patient feeling much better. Asked the patient to repeat an x-ray.	
7th Nov'00	X-Ray – KUB:- Nothing Abnormal detected urinary bladder shows no calculus or growth.	

Authenticity of Cure

CD Reference: U004-RENAL CALCULI-AD

5. A CASE OF RENAL CALCULI AND HYDRONEPHROTIC KIDNEY : MR. G.D.

Case No. U005

Age 20+.

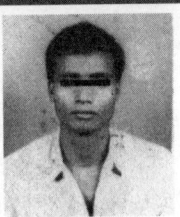

Photo of the patient
Mr. G. D.

Presenting Complaints

- Pain in the left side of back, severe cutting pain, felt like someone cutting with a knife. Pain started about 12 months ago; he has occasionally taken painkillers, but has had no proper treatment.
- Pain aggravates from rest, though he feels tired he has to move, which gives some relief. Occasionally he draws up the left leg towards the abdomen, which affords some relief. Rubbing his back ameliorates.
- Urine scanty, painful, takes a long time to complete. Burning pain during urination. Pain continues after passing water.
- Frequent urination.
- Feels tired +++ easily. Can't work long hours, feels weak.
- Loss of appetite. Anorexia.
- Constipation.
- Occasional headache, especially left side, cutting sensation there as well.
- Sleep: disturbed.
- Mind: Tendency to suppress feelings. Keeps himself to himself. Introvert. Strong views about religion and non-flexible. Rigid.
- Neat & tidy ++.
- Dwells on sexual thoughts. Hyper-sexuality.
- Desires: Salty ++, salt ++, cold food.
- Aversion: Vegetables.
- Does not like humid rainy weather at all. Hates rainy season, loves summer. Chilly ++.
- Family history: Father : Asthma. Mother: Rheumatism.
- Thirst: Average.
- Sweat: Profuse (++)

Investigations Carried Out Before/After Dr. Banerjea's Treatment

1st Nov'95: Urine: Albumin – Trace. Specific gravity: 1015. Red Blood Corpuscles – 1 hpf. Pus cell – 3-5 hpf

3rd Nov'95: Ultra sonography: Kidney, Ureter, Bladder: Hydronephritic left kidney. Left ureteric stone

6th Nov'95: Urea - 29mg%. Creatinine – 0.95 mg%

16th Nov'95: X-ray Kidney, Ureter, Bladder (Intra Venous Urogram). Remark:- Left ureterolithiasis with left sided hydronephrosis and left upper hydroureter.

15th Jan'97: Straight X-ray Kidney, Ureter, Bladder: Remark:- No radio opaque stone or abnormal calcification noted in either renal areas or ureteric region & urinary bladder area.

Everything has cleared.

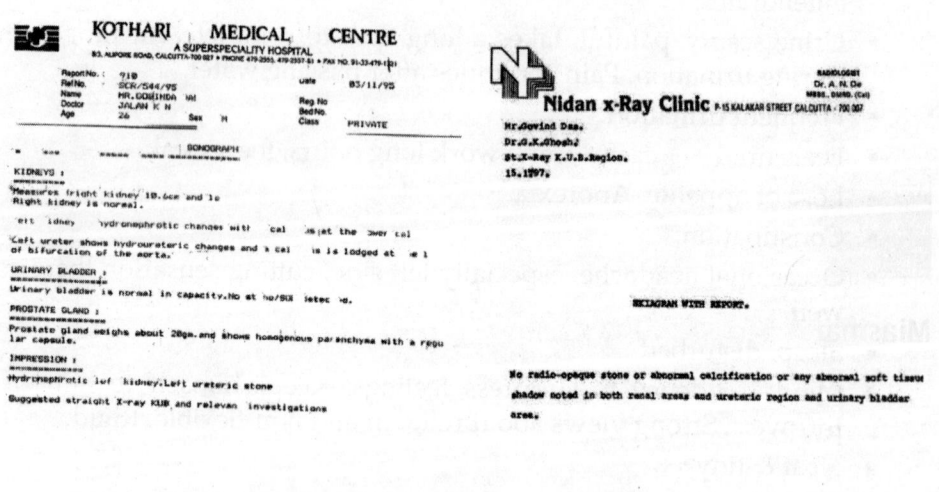

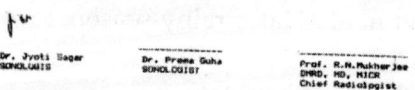
USG report of Mr. G.D. before treatment

X-Ray (K.U.B) report; 12 months after treatment

Rheumatological Diseases - Cured Cases

Final Note

(A) Before treatment by Dr. Banerjee

1. Vomiting & Pain abdomen Left side, for one year.
2. Burning pain during micturition for one year.
3. Less urination but long time to complete urination.
4. Frequent urination and pain in the penis during micturition.
5. Constipation.
6. Anorexia.
7. Weakness and on doing work.
8. Waist pain.

Above symptoms were persisting for one year.

(B) After treatment By Dr. Banerjee from 23-12-95.

1. Clear urination and no difficulty in urination.
2. No constipation.
3. No Anorexia.
4. Expulsion of stone per penis two pieces size about ground nut, one by surgical procedure and one spontaneously with urine.
5. No burning pain during micturition.
6. No weakness.
7. Left-side waist pain persisting.

Gobinda Das.

Patient's comments after treatment

CASE ANALYSIS, MIASMATIC DIAGNOSIS AND FINAL PRESCRIPTION

Miasmatic Analysis

- Pain: severe cutting pain: Sycotic.
- Pain: though feels tired has to move: Physically restless: Sycotic.
- Aggravation from rest: Sycotic.
- Draws up the left leg towards the abdomen, which affords some relief: Sycosis.
- Feels tired +++ easily: Psora.
- Urine scanty: Psora.
- Loss of appetite: Psora.
- Mind: Tendency to suppress feelings: Sycosis.
- Introvert: Sycosis.
- Neat & tidy ++: Sycosis.

- Hyper-sexuality: Sycosis.
- Desires cold food : Syco – tubercular.
- Aversion- Vegetables: Hydrogenoid: Sycosis.
- Hates rainy season: Sycosis.
- Family history: Father: Asthma. Mother: Rheumatism: Sycosis.
- It's a mixed miasmatic case with Syco-psoric preponderance.

Prescription Made on the Basis of

- Pain in the left side, like cutting with a knife.
- Pain aggravates from rest, though feels tired has to move, which gives some relief.
- Occasionally draws up the left leg towards the abdomen, which affords some relief. Rubbing back ameliorates.
- Burning pain during urination and continues after passing water.
- Feels tired +++ easily.
- Occasional headache, especially left side, cutting sensation there as well.
- Sleep: disturbed.
- Mind: Tendency to suppress feelings. Keeps himself to himself. Introvert. Strong views about religion and is non-flexible. Rigid.
- Neat & tidy ++.
- Dwells on sexual thoughts. Hyper-sexuality.
- Desire: Salty ++, salt ++, cold food.
- Aversion: Vegetables.
- Does not like humid rainy weather at all. Hates rainy season; loves summer. Chilly ++.
- Family history: Father: Asthma. Mother: Rheumatism.

The miasmatic breakdown of Thuja is Psora ++, Sycosis +++, Syphilis ++, Tubercular ++. This case was predominantly sycotic and was therefore covered well by this remedy.

Thuja covers the case miasmatically as well.

Final Prescription and Remedy Reaction

A detailed prescription chart is not available for this patient but I can provide details as follow:

I started the case with **Thuja 30 C** on 23rd December 1995 and the patient started improving right from the beginning; pain was much improved. The

30c potency was chosen for caution because of the pathological changes already present. I finished the case with Thuja 10M in just over a year. Expulsion of the stone occurred in two pieces via the penis: one via surgical procedure and the other spontaneously with urine. All other symptoms were cured, except the left sided pain which still persisted.

Authenticity of Cure

CD Reference: U005-RENAL STONE-GD

6. A CASE OF RENAL CALCULI IN 41 YEAR OLD MALE: MR. D.P.M.

Case No. U006

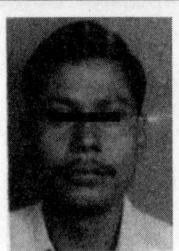

Photo of the patient, Mr. D. P. M.

Presenting Complaints

- Severe pain in lower abdomen and waist (more towards right). Pain++ from sitting to upright posture. Pain more towards the end of urination. Occasional burning on micturition. Only once blood comes through urination. Firstly pain occurred in abdomen with vomiting. Pain < jar, motion, damp weather, better by hot application.
- Pain neck and forehead < reading, exertion, damp weather, night, lack of sleep and thinking. Pain in sole and leg every day → Sleep disturbed. This burning started from childhood – at present it aggravates too much. Feels better by massage. Pain felt more in the bones.
- Feels weakness all the time.
- Acidity++. Heaviness of abdomen < evening.
- Mucous stool. Stool – not clear – uneasiness felt in the lower abdomen.
- Head:- Perspiration on forehead and back. Vertigo.
- Mouth:- Aphtha occurs in winter. Foetor oris. No salivation.
- Occasional palpitation, increases during heavy work, too much thinking, night watching.
- Abdomen:- Wind formation, whole abdomen and eructation – better by passing flatus. Pain in abdomen < empty stomach. Abdominal pain occasionally associated with backache.
- Pain lower abdomen. Felt pain constant right side of lower abdomen.
- Appetite – Poor. Heaviness of abdomen after little food, sour eructation.

Rheumatological Diseases - Cured Cases

- Profuse sweating on face, forehead and head.
- No odour.
- Urine:- Less, occasional white sediment, 8 – 10 times in a day. With odour like acid. Occasional burning. At present blood comes with urine. Occasional dribbling of urination at end with sharp pain in the urethra.
- Stool:- Constipated. White mucus.
- White discolouration all over the body → Swelling, < Sun heat, itching and burnng.
- < Summer, better by cold application.
- Tumour on right wrist joint, pain occurs in winter.
- Thirst Average.
- Delayed healing.
- Catches cold easily.
- Sleep – good, dreams – nothing.
- Thermal: Chilly patient.
- Food desire:- Sweet+++, Pungent, Salty, Veg & Spinach, Meat++, Spicy+, Luke warm food. Cold drinks. Aversion to Sour, Bitter.
- History of Scabies – Applied ointment.
- Mental:- Angry, fault finding; obstinate, silent habit, absent minded, desire for company, involuntary sighing. He gets more angry when critiscised, consolation aggravates. Fear of Snakes, incurable diseases.

Investigations Carried Out Before/After Dr. Banerjea's Treatment

2nd Mar'95: Ultrasonography whole abdomen – Nephrolithiasis right Kidney.

23rd May'01: X-Ray KUB (Kidney, Ureter, Bladder) – No radio opaque calculus in KUB (Kidney, Ureter, Bladder) region.

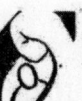

ULTRA SCAN, ENDOSCOPY AND X-RAY CLINIC
A DIAGNOSTIC UNIT OF
Dr. DAS's NURSING HOME
NEW TOWN, P.O. DIAMOND HARBOUR, 24 PARGANAS (S).
PIN CODE NO. 743 331, PHONE : 260 STD 63174

OPEN DAY & NIGHT

Name : DURGA PADA MANDAL   Age : 41
Referred by : DR. N. BHAR M.S   Sex : M
Parts Examined : UPPER ABDOMEN   Date : 2.3.95

REPORT OF ULTRA SONOGRAPHY

LIVER----The echogenicity of hepaticparenchymal tissue is normal. Intrahepatic bile channels are not dilated.
GALL BLADDER--It is shrunken as the patient has taken food. The wall is smooth. No calculus is seen in the lumen.
PANCREAS--The size and echogenicity are normal. No dilatation of CBD.
SPLEEN --The size and echogenicity are normal.
KIDNEY--Early hydronephrotic and hyfroureteric change is seen in the right Kidney. The left Kidney is normal.
IMPRESSION---Investigations are suggested to exclude any Nephrolithiasis in the RightKidney.

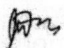

NOT VALID FOR MEDICOLEGAL PURPOSES

USG report of Mr. D. P. M. before treatment

Calcutta Medical Centre Ltd.
12, Loudon Street, Calcutta-700 017, Ph. : 240-1333/1337/2053

DEPARTMENT OF RADIOLOGY & IMAGING

CENTRAL CALCUTTA BRANCH
124/1, S. S. Ganguly Street, Calcutta-700 012, Phone : 227-7446

Name .... Durga Pada Mondal .... Age ... 47Y Sex .. M
Referred by .... Dr. S.K. Marjee .... Date .. 21.7.2001
Shielogram / Ultrasound of .... K.U.B.

REPORT

No radio - opaque calculus in KUB region.

Dr. A. N. Dey
Consultant Radiologist

Dr. S. Mondal
Consultant Sonologist

X-Ray (K.U.B.) of Mr. D. P. M. 23 months after treatment

CASE ANALYSIS, MIASMATIC DIAGNOSIS AND FINAL PRESCRIPTION

Miasmatic Analysis

- Renal stone: Sycotic.
- Severe pain in lower abdomen and waist, constant right side: Sycotic.
- Abdominal aggravated by damp weather: Sycotic.
- Burning micturition: Syphilitic.
- Pain felt more in the bones, aggravation: night: Syphilitic.
- Urine-white sediment: Sycotic.
- Dribbling of urination: Psora-Sycotic.
- Blood in urine: Tubercular. Acidic odour: Psora.
- Constipation: Psora. Mucous in stool: Sycotic.
- Abdomen- Heaviness: Sycotic. Acidity, gas, sour eructation: Psora.
- Skin-Profuse sweating: Sycotic.
- White discolouration all over body: Syphilitic.
- Itching and burning > by cold application: Syphilitic.
- Delayed healing: Syphilitic.
- Tumour on wrist: Sycotic.
- Desires: Sweet- Psora. Meat: Tubercular. Warm food: Sycotic. Cold drinks: Syphilitic.
- Mind-Angry: Psora-Sycotic. Obstinate: Tubercular. Absent minded: Sycotic. Mild-silent habit, desire company: Psora-Sycotic.
- Fears-Snakes, Incurable diseases: Psora.

It's a mixed miasmatic case with Syco-psoric preponderance.

Final Prescription Made on the Basis of

- Severe Pain in lower abdomen, more in the right side.
- Pain more towards the end of urination, aggravation:-damp weather.
- White sediment.
- Scanty Urine, blood in urine, burning, dribbling of urine towards the end.
- Pain felt in the bone aggravation:- night.
- Backache associated with abdominal pain.
- Profuse Sweat.

- Warm food, Sweet+++, Cold drinks, Appetite poor.
- Absent minded, Angry when critiscised, Obstinate.
- Acidity, gas, sour eructation.
- Delayed healing.
- Chilly patient.

The miasmatic analysis of Sarsaparilla is Psora ++, Sycosis +++, Syphilis++, Tubercular +

Sarsaparilla covers the case miasmatically as well.

Final Prescription

On the basis of the Sycotic preponderance and the totality, Sarsaparilla 30C was prescribed.

Prescription Chart

The patient came to see me in June 1999, with four years of suffering with off and on pain from kidney stone. I started the case with Sarsaparilla 30C and approximately within two years, patient got completely better.

23rd May, 2001:- X-Ray KUB – No radio opaque. Calculus in KUB region.

Authenticity of Cure

CD Reference: U006-RENAL CALCULI-DPM

7. A CASE OF RENAL CALCULI: MR. J.H.

Case No. U007

Age : 30 years old as on 3rd December, 2003
Sex : Male

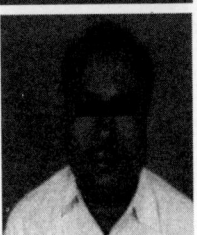

Photo of the patient
Mr.J.H.

Presenting Complaints

- Pain in lower abdomen (occasional), duration – 2 years, in this period – 4 attacks. Sonography report:- Left renal Calculus. Pain in left lower abdomen, pain better by bending double. Pain stitching in character, sometimes better by hard pressure.
- K.U.B. – X-ray – N.A.D.
- Catches cold easily. Breathing trouble due to severe cold infection.
- Occasional gas & acidity → occasional heart burn. Occasional pain in abdomen due to gas. Takes antacid regularly after attack of pain in abdomen.
- Occasional headache – during cold infection.
- Headache, aggravated by sunlight. Headache ends with blurred vision.
- Pain in lower abdomen.
- Winter < cough.
- Cold + Cough + Sinus. Sinus pain.
- Head:- Perspiration.
- Nose:- Blocked, both nostrils. Discharge from nose. Irritation, burning in the nose due to cold infection.
- Mucus in throat.
- Chest/Respiration:- Dry or moist cough. Aggravates in change of weather. Occasional breathing trouble. Thick expectoration.
- Stomach:- Appetite – Normal. Occasional burning.
- Abdomen:- Occasional distension. Passing flatus gives no relief to the discomfort.
- Bowels:- Stool clear, 3/4 times. Tendency towards Diarrhoea.

- Perspiration:- More on the upper part of the body.
- Appearance of Nails:- Thick. Ribbed..
- Skin:- Heals ok.
- Temperament:- Angry++; Introvert+; Irritable++; Positive+; Talkative+.
- Thermal Reaction:- Chilly patient.
- Food preference:- Salty+++; Warm food; Sweet+; Bitter++; Savoury++; Meat++; Fish++; Chicken+; Egg+; Green leafy+++; Spice+.
- Thirst Details:- Hot drinks. Long drinks at long interval. Medium thirst.
- Sleep:- Normal.
- Bleed easily. Heals quickly. Occasional aches and pains in the body or joints.
- Addiction:- Tobacco.
- Minimal prostatomegally. Urine – was frequent now cured.
- Catches cold easily. Cold allergy. Duration – 1 year. Causation – Nose block at night. Cold allergy. Allergic Rhinitis.
- Cold infection → breathing trouble → palpitation.
- Early ejaculation during coition. Duration – 4 years.
- Stool – Regular.
- Sleep – Sound.
- Sweat – More on whole body, on scalp.

Investigations Carried Out Before/After Dr. Banerjea's Treatment

16th Jun'03: Ultra Sonography (USG) KUB (Kidney, Ureter, Bladder) + Prostate:- Left Renal Calculus. Dilated pelvicalyecal system in right kidney – is due to passage of calculus.

9th Nov'05: Ultra Sonography (USG) – KUB (Kidney, Ureter, Bladder):- No calculus little prostate calcification.

29th Apr'09: Ultra Sonography (USG) whole abdomen:- Minimal hepatomegaly. Mild Prostatomegaly? Cystitis.

Rheumatological Diseases - Cured Cases

U.S.G report of Mr. J.H. before treatment

U.S.G report of Mr. J.H. 22 months after treatment

H-523.

Before Treatment
1. Gas Ulcer
2. KUB Stone.
3. Asma CORP.
4. Cold Nasal.
5. Pain Massal.

After Treatment
1. Nessorany Nasal cold-close
2. Something Ulcer
3. Physical Maintain.
4. Sexual weakens

Name - Zakir Hossain khan.

Comment of patient Mr. J.H.

CASE ANALYSIS, MIASMATIC DIAGNOSIS AND FINAL PRESCRIPTION

Miasmatic Analysis

- Pain in lower abdomen, Left renal Calculus: Sycosis.
- Pain in left lower abdomen, pain better by bending double. Pain stitching in character, sometimes better by hard pressure: Sycosis.
- Occasional headache – during cold infection: Psora.
- Headache, aggravated by sun light: Psora.
- Headache ends with blurred vision: Sycosis.
- Perspiration:- More: Sycosis.
- Appearance of Nails:- Thick. Ribbed: Sycosis.
- Temperament:- Angry++: Sycosis.
- Introvert+: Psora-Syphilis.
- Talkative+: Sycosis.

Final Prescription Made on the Basis of

- Pain in lower abdomen (occasional), duration – 2 years, in this period – 4 attacks. Sonography report:- Left renal Calculus. Pain in left lower abdomen, pain better by bending double. Pain stitching in character, sometimes better by hard pressure.
- Catches cold easily. Cold allergy. Allergic Rhinitis.
- Occasional headache – during cold infection.
- Headache, aggravated by sunlight. Headache ends with blurred vision.
- Perspiration:- More on the upper part of the body.
- Appearance of Nails:- Thick. Ribbed.
- Temperament:- Angry++; Introvert+; Irritable++; Positive+; Talkative+.
- Thermal Reaction:- Chilly patient.
- Food preference:- Salty+++; Warm food; Sweet+; Bitter++; Savoury++; Meat++; Fish++; Chicken+; Egg+; Green leafy+++; Spice+.

The miasmatic breakdown of Natrum mur is Psora+++, Sycosis+++, Syphilitic++, Tubercular++.

Final Prescription and Remedy Reaction
NATRUM MURIATICUM 200C

Prescription Chart

I started the case with Natrum Muriaticum 200C and gradually went up to 10M potency. Patient improved with Natrum Muriaticum and the follow-up ultrasonography report revealed the calculus has disappeared. Glory goes to Hahnemann and his wonderful Art and Science of Homoeopathy.

Authenticity of Cure:

CD Reference: U007-RENAL CALCULI-JH

SHORT CASE STORIES

(1) Acidity - Phosphoric Acid A middle aged man had flu for seven weeks and two months after this, he gradually developed apathy and acidity. After several more months he lost interest in life and the acidity was almost unbearable. His GP thought he lost the interest in life because of the acidity and then developed the apathy. Despite taking ample antacids and having an endoscopy which was negative he still had a tremendous discomfort. He was getting more and more depressed and apathetic. There is a line in Boericke's Materia Medica, "Whenever the system has been exposed to the ravages of acute disease, excesses, grief, loss of vital fluids, we obtain conditions calling for it. Pyrosis, flatulence, diarrhea, diabetes, rachitis and periosteal inflammation". As a consequence of these aetiologies, Phosphoric acid suffers from six types of debility

- Mental apathy, indifference, memory weakness
- Gastric acidity, pyrosis, flatulence
- Sexual weakness, lack of erection
- Profuse and frequent urination
- Cardiac weakness, irregular pulse with palpitation
- Ophthalmological, photophobia

Phosphoric acid in potency 30C followed by 200C restored the case dramatically.

I prescribe two potencies

- when I am prescribing on the basis of aetiology or NBWS
- when I am prescribing a medicine as prophylaxis
- when a patient was improving nicely with a polychrest and there was a sudden cessation of improvement, I drop two potencies and prescribe two potencies e.g., patient was improving nicely with Lycopodium and you went up to 10M potency and then there was a sudden cessation of improvement; so you drop two potencies from 10 M i.e., 10M → 1M → you give 200C and followed by 1M. Generally I will give these two potencies in the following way: One single poppy-seed sized globule of the medicine, dispensed in some sugar of milk in a sachet which is dissolved in a bottle of water, then shaken and sipped for 3 to 5 days. Then a gap of 7 days and thereafter the next potency in the same way.

(2) **Acne - Asterias Rubens** Recurrent pimples since age thirteen years were making this young adult very miserable. I tried Pulsatilla and then Berberis Aquifolium thinking this was the correct similimum, however there was no appreciable change. The patient was plump in appearance and the pimples were more on the left side of the face. I finally prescribed Asterias 200 considering disposition to pimples at adolescence, plump, flabby appearance with a left sided preponderance. All the pimples got better within one year. I finished with Thuja as this follows Asterias well.

(3) **cne - Bovista** Constant and recurrent pimples for three years drove this twenty four year old woman to my consulting room. She had been to many other doctors who has given different medicines, but there was no appreciable change. The patient had a rigid complex about her dark skin and was in a habit of using lots of cosmetics. She also mentioned that she do not like any tight fitting clothes and cannot wear polo-neck jumpers and even undoes the top button of her jeans. I prescribed her Bovista 30C considering acne from use of cosmetics and unable to bear tight clothing. Bovista cleared up her skin very quickly.

(4) **Acute Bronchitis - Bacillinum** This is a story of an eighteen years old boy who was suffering from recurrent attacks of acute bronchitis associated with suffocative cough, hot feeling and night sweats. The patient also has some wheeze which always aggravates from strong odours such as perfume and paint which is a tubercular manifestation. Bacilinum restored the case and stopped the recurrence.

(5) **Agalactia - Asafoetida-** A young woman with her first child, had poor milk production and the baby was crying a lot which made the mother extremely anxious. Whenever the baby was sucking the breast, there was extreme soreness of the nipple. Since delivery, the woman developed lot of gas and distension with loud belching. I prescribed Asafoetida 200 and one single dose allowed the mother to successfully breast feed. The clue of the prescription was agalactia with sensitiveness, hysterical belching with loud eructation.

(6) **Allergic Asthma - Pothos Foetidus** This is a case of my uncle, who was treating a rich industrialist suffering from asthma precipitated by a dust allergy. My uncle was treating him for eight months without appreciable change. Finally he decided to bring his Guru, Tarak Palit, a physician, who had never been to any medical institution but had a prolific control over his Materia Medica. At that time Tarak Palit was old and did not see many patients any more, but on my uncle's insistence, he went to see this industrialist at home. They arrived at a marble house where the patient was on

the fourth floor and Tarak Palit climbed up to the 1st floor and sat on the staircase, refusing to go any further! This did not look good in such house, that the 'super-consultant' was sitting on the stair case with his dhoti (a traditional Indian wrap), instead of trousers and ragged shirt. He said, "I am not going to climb up to the top floor, where the patient is." He read the case notes sitting in the stair case and said, "bring your patient down here and I will make him fit to climb upstairs within a week." He was so confident, that even is such circumstances, my uncle requested the patient to come down and Palit prescribed Pothos on the basis of asthma excited by dust, even if someone dusted the blanket in the next room, he was affected. Asthma is better by sitting in the toilet and even passing flatus, which he interpreted as better by passing stool. Pothos 30 made the patient fit within seven days. This is the confidence of a great master and Homoeopathy can work so well when there is such clinical acumen!

(7) **Amyotrophic Lateral Sclerosis (ALS) - Cyclamen** A Professor of Economics visited my Harley Street clinic in Central London suffering from ALS. He was in a wheel chair with emaciation and spasms of muscles especially of the lower extremities. I went through the case taking as detailed by the patient. After reading 75% of the case, I was coming to the conclusion that it was a Lycopodium case. At that stage, there was a question in my case taking form/book, "What is saddest incident in your life?" He wrote in the form, "when Jasper died". Obviously I asked, "Who is Jasper?" As soon as I asked this question, he started crying loudly, which I was not expecting from a Professor in his late fifties.

So I said that I am sorry to raise this question but I have to be clear. He said "Jasper is our German Shepherd dog and about four years ago he was ill. My daughter is a vet and she took the dog away from us and looked after him and made him better and brought him back to us few days before Christmas. She told us, "Mum and Dad, Jasper has a clean bill of health, look after him". On Christmas Eve, I was going through the examination papers of the University and at that time my wife told me she was going for some last minute's shopping for Christmas lunch, she informed me that Jasper was in the garden and would I please take him for a walk. After an hour or so, I suddenly remembered what my wife said and absent mindedly opened the garage door. Jasper came from the garden through to the garage and as soon as I opened the door, he saw a fox in the drive way and chased it. Unfortunately, he ran to the main road and was run over by a truck and was killed instantly.'

I clarified that the weakness of the lower extremity was the first symptom and started six months after the above incident. Rather than me interpreting his reaction to the situation incorrectly, I clarified his response in the following way. I offered him eight different possible responses:

- Anger, suppressed
- Grief
- Bad News, tragedies
- Mortification, reserved displeasure
- Guilt
- Duty not done
- Terrors of conscience
- Anger to indignation;
- Anger to disappointment;
- Love to disappointment;

He said that he felt it was duty not done, a bite of conscience, as his daughter said, "Jasper has a clean bill of health; look after him". I prescribed on duty not done, guilt, bite of conscience and gave Cyclamen 30 followed by 200 and the case has improved about 25% to 30% as you know in a Motor Neurone Disease like ALS the prognosis is restricted. The patient is still with me and I am maintaining a standstill status which I believe is a great achievement.

(8) **Anaemia - Cyclamen** Undefined weakness with anaemia and headache which is better in warm room, worse in open air, was the complaint of a woman in her mid twenties who had been suffering for the last three years, since her mother died. She had been to other Homoeopaths who have given grief medicines, e.g., Causticum, Natrum Mur, and Phosphoric Acid. I always give a patient hearing about the chronological development of symptoms, which Kent refers to as anamnesis, which is a bridge linking the present complaint with that of the past history and the family history. The patient said, she was the only daughter of her mother. She lost her Dad when she was two years old. Mum brought her up with extreme hardship. She got married three years back and went for a honeymoon for two weeks. On the third day of the honeymoon, she received a phone call that her mother was not well. She ignored this and stayed on her honeymoon. On the fifth day she was informed that her Mum was in hospital, she made a decision to return from her honeymoon on the tenth day. On the eighth day, her mother

died. I asked the patient whether it was the grief and bereavement or something else. I gave time to the patient and asked her to reflect to the situation. The patient said that she felt that she has not done her duty as her Mum was so caring for her and in her last moments, she could not be at her bed side. I interpreted this as guilt, duty not done and prescribed Cyclamen 30 followed by 200 and the patient reported cured within six months.

(9) **Angina - Naja** This is a case of angina with palpitation in a middle aged man in his fifties. The patient also had tremendous perspiration in his palm which almost preventing him from writing. During the consultation, it was typical English weather and was raining outside. The patient revealed he has tremendous aggravation of his angina pain from rain which I excluded whether damp aggravation or not and the patient almost has a fear of rain. This gave me the clue and I prescribed Naja 30 which also covers perspiration+++ in palms. (Ref. Clarke).

(10) **Anorexia after 'Flu - Natrum Ars** I have prescribed Natrum Ars in 30C followed by 200C potencies, as you are prescribing on the basis of aetiology, NBWS 'flu, several times to conserve the strength and appetite after 'flu and to terminate the cold.

(11) **Anorexia - Alfalfa** This was a patient around her menopause, she developed anorexia and was also losing weight. She was missing her main meals but constantly nibbling comfort food such as chocolates. I prescribed Alfalfa 200 and the patient got better within few months.

(12) **Anxiety Neurosis - Dysenteri Co** A middle aged man, who works in a very stressful job, he developed angina with palpitation with lot of anxiety and tension; cannot relax at all; always stressed. The wife of the patient gave me the clue that even during holidays he takes phone calls from work and as a consequence of this prolonged stress he gradually developed that undefined pain in the chest associated with palpitation. I prescribed the heart nosode for stress, Dysenteri Co, a bowel nosode, which is one of our leading medicines for anticipation, nervous tension, stress, which manifests as a cardiac malfunction including myocardial ischaemia. Dysenteri Co restored the patient to normal.

(13) **Aphonia - Hypericum** This is a remarkable story of one of my English patients in the U.K who had developed some hoarseness and the consultant found a small benign nodule in the vocal cord and operated accordingly. Unfortunately after the surgery, the hoarseness got worse and a laryngoscopy, revealed no abnormality.

The patient was extremely upset and had no faith in Homoeopathy but was almost dragged down to my clinic by one of my previous patients, who was his nephew. I prescribed Hypericum 200 followed by 1M, considering surgery could have injured the sentient nerves and as the prescription was based on aetiology, two potencies were given. There was 50% improvement during the first follow-up after eight weeks. I finished the case with 10M followed by 50M with complete recovery.

(14) **Arthritis - Kali Iod.** This was a case of degenerative Osteo-arthritis of both knees in a woman in her sixties. She was on the waiting list of the NHS (National Health Service) in the United Kingdom for a knee replacement. She came to me for extreme soreness and swelling of both her knees and would not allow anybody to touch her knee even the touch of clothes was almost unbearable. She also revealed that the pain was coming from the shaft of the bone. I prescribed Kali Iodatum 30 considering degenerative osteo-arthritis (which is Syphilo-Sycotic and Kali Iod is also a Syphilo-Sycotic medicine). Patient would not allow knee to be touched, sensitive and sore with oedema. Kali Iod. also covers bone pains and contracted joints.

(15) **Asthma - Caladium** This was a case of asthma associated with eczema. The patient habitually used allopathic cream and an inhaler constantly, therefore the modalities of the case were not clear. As soon as patient had an attack of asthma or itching skin the patient would take the inhaler or apply ointments. So it was almost a one sided case with scarcity of symptoms §173, Organon. The only remarkable thing was, itching of eczema alternated with asthma. I prescribed Caladium 200 on the basis of itching rash alternates with asthma and case has magically improved. Thereafter, I asked the patient to reduce the conventional medication gradually and subsequently modalities and sensations became clearer. I changed the plan of treatment and finished the case with Nitric Acid which is complementary of Caladium.

(16) **Asthma - Ferrum Met** This is a story of a middle aged man suffering from asthma and his wife said that whenever her husband engages himself in a conversation, his asthma is remarkably better. Initially I took that as asthma better while speaking which I interpreted as motion and gave Kali Carb. But unfortunately there was absolutely no change. Then I suddenly remembered the line in Ferrum Met, asthma better from talking, though feels weak but looks strong and prescribed Ferrum Met 200 with a remarkable result.

(17) **Asthma - Hypericum** Asthma of six years duration in a middle aged man who lives in Scotland, used to consult me over the telephone

and video conference. His asthmatic manifestation was better by leaning his head backwards and accordingly a homoeopath from Glasgow prescribed Hepar Sulph but there was no appreciable change. One day he was doing a video conference consultation with me, sitting in his conservatory, a room with large glass windows, and I could see it was very foggy outside and the patient was really suffocating. I asked about the weather and he confirmed that in foggy weather, his asthma gets worse. I prescribed Hypericum 200, which covers asthma, aggravation foggy weather, cold and damp, better leaning the head backwards.

(18) **Asthma - Nat Ars.** Asthma which was only relieved by urination was presented by an elderly woman and I prescribed Natrum Ars. 30 with a remarkable result.

(19) **Asthma - Ranunculus Bulbosus** This was a case of a middle aged man suffering from asthma which is caused and aggravated in cold air and the only way he found that the asthma improves, is when when he climbs stairs in his office or home which gave me the clue to prescribe Ranunculus Bulbosus 30C which covers asthma better from ascending Ref. Boger, as well as asthma caused and aggravated in cold air.

(20) **Asthma - Syphilinum** I have prescribed Syphilinum in 30 and 200C potencies several times for summer asthma.

(21) **Asthma - Tarentula Hispania** This was another very interesting case of a young man in his mid thirties suffering from asthma. Initially I prescribed Bacilinum for the apparent totality without any appreciable change. In one of the follow up visits, I noted that he was waiting on my patio and smoking, as no smoking is permitted in my consulting and waiting rooms. I observed through my window that he was not suffocating. When his turn came, he entered my consulting room with severe bouts of suffocation, which surprised me. I asked him that while he was on the patio and smoking, there was no suffocation. He confirmed, during smoking he never suffers from any suffocation which immediately prompted me to prescribe Tarentula Hispania in 30C potency as Clarke mentions asthma better from smoking.

(22) **Autism - Oxytropis Lamberti** Several times I have prescribed of Oxytropis Lamberti in 30 and 200 potencies for lack of awareness in autistic children when medicines like Baryta Carb or Baryta Iod have failed.

(23) **Bile vomiting - Homarus** When Nux vomica has failed in biliousness Homarus can be prescribed, patients have aggravation from milk or milk products, Homarus 30C is the best potency.

(24) Bipolar Depression - Lyssin It was a case of an extremely jealous and suspicious person suffering from bipolar depression with bouts of extreme and violent rage during which things are broken and destroyed, on the other hand he is extremely introverted with depression. I have noted from the case history that the nature of symptoms was intermittent and in the past history, the patient had extreme oversensitivity of hearing and smell. The patient could not be in any noisy place including the town centre. The patient almost went into spasm from smelling a flower. This made the person gradually withdraw from the exterior world and he became self-centered and selfish because he could see other people were enjoying life and the music, flowers but he could not. This carried on for six years and finally the patient entered into this state of bipolar depression. I prescribed Lyssin 200 followed by 1M to the case, to start with, considering extreme hypersensitivity relating Doctrine of Signature to that of a dog, selfish and violent rage, like the mad dog alternating with introverted depression. It took about two years and Lyssin completely restored the case.

(25) Brain Injury - Helleborus A slow, sluggish boy aged twelve years, was brought to me with lack of coordination of muscles, he could not grip tightly or button his shirt and his gait was unstable. Emotionally he was slow and with a mental age of about three years behind his actual age. His previous Homoeopath had given Calcarea Carb and Baryta Carb without any noticeable change. I meticulously investigated the development of symptoms and accordingly it transpired that the patient had a fall on his head from about 8 feet onto a concrete playground when he was eight years old. The problem gradually developed six months after the fall. I prescribed Helleborus 30 followed 200, considering sensorial depression, interpreted from slow and sluggish, muscular weakness, interpreted from lack of muscular coordination and defective gait, I am delighted to report Helleborus has completely restored the patient.

(26) Cancerous Ulcer - Latrodectus Hasselti This is a magnificent case of my grandfather who was treating a patient, aged about thirty eight years, suffering from an ulceration on the lower lip which was had not healed for three years. This was in the 1940s and therefore there was no proper diagnosis in India for Cancer. My grandad was treating with apparently indicated medicines but there was no apparent change for the eight months. One day this patient visited the clinic with his ten years old son. His son saw a spider on the wall and started pushing his Dad, whispering constantly, "Dad,

Dad there is a spider on the wall". He kept repeating this gesture which finally made my grandad task, "I am sorry that there is a spider on the wall, as this is an old house we often find them, but why is your son repeatedly bringing your attention to this?" The patient got embarrassed and replied "sorry, we live in an old house as well and there are quite a few spiders in our house too. Whenever I smoke, my son asks me to touch the lighted end of the cigarette on the legs of the spider and in that way the spider runs up the wall away from the cigarette. Unfortunately my son enjoys this." What a syphilitic boy! My grandfather asked one more question after this and made the prescription. What was the question?

He asked, "do you continue to smoke the same cigarette after touching the end of the cigarette on spider's leg?" The patient replied, "yes" That made my grandfather to prescribe Latrodectus Hasselti, which is a New South Wales Spider and covers the type of ulceration on the patient's lips. My grandfather's interpretation was, let likes be treated by likes. Through smoking the same cigarette, he was inhaling the fluid of the burnt spider which probably caused the ulceration, accordingly he prescribed the medicine prepared from spider. Glory goes to Hahnemann and his beautiful art and science of let "likes be treated by likes!" The patient got better within six months.

(27) **Chronic Fatigue Syndrome - Ambra Grisea** This was a case of a middle aged man who was a workaholic but was gradually getting weaker without any apparent reason. He was also withdrawing from his family and friends and getting more and more closed and introverted, even was getting irritable from listening to music. His wife thought he was suffering from some serious disease and took him to a big private hospital and was investigated head to foot, including CT scan and MRI, nothing abnormal was detected. They spent huge amounts of money and nothing was resolved. Finally they got frustrated and tried homoeopathy. I prescribed Ambra Grisea on the basis of weakness from overwork, desire to be alone, introverted, depressed and it has even aggravation from music. The beauty lies in the similimum.

(28) **Chronic Fatigue Syndrome - Kali Carb** A woman in her mid forties. Her husband left her eighteen years ago when her pregnancy was full term. This man never contacted her or the child. The daughter, now eighteen years old suddenly made some contact with her Father, whom she had never seen. She left her Mum and went to live with her Dad. The weakness of my patient started six months after the above incident. The weakness was aggravated

in the early morning and after eating, especially lunch. She also developed some water retention in the foot which improves with movement. I prescribed Kali Carb 30 followed by 200 considering disappointment from bad news and love (daughter moved away) as described above. The weakness started then and is aggravated in the early morning, which is a Kali Carb symptom. Throughout the nine months I treated this patient her emotional strength improved alongside her physical energy.

(29) **Chronic Fatigue Syndrome - Lycopodium** This is a case of a man in his mid fifties suffering from undefined weakness associated with pain in the renal area, aggravated around 6.00 p.m. The patient has a very pleasant, courteous personality. The past history revealed two episodes of hepatitis. I prescribed Lycopodium 30C. Please remember the sphere of action of a polychrest, in Lycopodium it is the gastric including liver, renal and throat this is a part of the totality and when these areas are affected in a patient that becomes a very strong indication of the medicine.

(30) **Chronic Fatigue Syndrome - Mag Carb** I am going to share with you the story of a competitive, ambitious, workaholic woman in her late thirties. In order to commute to London every day she has to leave home by 7.30 a.m.. She returns around 10.00 p.m. because her job includes taking her business clients to dinner. Her main complaint was undefined debility, a sort of worn out feeling. She also suffers from headache which is worse from concentration and better in open air. She has occasional acidity because of the frequency of dining in restaurants; she often has heavy lamb dishes, which she loves. This over consumption of meat results in constipation. She loves citrus drinks, grapefruit and fresh orange juice especially. This is the story of a case that looks like Nux Vomica which is actually Mag Carb., who is an achiever and committed to success and I say they are Mrs. Nux Vom. Mag Carb 200 restored the patient completely and now she is a dedicated to Homoeopathy.

(31) **Cicatrical Tissue – Graphites** An ugly scar was troubling a woman, in her mid thirties who has had an abdominal hysterectomy following which there was incisional scar, which she hated. The scar was gradually getting bigger and turning blackish which is unusual in a Caucasian skin. One of the interesting aspects of the case was the surrounding skin of the scar was extremely dry, almost parchment dry. I prescribed Graphites, which is in Dr. Margaret Tyler's trio of scar tissue medicines, others are Causticum and Silicea. In such cases, topical application of Anagallis tincture. 10 drops, soaked in cotton wool, to be applied on the affected scar

tissue or keloids, three times daily for three – five months will give good results.

(32) **Claustrophobia - Calcarea Carb** This is a story of a middle aged woman who was trapped in a lift for six hours from this she developed an extreme degree of claustrophobia with anxiety and fear. When she is anxious and scared, she sweats profusely. I considered the event of being trapped in the lift as a tragedy and looked upon her subsequent fears and claustrophobia as Post Traumatic Stress Disorder. Calcarea Carb 200 followed by 1M restored her.

(33) **Cold Allergy - Dulcamara** I have prescribed Dulcamara enumerable times, in cases of cold allergy, e.g. touching a chilled bottle in the fridge which results urticarial blebs at the point of contact.

(34) **Colic - Staphysagria** Repeated attacks of abdominal colic instigated a forty three year old man to try homoeopathy because after investigations nothing abnormal was detected. While taking the history I found multiple griefs in a period of sixteen months, his grandfather, mother and brother died. Another interesting clue narrated is that he gets loose bowels as soon as he drinks chilled water, which he is fond of. This confirmed my choice of Staphysagria which not only covers the history of multiple grief but also the loose stool from chilled water.

(35) **Colicky Baby - Senna** I have prescribed Senna 30C many times for young babies for infantile colic. The baby is full of wind which is aggravated at night.

(36) **Convalescence - Psorinum** Here comes a story of a man in his mid forties, who unfortunately suffered from three or four chest infections every year for the last three years, every infection was associated with cold and cough, which lasted almost six – eight weeks. For the last two years, he was treated with antibiotics and every time the suffering was prolonged. So this year after antibiotics failed again, he decided to come to me. He is an extremely chilly patient, nervous and anxious. He does not have lot of verve, rather pessimistic and withdrawn, even though his life was secure both in relationships and financially. I prescribed Psorinum 200 considering 'lack of reaction' of the body's immune system, the body is not recovering after an acute illness leading to weakness and weak immunity. The weakness from defective phagocytosis giving rise to lingering infection in a person who is pessimistic, anxious, lack of positive thoughts, lack of will power and ambition.

(37) **Convulsion - Artemisia Vulgaris** The interesting part of this story of convulsions, is that whenever he used to sit in the car, in bright

sunshine with closed tinted windows, he used to get attack of seizure. I took this as coloured light produces dizziness leading to convulsion. Therefore, I prescribed Artemisia Vulgaris 30 and there was remarkable improvement. I finally finished the case with 1M.

(38) **Convulsion - Opium** This is a wonderful story of one of my patients, aged seven years who was brought to me with convulsions. The boy has been treated by other Homoeopaths before without any convincing change. The convulsions were very occasional since birth, once in six months. When the boy was aged three years, the convulsions aggravated and now occurred two or three times every month. Initially patient had conventional medicines but after six months of treatment, the patient was becoming a vegetable, losing all interactions. Therefore, the parents stopped the conventional medication and started Homoeopathy. Whenever I see a patient under twelve years, I ask the pregnancy and delivery history. Following this question the Mother told me the following: she (the patient's mother) was staying in her maternal village house, during the last trimester of pregnancy. One evening, at twilight, she was putting her washing on the washing line, in the terrace. She saw an image in the corner of the terrace, which was nothing but the reflection of a big tree, growing in the back garden and the shadow of the branches were moving on the terrace. On seeing that image, she fainted, as she thought it was a ghost. Since then, whenever she used to go to the terrace, she felt scared ++ and tried to avoid looking that corner. I took this, as fear of fright still remaining which affected the foetal circulation. The child was affected and developed convulsions. Hence, Opium was prescribed to the child. I started with 200 followed by 1M as the prescription was based on aetiology. There was remarkable improvement. I finally finished the case with 10M followed by 50M. Glory goes to Hahnemann and his beautiful Homoeopathy!

(39) **Cough - Alumina** A chilly elderly woman suffered from intermittent bouts of chronic cough for the previous four years. Cough aggravated from spicy foods, garam masala, and cardamom. I prescribed Alumina 200 and the patient got better within three months. Alumina covers cough from irritating food.

(40) **Cough - Capsicum** I saw this very interesting case, just after I graduated, when I was alongside my uncle, late Dr. N. K. Banerjee. A person was coughing loudly in the waiting room. It was one of the loudest coughs you can imagine. As there was a long queue of patients in the waiting room and the patient had to wait and

during this time, the patient coughed persistently. Suddenly my uncle asked me to visit in the waiting room and check whether that patient experience any pain during the cough? The patient replied, yes, every time he coughs, he has some pain in his thighs. I came back to my uncle and reported the symptom. My uncle told me to give the patient Capsicum 200, even without seeing the case. To be honest, I was not very happy that this patient has travelled 200 miles to see my uncle, and he was prescribing in this way. With mild protest, I dispensed the medicine. The patient came back after a month, and reported 90% improved. This is true classical homoeopathy. You do not always need to spend a long time with your patient but the qualities of the symptom should match with the qualities of the medicine. He prescribed Capsicum on the basis of explosive cough, during which there was pain in the distant parts.

(41) **Crack and Fissures of Skin - X-Ray** Deep cracks with thickening were giving a thirty eight year old woman a lot of pain during walking and her toe nails are also quite deformed and thick. The patient was in a habit of taking over the counter medicines for acidity, pain-killers for headaches and analgesics for 'flu. I considered this as prolonged history of suppression from iatrogenic cause which manifested in the skin and nails causing cracks and deformities and consequently prescribed X-Ray 200 with remarkable results.

(42) **Depression - Carcinosin** I prescribed Carcinosin for an extremely unhappy woman in her mid-forties with a prolonged history of domination by her husband and suppression of any feelings she had. She suffered from periodic depression but concealed how she was feeling from her children. She behaved like a door mat and took the insults and domination and suffered in silence. Occasionally she exploded with anger when she was being pushed to the limit. I prescribed Carcinosin 200 followed by 1M, considering the prolonged history of unhappiness, suppressed anger and the domination from her husband which resulted in her depression. Doctrine of Signature for Carcinosin is to think of it as a cancer cell which tries to localise in less important organs, while keeping the vital organs healthy as long as possible. So the part affected by the cancer, silently suffers while the vital organs perform well. If you consider the above story, where the woman was silently suffering, keeping the family happy and her body finally explodes when she is pushed to the limit. I have given a wonderful picture of Carcinosin in my book, "Classical Homoeopathy for an Impatient World".

(43) Depression - Staphysagria Through our patients we learn of other cultures and this story of an eleven years old Slovakian girl shows us how a slight change of location had such a devastating effect. She had introverted depression and stopped going to school. The family is Slovakian, although now they live in Prague, Czech Republic. At home, they speak Slovakian and the girl used to go to a school with predominantly Slovakian children. For the last six months, she has changed to a different school in Prague where the language is predominantly Czech. At the new school the teacher asked some questions, and my patient replied immediately, but unfortunately and accidentally in Slovakian. The teacher was extremely rude and told her off in front of the class for speaking Slovakian. Since then, this bright and intelligent girl, totally withdrew and stopped going to school with introverted depression. Another Homoeopath prescribed her Natrum Mur on the basis of grief, mortification, ridicule and humiliation. When I took the case, I asked the girl her reaction and feelings to that unfortunate situation. Even after spending reasonable amount of time, she kept quiet and could not say. At that stage, in order to assist her, I put seven different possible reactions and she said that she felt it was an injustice and as a consequence, she is angry for being told off for speaking her mother language by accident. She also felt her teacher was extremely rude. So I prescribed Staphysagria considering the aetiology from injustice, rudeness of others, with anger after. The choices I offered the girl, which helped her define how she felt are listed below, with the relevant medicine choices.

- **Abused, from being-** ANACARDIUM, Argentum nitricum, Aurum, Bryonia, CARCINOSIN, Chamomilla, COLOCYNTH, Conium, IGNATIA, Lachesis, LYCOPODIUM, Lyssin, NATRUM MUR., Nux vomica, PALLADIUM, PHOS. AC., PULSATILLA, STAPHYSAGRIA, Sulphur (ref. R.Morrison).
- **Anger, after-** OPIUM, Phosphoric acid, Phosphorus, PLATINA, Pulsatilla, Ranunculus, Sepia, STAPHYSAGRIA, Tarentula hispania (ref. R.Morrison).
- **Embarrassment & humiliation-** Gelsemium, Ignatia, Phosphoric acid.
- **Humiliation-** Aconite, ANACARDIUM, Argentum nitricum, Arsenicum album, Aurum, Bryonia, Calcarea, CARCINOSIN, Chamomilla, COLOCYNTH, IGNATIA, Lachesis, LYCOPODIUM, Lyssin, NATRUM MUR, Nux vomica, Palladium, PHOSPHORIC ACID, Pulsatilla, STAPHYSAGRIA, Sulphur, (ref. R.Morrison).

- **Injustice-** Calcarea phos, Causticum, Hepar Sulph, Ignatia, Kali Iod., Mag Carb, Mag Mur, Nux vomica, Phosphoric acid, *Staphysagria*, Sulphur, Veratrum Album.
- **Rudness, of others-** Calcarea carb., Colchicum, Ignatia, Lycopodium, Medorrhinum, Natrum mur., STAPHYSAGRIA (ref. R.Morrison).
- **Wounded pride-** Silicea.

(44) **Diarrhoea - Chininum Ars.** A patient suffered from periodic episodes of diarrhoea and although he thinks it is related to some food or stress, he is unclear of which affects him. I asked him to be more vigilant and subsequently he concluded it is definitely eggs, which he likes, but his body does not. I prescribed Chininum Ars 30 on the basis of diarrhoea from eggs.

(45) **Drug addiction - Calcarea Phos.** A boy of thirteen years was brought to me by his distraught Mother who discovered her son was regularly smoking Marijuana. His mother was clear in telling that she is separated from his father and her son cannot tolerate his Mum's new man. While asking questions and trying to clarify the chronological development of symptoms, I understood that the boy is extremely unhappy about his parent's separation and experienced it as lack of love from his parents towards him. As a consequence of that he lost all his motivation, dropping out from school and became reckless and rebellious. He started drugs which gave him some temporary relief from his unhappiness. This is a classical picture of Calcarea Phos. For clarification you may consult my book, "Classical Homoeopathy for an Impatient World". I prescribed 200 followed by 1M as the prescription was based on the aetiology. Homoeopathy has presented a normal boy back to his mother in fourteen months. Glory goes to Hahnemann and his beautiful art and science of Homoeopathy!

(46) **Dry Lips - Pulsatilla** In the slum clinic in Calcutta, fast prescribing is necessary in order to expedite prescriptions for, often a very long queue of people. A young girl in her mid twenties was perturbed by extreme dryness of her lips. As a homoeopath you should have very observant eyes and I noted that she was frequently licking her dry lips. A dose of Pulsatilla 200 completed the case.

(47) **Dysfunctional Uterine Bleeding - Lachesis** A woman approaching her menopause, was suffering from profuse menorrhagia, with no clots. As a consequence of bleeding, she developed extreme weakness with bouts of depression. The periods were still normal and occurring every month. The bleeding is more profuse at night.

One of the interesting points that drew my attention was the menstruation was regular and exactly on the right time, on which I prescribed Lachesis which resolved not only the menorrhagia but also the debility and depression.

(48) **Dysmenorrhoea - Pulsatilla** I have prescribed Pulsatilla repeatedly with success in cases of dysmenorrhoea with irregular, intermittent flow; pain associated with chilliness and restlessness, aggravation in the evening, better by lying on painful side and cold application. Pulsatilla 200 will restore such cases.

(49) **Eczema – Morgan** A young boy of nine, had been suffering from eczema since he was two years old. Initially conventional medication was tried and unfortunately later on the patient developed asthma. Then the conventional medication was stopped and Homoeopathy was tried. The asthma improved but no appreciable change for the eczema. His skin was very dry with lots of itching, aggravated by the warmth of the bed, at night. From his prolonged suffering, the skin had become a little thickened and rough. The boy was extremely frustrated and I saw a long list of Homoeopathic medicines had been tried by other Homoeopaths, including Arsenicum alb; Graphites, Kali Silicata, Psorinum, Sulph Iod; and Tuberculinum. I prescribed Morgan Pure (Bach) 30C considering the infantile eczema with dryness and itching, aggravation from heat, night with thickened skin. This also includes the past history of congestion in the lungs as consequence of conventional suppression. I went up to 10M over a period of a year and finished the case with Tuberculinum.

(50) **Eczema - Thuja** This is a case of a woman in her mid-fifties suffering from eczema, mostly in the groin and buttock area associated with dry skin, itching worse after scratching. The interesting clue in the case was perspiration mostly during sleep which she regarded as menopausal hot sweat. She was generally constipated and had urging especially after a cup of tea in the morning. I prescribed Thuja 30 and finished the case with Thuja 10M.

(51) **Epistaxis - Phosphorus** A young girl aged eleven years, suffered from recurrent episodes of epistaxis for a period of 10 months. She was a bright young girl and there was no history of fall or injury. The interesting aspect of the case was that the bleeding occurs very, very suddenly without any reason. I took the suddenness in consideration and prescribed Phosphorus on the basis of the personality of the girl which was bright, intelligent, caring and sympathetic, popular with friends and a strong desire for company. Phosphorus 200C restored the case.

(52) Fibromyalgia - Actea Racemosa I have successfully prescribed Actea Racemosa many times for I. T. people, who spend long time in typing, using the mouse and entering data and thereafter suffer from excruciating pain in the deltoid muscles with soreness and heaviness, almost incapacitating the person for work the next day. Actea Racemosa covers muscular soreness, heaviness and pain as a consequence of typewriting, piano playing, and sewing. As the prescription is based on the aetiology, so, I prescribe 30 followed by 200.

(53) Fibromyalgia - Helonias Dioca I find this medicine useful for people after over exertion. For example excessive Christmas (England) or Puja (India) shopping and thereafter in the evening or the next day, the over tired muscles which burn and ache. Helonias 30 followed by 200 will restore such cases.

(54) Fibromyalgia - Radium Bromide A busy I.T. consultant developed aches and pains in his arms and thighs which were aggravated by first motion and better by continued motion. Pains of the muscles are relieved by warmth. Just prior to the development of the aches a lot of moles and skin tags appeared which I interpreted as a consequence of radiation from the computer screen over long hours. This is exactly covered by Radium Bromide. Accordingly I prescribed Radium Bromide 30 followed by 200, two potencies because the prescription was based on aetiology. Radium Bromide not only took care of the fibro-myalgia but also of the moles. I have given an extensive picture of Radium Bromide and X-Ray in my book, "Classical Homoeopathy for an Impatient World".

(55) Fibromyalgia - Squilla This was a remarkable case of a young, attractive woman in her early twenties working as shop assistant in duty free perfume shop in a London Airport. Her job requires her to stand on her feet during the entire period and show customers different perfumes in one of the world's busiest airport. She developed fibromyalgia, sore and tender feet from standing a long time. She had been to other homoeopaths who have tried Rhus Tox, Causticum and Arnica. without any appreciable change. I prescribed Squilla 30 which has exactly this symptom mentioned in the Boericke's Materia Medica. The patient got better within three months. Once again, the qualities of the symptoms should exactly match with qualities of the medicine.

(56) Fractured Bone pains - Symphytum I have frequently prescribed Symphytum in 200C followed by 1M potencies for pain in fractured bone, aggravation from touch.

Short Case Stories

(57) Gastric Ulcer – Bryonia A middle aged single woman, was working in the financial sector, but unfortunately due to circumstances beyond her control, she lost her job and was extremely fearful about her financial security. Her parents gave her a lump sum of money and said not to worry. She was extremely angry and indignant about her life and was insecure about her future despite the investment of the lump sum. Her anxiety was reduced by practicing meditation; her gastric pains were aggravated by warm drinks and after eating. I prescribed Bryonia 30 followed by 200 considering the loss of security leading to anger and anxiety. Although she had a large sum of money invested, fear of poverty was still present, which is incordination, sycotic. Her anxiety reduced by being still and aggravation from eating can be interpreted as aggravation from motion, characteristic symptoms of Bryonia which is why she reported full recovery quite quickly.

(58) Gastritis - Abies Nigra This is about a patient in his mid-fifties suffering from chronic gastritis with constipation and poor appetite. There was pain in the stomach, which always came on after eating. However the remarkable thing in the case was a feeling of a solid lump in the oesophagus, behind the sternum. I interpreted this as a "hard boiled egg lodged in the cardiac end of the stomach and all complaints are aggravated after eating". I prescribed Abies Nigra 30C and ended the case with 1M. This was a wonderful example of a small medicine completing the case, if the symptoms corroborate.

(59) Gastritis - Angustura V. This patient suffered from acute gastric pain and could not report any modalities or characteristics as pain-killers and antacids were taken regularly. I discovered that the patient drank an excessive amount of coffee and so far he remembers, the pain gradually developed as his coffee consumption increased. I prescribed him Angustura Vera which covers gastric pains in coffee drinkers.

(60) Gastritis - China A patient in his mid-forties, was suffering from chronic gastritis with acidity with a lot of bloating and distension. The patient was very fond of fruit, especially banana and guava, which he used to take as a snack in the afternoon at his work. Unfortunately the fruit gave him sour eructations and acidity. The patient reported that by evening around 7.30 p.m. the bloating and acidity disappeared. He used to leave his office around 6.30 p.m. and walked about a mile to reach home. This gave me the clue and I prescribed Cinchona 200C considering acidity worse after fruit, gas better by movement. The patient was totally better within three months.

(61) **Giardiasis - Homarus** This case of giardiasis presented with tingling pain in lower abdomen with frothy, stool with mucus. There was occasional pain while passing stool. All complaints were aggravated after taking milk or milk products, which he liked. The patient has reduced appetite although he feels a little better after taking solid food. When he doesn't eat, he gets a headache. I prescribed Homarus 30 for this case and once again it was a wonderful experience for me that even this small medicine has completely cured the patient because it covers the totality.

(62) **Impotency - Onosmodium** A man, in his mid thirties had lost confidence in his sexual ability because his ex-wife humiliated him and voiced her dissatisfaction publicly and announced his inability to sustain an erection. She divorced him and as a consequence he almost developed a phobia about any future relationships. His erection when alone confirms his physical ability but his ex-wife made him feel impotent. I prescribed Onosmodium 1M on the basis of psychical impotence.

(63) **Impotency - Titanium Met** Titanium Met 200C is successful for pre-mature ejaculation, when well selected medicines fail.

(64) **Insomnia - Agaricus** An Accountant by profession who does sedentary work for seventy hours a week with his high profile accounting job suffered from insomnia. He had been to another Homoeopath who prescribed Nux Vomica without any appreciable change. I prescribed Agaricus 200, followed by 1M as Agaricus is an interesting medicine for insomnia after working long hours at a desk.

(65) **Insomnia - Kali Phos** I find Kali Phos useful, in potencies like 200 and 1M for insomnia after anxiety and worry with restless legs.

(66) **Insomnia - Secale Cor.** I find Secale Cor in 30 and 200C potencies useful for insomnia of alcoholics.

(67) **Lumbago - Cobaltum** This was a case of chronic lumbago of five years duration and the patient was unable to share with me any particular aetiology or modalities. The only characteristic was that the back ache was almost unbearable while sitting at work and almost on the verge of making him incapable of continuing his normal schedule. One day he shared an interesting story with me. He was driving from London to Manchester and every hour he had to stop in the lay-by and stretch and walk for five minutes. This gave me the clue and I prescribed Cobaltum 200 on the basis of back ache aggravated while sitting, better walking. In seven months the patient was absolutely normal.

(68) **Menopausal syndrome - Sanguinaria Canadensis** A woman suffered from hot flushes, swelling and tenderness of the breasts during her menopause. The patient had a very interesting symptom that sugar tastes bad in the mouth and when I pressed about the exact nature of the taste, she mentioned it tastes almost bitter. This immediately gave the clue to prescribe Sanguinaria Canadensis 200 which completely cured both the symptoms. Dr. Clarke mentions this symptom in his 'Dictionary of Practical Materia Medica'.

(69) **Menopausal Syndrome - Sulphur** I have treated menopausal syndrome associated with hot flushes and bleeding per vagina, with Sulphur several times. This has been associated with a congestive feeling in the lower abdomen associated with heat and burning especially in self-centered, introverted women.

(70) **Milestone Delayed - Silicea** This was one of my Indian patients, a boy of four years old, all milestones delayed, especially walking, he can hardly walk, he totters and finds it difficult to remain firm on his legs. As part of the case taking in a child under twelve years, I always ask the pregnancy history and it became apparent that his mother was verbally abused by her in-laws who she lived with. This was further compounded by the abuse and insults given by her in-laws to her own parents. This immediately gave me the clue of wounded honour and being ridiculed which led to a feeling of inadequacy which transmitted to her child during intra-uterine life which caused the delayed milestones. I prescribed Silicea to the child and within weeks he was walking quite steadily and confidently.

(71) **Myalgic Encephalopathy (ME) - Curare** A case of Never Been Well Since Influenza and since then the patient was suffering from extreme weakness with lack of strength of the muscles. Walking a short distance was difficult and even after walking 50 metres there was trembling of the legs in a man in his forties. The patient was treated by other Homoeopaths with Gelsemium and Causticum but without any appreciable change. I prescribed Curare 30C considering NBWS flu followed by ME, well selected medicines, like Gelsemium had failed.

(72) **Myalgic Encephalopathy (ME) - Gelsemium** Another story of Never Been Well Since Influenza; this time the patient was suffering from extreme drowsiness and heaviness of the muscles. The muscles of the hand and legs felt so heavy that the patient was almost unable to move or raise them. There was a feeling in the patient that he was unable to cope with this situation and he had a fear of losing control. I prescribed Gelsemium which has 4D's.

Dull, Dizzy, Drowsy, and Debility and H -Heaviness. To confirm the choice Gelsemium has the feeling of cannot cope. 30 followed by 200 took care of the problem.

(73) **Nasal Catarrh - Medorrhinum** Large swollen tonsils and a blocked nose with thick yellow profuse mucus was the presenting complaint in a six year old restless boy. His mother said he can be quite aggressive one moment and then becomes very affectionate. I prescribed Medorrhinum 200 and a single dose restored the case. The extreme, erratic personality with contrasting moods from one moment to the next is the personality and Dr. Burnett mentions the medicine as "The Mother of pus and catarrh".

(74) **Obsessive Compulsive Disorder - Causticum** A promising young man developed OCD with fear. He behaved as if he had committed a crime and would not go out of his house in case the police were there to catch him. The problem started when he was unjustifiably sacked from his job with the accusation that he was a slow worker. Since then he is very opinionated about any injustice and will dwell on any injustice with a very dark mood of depression and hopelessness. Dark can aptly summaries his mental state, dark mood, hopeless, world goes dark around him, pessimism, fears as if he had committed a crime. He is extremely inflexible, which I implied as stiff and rigid. Considering the aetiology of injustice and manifestation of dark mood and temper, hopelessness, stiff and rigid and the sycotic OCD led me to prescribe the tri-miasmatic Causticum and the patient improved within six months.

(75) **Obsessive Compulsive Disorder (OCD) - Nitric Acid** It was a striking case of a woman in her late thirties who developed OCD about infectious diseases. She was under extreme stress of looking after her autistic child as a consequence there was a lot of anxiety, being up at night watching over her son who did not go bed till 1 a.m. I interpreted this as over exertion of body and mind, worry and anxiety leading to fear of infectious diseases and accordingly I prescribed Nitric acid 200 followed by 1M which totally restored the case in approximately twelve months.

(76) **Obsessive Compulsive Disorder - Opium** This is a curious case of an American woman who consulted me over the phone. She is eighty six years old and had an accident whist attending her chair exercise class for elderly people, to maintain strength in the muscles and improve circulation. Another elderly woman lost her balance and fell against my patient, knocking her down. Ever since then, she has had a very strong fixation on her bowels, thinking she is constipated. Along with this, she has made some unusual phone

calls, calling her doctor three times in twenty minutes saying she was remembering her appointment later that day, and would be coming on the bus, even though she never rides on the bus!

She have had lifelong constipation, and frequently uses a small enema to move her bowels in the morning, but since this accident she believes she is totally constipated, to the point that she takes laxatives, then forgets she has taken them and takes some more. I prescribed for this case Opium 200 followed by 1M considering the accident as mental shock resulting fixation of mind and obsessive compulsion about constipation. This patient improved dramatically!

(77) **Oedema - Natrum Mur** This is an interesting case of a young girl, age twelve suffering from huge water retention in her both feet for the last two years. All the investigations, including assessment of the kidneys were normal. The nephrologist could not diagnose the cause of the oedema and wanted to start steroids which the parents refused. In order to obtain a true picture of the chronological development, I felt I needed to speak to the girl privately and asked the girl about her emotional status. She stated that her parents have six children and she is the youngest. All six are girls and she feels left out. That there is a total lack of affection towards her and this leaves her feeling abandoned. Her first symptom was extreme constipation, visiting toilet even once in ten days and thereafter gradually the oedema developed. I analysed the case as, absence of mother's affection leading to a sense of abandonment along with disappointment of not having parent's love. This resulted in retention both as constipation and water retention. Interpretation of the case is always very important but may I take the opportunity to caution you that you should never, never interpret what you think but try to understand what the patient's reaction is to the situation. In this regard please refer to my case story of Amyotrophic Lateral Sclerosis (ALS) treated with Cyclamen and also the case of Depression cured by Staphysagria.

(78) **Osteo-Arthritis - Apis** A girl in her late teens reported osteo-arthritis with stiff joints and stinging pains, a lot of swelling, with aggravation on warm application, better by cold. The pain made her extremely restless. As I always give emphasis on the past history and anamnesis, I discovered that the patient had a very strict upbringing. Dominating parents, with a life full of rules. I prescribed Apis Mel 30 followed by 200, considering the aetiology and stiff joints with stinging pains, swelling, aggravation from warm application, and better by cold (reverse of Rhus Tox). She

was extremely restless from pain and the emotional aspects are also covered by Apis. Patient showed remarkable improvement in few months.

(79) **Ovarian Cyst - Conium** This young woman in her mid-twenties had been to many other homoeopaths with a diagnosis of Poly Cystic Ovarian Disease (PCOD) for the last three years. The patient had lot of physical weakness and was of very forgetful nature. She told me that her husband works in Dubai and only visits her once a year. I interpreted that as sexual suppression because of abstinence and prescribed Conium Mac 30 followed by 200.

The patient improved within a short period of time. I prescribed Conium on the basis of cysts in the ovary (Conium is a scrofulous or glandular medicine, as it affects the breast as well), sexual abstinence, physical weakness, and mental weakness portrayed by lack of concentration, poor memory, lack of focus and motivation.

(80) **Ovarian Cyst - Medorrhinum** A workaholic, working in the city of London in a busy recruitment office suffered from Poly Cystic Ovarian Disease (PCOD) for the last four years. She had lot of pain in the lower abdomen which aggravated in the early morning and was unable to wear tight clothing. She also suffered from sinusitis with thick yellow discharge. She relaxes at the weekend by walking by the sea with her dog. I prescribed her Medorrhinum 200 on the basis of PCOD with pelvic inflammatory diseases. Pain < 4 a.m., < touch of clothing, thick yellow catarrh, better by the sea side. Patient is a workaholic, which is strongly sycotic along with other predominantly sycotic symptoms of yellow discharge, and ovarian incoordiantion.

(81) **Panic Attacks - Arsenic Album** An adolescent girl was suffering from severe panic attacks at night especially around 1.00 – 2.00 a.m. While taking the history, I came to know that there is a strong feeling of being neglected by her parents as Dad is always busy and frequently travelling and Mum is a nurse and works night shifts. As a result of this, she felt uncared for. She was also being bullied which wasn't being handled very well at school. I prescribed Arsenicum Album 200 which covers humiliation, being bullied as well as indignation from feeling uncared for, which gradually built up in the psyche of the patient, resulting in panic attacks in the night. Arsenicum album restored the case in nine months.

(82) **Pessimism - Carbo Vegetabilis** This is a combination of an extreme degree of pessimism with anxiety, aggravated around 5.00 p.m. to 6.00 p.m. There was also apathy and depression present in this patient, who also suffered from distention with some burning in the

abdomen, made better by eructation. When the patient was bloated, he felt weak and had coldness of the extremities with offensive diarrhea. I prescribed Carbo Vegetabilis to this case. Carbo veg covers the pessimism and apathy too. Ref. "Classical Homoeopathy for an Impatient World" by this author.

(83) **Pneumonia - Hippozaenum and Tuberculinum Aviare** In England, I get lot of elderly patients around Christmas time who suffers from recurrent and persistent cough and cold and many times there is congestion and consolidation in the base of the lungs with rattling mucus. To clear this rattling in the base of the lung, I prescribe Tuberculinum Aviare in patients with the preponderance of Tubercular miasm. The other useful medicine is Hippozaenum, which I call Antim Tart for the Syphilo-Tubercular elderly patients.

(84) **Post Natal Depression - Cinchona** After this patient delivered her second child she suffered from post partum haemorrhage (PPH) followed by extreme depression associated with apathy and indifference. She had no desire to live, with an unfortunate feeling. I prescribed Cinchona 30C followed by 200C (two potencies because the prescription is based on the aetiology). It took about three months to restore the patient to her old happy self. Here the clue was haemorrhage followed by depression.

(85) **Pre-Menstrual Tension (PMT) - Sepia** A young girl came with her Mother and began the consultation by telling me her Mother is almost getting impossible to live with, especially during pre-menstrual time. She gets an extremely negative attitude, nagging and complaining and yells a lot of the time! It is a case of an extremely irritable, critical, spiteful woman. This is the Margaret Tyler's description of Sepia and Sepia only! I gaave Sepia to the mother.

(86) **Pre-Menstrual Tension (PMT) Thyroidinum** This consultation began with a declaration of love for chocolate! The woman was obese, plump, easily fatigued, puffed out woman and came to see me for extreme breast tenderness before menses with irritability, the least opposition would upset her. She was approaching her menopause and quite unbalanced with this change of life and felt an imbalance of hormones including low energy, swelling of the breasts, and water retention before menses and episodes of depression. I prescribed Thyroidinum 200 to the case. Thyroidinum is a medicine for mal-adjustment, strain during some particular period of development, hormonal imbalance during puberty, pregnancy and menopause. The mal-adjustment is manifested in the metabolic area which can result in obesity or emaciation; the vascular area reflecting variation

in blood pressure and temperamental mal-adjustment, irritability, temper tantrums.

(87) **Prolapse Rectum - Ruta** After her third delivery a woman in her thirties opted to try homoeopathy for her rectal prolapse with stitching pain. She also gave me an interesting symptom of nausea felt in rectum, while straining at stool. The desire to pass stool was often unsuccessful and this gave me the clue to prescribe Ruta 200C with an amazing result. Please note, homoeopathy can only help very early first degree prolapse. If the prolapse is advanced, it is a structural problem and homoeopathy cannot help. You should be very clear and explain the limitations of homoeopathy to your patients and in this way homoeopathy will not be misunderstood.

(88) **Post Traumatic Stress Disorder - Stramonium** A man crossed the White Chapel underground station 5 minutes before the bombing terror attack of 7-7 and since then he became almost maniacal with fears. His night terror alternates with some violence during the day, manifested as violent rage with the destructive impulse of throwing things and breaking crockery. I prescribed Stramonium 200 followed by 1M considering the aetiology Fear of violence causing rage, fright at night resulting in night terrors then rage and violence. Stramonium removed the effect of this frightening incident.

(89) **School Going Fear - Natrum Sulph** A young girl of six years age developed tremendous fear about school. She has become withdrawn, unable to mix with her friends or even visit them in their homes. In the history, I found there was repeated history of fall between age 1 and 3 from the sofa unto the carpet. My interpretation was that as a consequence of such repeated falls there was mental traumatism causing incoordination of mental harmony which manifested as an inability to socialize. Accordingly I prescribed Natrum Sulph 200 followed by 1M. It took about nine months before the child was able to socialise comfortably.

(90) **Sciatica - Indigo** Eating was a simple pleasure for a sixty year old woman who came to me for sciatica. She enjoyed her meals but was convinced that every time she ate her sciatica pain increased, which was bewildering, but she felt accurate. She was a woman of simple pleasures and was becoming quite low, as her social life revolved around lunches and coffees with friends. I prescribed Indigo 1M. Indigo covers sciatica < from eating. It also covers depression in neurological diseases. The patient was better in a very short time.

(91) **Sciatica – Nyctanthes** Sciatic pain was incapacitating a middle aged man which was making him extremely sad. He had tried various

means of helping himself but he could find no relief or aggravating factors. I spent a good deal of time with him and he was unable to relate any modalities to characterize the case. Considering sciatica with sadness, I prescribed Nyctanthes 1M which covers sciatic pain with sadness.

(92) Senile Dementia – Conium Mac An extremely forgetful man in his late seventies was showing signs of senile dementia. There was aversion to company, no inclination to do anything, closed and introvert, indifferent and withdrawn. While taking the history I found that the patient has lost a large amount of money in shares about six years back. This led me to Conium which covers the loss of property, finance and fortune as a mental aetiology. The patient has improved to certain extent but obviously considering his age there were limitations. In such cases, I have also seen the wonderful action of Withania Somnifera in tincture, 10 drops in half cup of luke warm water, three times daily, for three – four months, gives some stability to the case.

(93) Sneezing - Merc. Sulph. Due to the enormous patient queue, in the slums of Calcutta I have to make prescription decisions very quickly and when 'sneezing from sun's rays' is reported Merc Sulph 30C is my prescription of choice.

(94) Tonsillitis - Calcarea Iod. I have successfully prescribed Calcarea Iod 200C for huge swollen tonsils with a honey comb appearance. These tonsils have crypts or lacunae on the surface Ref. Dr. Bhanja. My experience has taught me these types of tonsils react with the cold. In Calcarea Iod. you have some symptoms of Calcarea Carb. and some symptoms of Iodum in a hot patient with a strong desire for open air.

(95) Toothache - Merc. Sol. My experience in the slum clinic of Calcutta has taught me to refine the modalities of a case. So when a patient comes to me with a toothache which is better by rubbing, I prescribe Merc. Sol., with very positive results.

(96) Tremor - Argentum Nitricum This case has stayed in my memory for twenty five years. There was a coal mine disaster in Chasnala, Bihar and the patient was a miner and was trapped under the coal mine over seventy two hours. While being trapped, he gradually lost all hope of being rescued. His battery lamp gradually dimmed and he was in complete panic. Finally he was rescued. Six months after the accident, the man in his forties suffered from un-defined tremor and had consulted various neurologists, who negated Parkinson's Disease but could not diagnose the condition. Meanwhile the tremor of arms and legs were increasing gradually. The tremor started in both arms then progressed to the legs and the patient could not walk with his eyes closed and was trembling continually with profound weakness. I tried Zincum on the presenting features but this did not make any difference. I decided to go back to the aetiology and here I took the cause as being trapped in the coal mine for seventy two hours and losing all hope of rescue. I inferred this as "long continued mental exertion" and prescribed Argentum Nitricum 200 followed by 1M. Argentum Nitricum gradually restored the patient completely.

(97) **Trigeminal Neuralgia - Chamomilla** The patient was extremely irritable and snappy in the consultation and demanded to know 'how fast you can make me better?' This struck me as extreme as this was his opening line, I had no idea what was wrong! He was a young man in his mid twenties suffering from trigeminal neuralgia with pain and numbness, on the right with tremendous aggravation of pain from warm application and to a certain extent better by cold. This is a classical indication of Chamomilla where we have impatience, demanding, anger and rage. Also I always refer "hot" to Chamomilla. It has hot head, hot aggravation, hot diarrhoea. I prescribed Chamomilla 10M straight and it worked like magic!

(98) **Urinary Tract Infection - Tuberculinum** I have treated many cases of recurrent UTI with Tuberculinim, when well selected medicines have failed to improve. Generally you will find tubercular emotional components like dissatisfaction and impatience present and also may be the reckless and rebellious nature, who loves travelling. The patient will be chilly, who catches cold easily but loves fresh air. The other medicine you can think in this regard, for recurrent UTI is B.Coli in potency.

(99) **Uterine Haemorrhage – Hamamelis Ver.** A woman in her mid thirties was trying to conceive for eight years and was not interested in IVF, so tried various therapies to no avail. I was treating her for about nine months but not having any success and she was by now, desperate, so decided to participate in a Hindu ritual which consists of making a pilgrimage, while carrying two brass pots of Holy Ganges water, balanced on a long bamboo stick across the shoulder, from the bank of Kolkata's Ganges to Tarakeswar which is about fifty miles. The aim is to pour the carried water onto Lord Shiva in the Tarakeswar Temple for blessings. She was not used to such strenuous activity as her travelling usually consisted of a chauffeur driven car. Unfortunately she started to bleed after the prayer was offered. An ambulance rushed her back to Calcutta as the bleeding was profuse and she was admitted to one of the newest

private hospitals in the city. Two eminent gynecologists could not stop the haemorrhage and after three days struggling, suggested a pan-hysterectomy to stem the bleeding. After these three days the woman was ailing and there was fear for her life. At this juncture I was called, the haemorrhage was profuse, and she was receiving blood transfusion. I went to the hospital straight after my evening clinic and listened to the story from her husband and understood that she walked these 50 miles with a rhythmic bouncing gait to the chant of Om Shiva, in a crowd. I prescribed Hamamelis Ver 30 followed by 200 on the basis of her jolting motion. In Materia Medica text it says 'Uterine haemorrhage from riding or jolting over rough roads.' The haemorrhage had stopped by the morning and the gynecologists had no surgery to perform.

(100) **Vocal Cord Nodule - Rhus Tox.** I have successfully treated many cases of nodules in the vocal cords which result in a hoarse and husky voice with Rhus Tox. Here one of the most important modality is aggravation of hoarseness from first talking, almost inaudible at first, but gets better from continued talking. The aetiology would be straining of vocal cord in public speakers.

(101) **Worm Infestation - Kousso** Extreme undefined debility was preventing a nine years old girl going to school. There were no other apparent symptoms except her mother said that she had to be regularly de-wormed as she has frequent tape worm infestation. This gave me the clue and I prescribed Kousso 30C which covers worms with extreme prostration.

Other Books From Dr. Subrata Kumar Banerjea

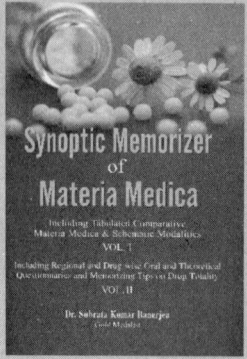

978-81-319-0265-3

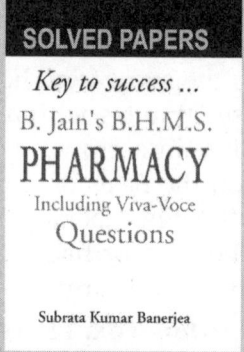

978-81-319-0612-5

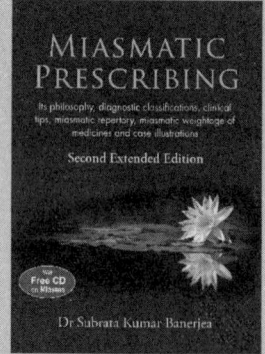

978-81-319-0943-0

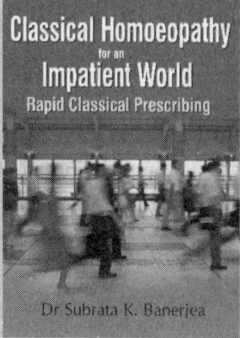

978-81-319-0339-1

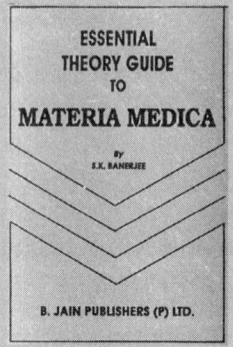

81-7021-671-0
BB2039

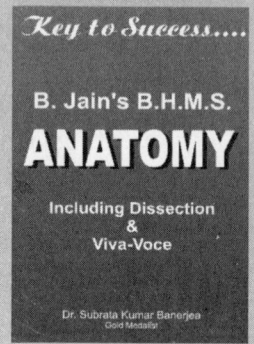

81-7021-386-X
BB2040

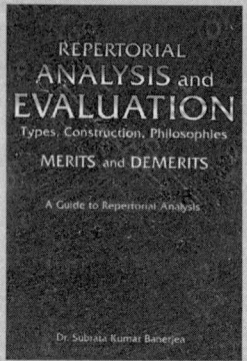

81-8056-062-7
BB3874

www.bjainbooks.com